# Molecular Detection, Characterization, Antimicrobial Resistance and Genomic Epidemiology of Pathogenic Bacteria

# Molecular Detection, Characterization, Antimicrobial Resistance and Genomic Epidemiology of Pathogenic Bacteria

Andrey Shelenkov

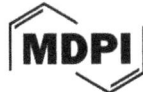

Basel • Beijing • Wuhan • Barcelona • Belgrade • Novi Sad • Cluj • Manchester

Andrey Shelenkov
Molecular Diagnostics and
Epidemiology Department
Central Research Institute
of Epidemiology
Moscow
Russia

*Editorial Office*
MDPI AG
Grosspeteranlage 5
4052 Basel, Switzerland

This is a reprint of the Special Issue, published open access by the journal *Antibiotics* (ISSN 2079-6382), freely accessible at: www.mdpi.com/journal/antibiotics/special_issues/pathogen_antibiotics.

For citation purposes, cite each article independently as indicated on the article page online and using the guide below:

Lastname, A.A.; Lastname, B.B. Article Title. *Journal Name* **Year**, *Volume Number*, Page Range.

ISBN 978-3-7258-1718-4 (Hbk)
ISBN 978-3-7258-1717-7 (PDF)
https://doi.org/10.3390/books978-3-7258-1717-7

© 2024 by the authors. Articles in this book are Open Access and distributed under the Creative Commons Attribution (CC BY) license. The book as a whole is distributed by MDPI under the terms and conditions of the Creative Commons Attribution-NonCommercial-NoDerivs (CC BY-NC-ND) license (https://creativecommons.org/licenses/by-nc-nd/4.0/).

# Contents

About the Editor . . . . . . . . . . . . . . . . . . . . . . . . . . . . . . . . . . . . . . . . . . . . . . . . . . . . . vii

**Andrey Shelenkov**
Molecular Detection, Characterization, Antimicrobial Resistance and Genomic Epidemiology of Pathogenic Bacteria
Reprinted from: *Antibiotics* **2024**, *13*, 494, doi:10.3390/antibiotics13060494 . . . . . . . . . . . . . . . 1

**Katja Šuster and Andrej Cör**
Induction of Viable but Non-Culturable State in Clinically Relevant Staphylococci and Their Detection with Bacteriophage K
Reprinted from: *Antibiotics* **2023**, *12*, 311, doi:10.3390/antibiotics12020311 . . . . . . . . . . . . . . . 5

**Rima El Hage, Jeanne El Hage, Selma P. Snini, Imad Ammoun, Joseph Touma and Rami Rachid et al.**
The Detection of Potential Native Probiotics *Lactobacillus* spp. against *Salmonella* Enteritidis, *Salmonella* Infantis and *Salmonella* Kentucky ST198 of Lebanese Chicken Origin
Reprinted from: *Antibiotics* **2022**, *11*, 1147, doi:10.3390/antibiotics11091147 . . . . . . . . . . . . . . . 17

**Eugene Sheck, Andrey Romanov, Valeria Shapovalova, Elvira Shaidullina, Alexey Martinovich and Natali Ivanchik et al.**
*Acinetobacter* Non-*baumannii* Species: Occurrence in Infections in Hospitalized Patients, Identification, and Antibiotic Resistance
Reprinted from: *Antibiotics* **2023**, *12*, 1301, doi:10.3390/antibiotics12081301 . . . . . . . . . . . . . . 36

**Amani H Al Fadhli, Shaimaa F. Mouftah, Wafaa Y. Jamal, Vincent O. Rotimi and Akela Ghazawi**
Cracking the Code: Unveiling the Diversity of Carbapenem- Resistant *Klebsiella pneumoniae* Clones in the Arabian Peninsula through Genomic Surveillance
Reprinted from: *Antibiotics* **2023**, *12*, 1081, doi:10.3390/antibiotics12071081 . . . . . . . . . . . . . . 51

**Mohammad Riaz Khan, Sadiq Azam, Sajjad Ahmad, Qaisar Ali, Zainab Liaqat and Noor Rehman et al.**
Molecular Characterization and Epidemiology of Antibiotic Resistance Genes of $\beta$-Lactamase Producing Bacterial Pathogens Causing Septicemia from Tertiary Care Hospitals
Reprinted from: *Antibiotics* **2023**, *12*, 617, doi:10.3390/antibiotics12030617 . . . . . . . . . . . . . . . 65

**Samia Habib, Marjorie J. Gibbon, Natacha Couto, Khadija Kakar, Safia Habib and Abdul Samad et al.**
The Diversity, Resistance Profiles and Plasmid Content of *Klebsiella* spp. Recovered from Dairy Farms Located around Three Cities in Pakistan
Reprinted from: *Antibiotics* **2023**, *12*, 539, doi:10.3390/antibiotics12030539 . . . . . . . . . . . . . . . 76

**Angelina A. Kislichkina, Nikolay N. Kartsev, Yury P. Skryabin, Angelika A. Sizova, Maria E. Kanashenko and Marat G. Teymurazov et al.**
Genomic Analysis of a Hybrid Enteroaggregative Hemorrhagic *Escherichia coli* O181:H4 Strain Causing Colitis with Hemolytic-Uremic Syndrome
Reprinted from: *Antibiotics* **2022**, *11*, 1416, doi:10.3390/antibiotics11101416 . . . . . . . . . . . . . . 88

**Akela Ghazawi, Nikolaos Strepis, Febin Anes, Dana Yaaqeib, Amal Ahmed and Aysha AlHosani et al.**
First Report of Colistin-Resistant *Escherichia coli* Carrying *mcr-1* IncI2(delta) and IncX4 Plasmids from Camels (*Camelus dromedarius*) in the Gulf Region
Reprinted from: *Antibiotics* **2024**, *13*, 227, doi:10.3390/antibiotics13030227 . . . . . . . . . . . . . . . 104

**Srinivasan Vijaya Bharathi and Govindan Rajamohan**
Biocide-Resistant *Escherichia coli* ST540 Co-Harboring ESBL, *dfrA14* Confers QnrS-Dependent Plasmid-Mediated Quinolone Resistance
Reprinted from: *Antibiotics* **2022**, *11*, 1724, doi:10.3390/antibiotics11121724 . . . . . . . . . . . . . **120**

**Andrey Shelenkov, Lyudmila Petrova, Anna Mironova, Mikhail Zamyatin, Vasiliy Akimkin and Yulia Mikhaylova**
Long-Read Whole Genome Sequencing Elucidates the Mechanisms of Amikacin Resistance in Multidrug-Resistant *Klebsiella pneumoniae* Isolates Obtained from COVID-19 Patients
Reprinted from: *Antibiotics* **2022**, *11*, 1364, doi:10.3390/antibiotics11101364 . . . . . . . . . . . . . **131**

# About the Editor

**Andrey Shelenkov**

Andrey Shelenkov is a senior scientist at the Laboratory of Molecular Mechanisms of Antibiotic Resistance in the Central Research Institute of Epidemiology of the Federal Service for Surveillance on Consumer Rights Protection and Human Wellbeing (Rospotrebnadzor), Moscow, Russia. He has a Ph.D. degree in Applied Mathematics and Bioinformatics. His general research interests include the genomic epidemiology of ESKAPE and other bacterial pathogens of clinical, food, and environmental origin. He is responsible for computational analysis of whole-genome sequencing data, developing annotation pipelines for bacterial genomes, performing investigations in the fields of infection outbreak detection, and revealing the mechanisms of antimicrobial resistance acquisition in various bacterial populations. He is a member of the European Society of Clinical Microbiology and Infectious Diseases (ESCMID) and a member of the Reviewer Boards of MDPI and Elsevier journals. He is an author of more than 70 publications in peer-reviewed journals.

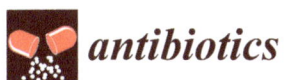

*Editorial*

# Molecular Detection, Characterization, Antimicrobial Resistance and Genomic Epidemiology of Pathogenic Bacteria

Andrey Shelenkov

Central Research Institute of Epidemiology, Novogireevskaya Str., 3a, 111123 Moscow, Russia; fallandar@gmail.com

In recent decades, growing attention has been directed worldwide toward antimicrobial-resistant (AMR) bacterial pathogens causing infections in clinical, environmental, and food chain production settings. The healthcare-associated infections (HAIs) caused by multidrug (MDR)- or pandrug-resistant bacteria have already been declared a 'silent pandemic' [1] and have raised a global concern due to increased patient morbidity and mortality associated with such agents [2]. In order to develop advanced prevention measures and treatment plans to combat such infections, specialists in various fields, including microbiology, medicine, molecular biology, and bioinformatics, need to work together. This will ensure a better understanding of the mechanisms driving resistance development and dissemination within bacterial populations.

It is well known that resistance spreading in clinically relevant bacterial species like *Klebsiella pneumoniae* or *Acinetobacter baumannii* is usually driven by several lineages called 'global clones' or 'international clones of high risk', and thus the detection and surveillance of the isolates belonging to such clones represents an important epidemiological task [3,4]. In addition, the continuous monitoring of AMR gene presence within clinical, environmental, veterinary, and food samples is essential for tracking the underlying mechanisms of resistance acquisition and developing proper control measures, especially considering the One Health paradigm [5,6]. Currently, molecular and whole-genome sequencing (WGS)-based methods are the gold standard for global clone detection or investigations of the AMR genes, virulence factors, and plasmids for bacterial isolates, even in time-critical situations [7,8].

Given the above findings, this Special Issue was contemplated as a collection of high-quality papers describing various applications of molecular biology, WGS, and genomic epidemiology methods for investigations of bacterial pathogens, with additional focus on population structure and AMR gene detection.

The papers published in this Special Issue describe various aspects of antimicrobial resistance and whole-genome analysis of pathogenic bacteria. The first aspect includes the genomic analysis of particular *Escherichia coli* and *Klebsiella pneumoniae* strains, providing valuable insights into mechanisms of AMR acquisition and dissemination of the studied isolates (Contributions 2, 3, 4, and 10). The second aspect refers to more general molecular and genomic epidemiology studies elucidating the structure of bacterial populations of *K. pneumoniae*, *Acinetobacter*, non-*baumannii*, and other species in clinical and agricultural environments (Contributions 6, 7, 8, and 9). The third aspect pertains to the caveats within molecular diagnostics and infection prevention, namely, the detection of viable but non-culturable bacteria (contribution 5) and the revelation of potential probiotic agents against *Salmonella* infections (contribution 1). A brief description of all these reports is provided below.

Contribution 1 is dedicated to the detection of *Ligilactobacillus salivarius* bacterial strains, which can serve as a potential preventive probiotic against *Salmonella* infections in poultry, in particular, for the ones caused by *S.* Enteritidis, *S.* Infantis, and *S.* Kentucky. Since *Salmonella* is the leading cause of foodborne disease globally [9], the development of

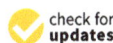

Citation: Shelenkov, A. Molecular Detection, Characterization, Antimicrobial Resistance and Genomic Epidemiology of Pathogenic Bacteria. *Antibiotics* **2024**, *13*, 494. https://doi.org/10.3390/antibiotics13060494

Received: 0 May 2024
Revised: 17 May 2024
Accepted: 23 May 2024
Published: 27 May 2024

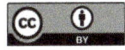

Copyright: © 2024 by the author. Licensee MDPI, Basel, Switzerland. This article is an open access article distributed under the terms and conditions of the Creative Commons Attribution (CC BY) license (https://creativecommons.org/licenses/by/4.0/).

suitable prevention measures against its spread among poultry and other food-producing animals becomes crucial.

Contribution 2 reveals the possible mechanism of amikacin resistance in clinical isolates of *K. pneumoniae*. Hybrid long- and short-read WGS revealed the precise sequence of a small plasmid carrying an amikacin resistance gene in only one member of a group of isolates with identical cgMLST profiles and thus possessing very similar genome structure. This small plasmid made a difference in the AMR of these isolates, which was confirmed by susceptibility testing.

Contributions 3 and 4 involve the genomic analysis of *E. coli*. The former describes the diarrheagenic hybrid strain and includes a comparative analysis of its genome and plasmids with previous outbreak isolates. The latter reveals the possible mechanism of quinolone resistance in an MDR isolate. Although *E. coli* is usually considered to be less dangerous in a hospital than, for example, *K. pneumoniae*, it can also cause serious outbreaks [10] and thus requires special attention.

Contribution 5 proposes a method for the detection of nonculturable *Staphylococci* using bacteriophages. This approach facilitates effective distinction between viable and dead bacteria in a sample, which can be very beneficial since most bacterial analysis approaches rely on culturing methods and fail to produce accurate results for nonculturable strains [11].

Contribution 6 provides epidemiological data regarding the diversity and resistance gene presence for *Klebsiella spp.* samples isolated from dairy farms in Pakistan. The presence of multiple resistance genes, especially the ones encoding beta-lactamases CTX-M-15 and CTX-M-55, highlights the need for continued surveillance.

Contribution 7 involves a molecular analysis of beta-lactamase-producing *E. coli* and *Pseudomonas aeruginosa* in Pakistan tertiary care hospitals. The authors noted a general increase in AMR. Contribution 8 presents the in silico genomic epidemiology analysis of carbapenem-resistant *K. pneumoniae* (CRKP) in countries belonging to the Gulf Cooperation Council. The study revealed a wide distribution of high-risk clones and other epidemiologically valuable data.

Contribution 9 describes the wide-scale analysis of *Acinetobacter* non-*baumannii* species in hospitalized patients. Although most *Acinetobacter* studies are usually focused on *A. baumannii*, other members of this genus are becoming increasingly more important as opportunistic pathogens in clinical settings. The authors discuss the infections caused by these pathogens and the mechanisms of AMR, especially to carbapenem antibiotics.

Contribution 10 presents a genomic analysis of colistin-resistant *E. coli* isolates from camels and provides valuable insights into plasmid-mediated mechanisms of AMR transfer.

Taken together, the papers presented in this Special Issue highlight the importance of molecular, WGS, and genomic epidemiology methods for studying the clonal structure and AMR gene content within bacterial populations in clinical, environmental, and food production settings. In particular, WGS-based studies allowed researchers to capture the diversity of particular species and reveal possible AMR and virulence acquisition mechanisms in the studied isolates. Additionally, novel methods for *Staphylococci* detection and *Salmonella* spread prevention are presented.

The data provided in this Special Issue will be useful for researchers in various fields involving bacterial pathogen surveillance, detection, and treatment, especially in the emerging field of genomic epidemiology.

**Acknowledgments:** As a guest editor, I would like to express my deep appreciation to all authors whose work was published in this issue, as well as to all those involved in the peer review and manuscript publication processes, for their valuable contribution toward the success of this Special Issue.

**Conflicts of Interest:** The author declares no conflicts of interest.

List of Contributions

1. El Hage, R.; El Hage, J.; Snini, S.; Ammoun, I.; Touma, J.; Rachid, R.; Mathieu, F.; Sabatier, J.; Abi Khattar, Z.; El Rayess, Y. The Detection of Potential Native Probiotics *Lactobacillus* spp. against *Salmonella* Enteritidis, *Salmonella* Infantis and *Salmonella* Kentucky ST198 of Lebanese Chicken Origin. *Antibiotics* 2022, *11*, 1147. https://doi.org/10.3390/antibiotics11091147.
2. Shelenkov, A.; Petrova, L.; Mironova, A.; Zamyatin, M.; Akimkin, V.; Mikhaylova, Y. Long-Read Whole Genome Sequencing Elucidates the Mechanisms of Amikacin Resistance in Multidrug-Resistant *Klebsiella pneumoniae* Isolates Obtained from COVID-19 Patients. *Antibiotics* 2022, *11*, 1364. https://doi.org/10.3390/antibiotics11101364.
3. Kislichkina, A.; Kartsev, N.; Skryabin, Y.; Sizova, A.; Kanashenko, M.; Teymurazov, M.; Kuzina, E.; Bogun, A.; Fursova, N.; Svetoch, E.; et al. Genomic Analysis of a Hybrid Enteroaggregative Hemorrhagic *Escherichia coli* O181:H4 Strain Causing Colitis with Hemolytic-Uremic Syndrome. *Antibiotics* 2022, *11*, 1416. https://doi.org/10.3390/antibiotics11101416.
4. Bharathi, S.; Rajamohan, G. Biocide-Resistant *Escherichia coli* ST540 Co-Harboring ESBL, *dfrA14* Confers QnrS-Dependent Plasmid-Mediated Quinolone Resistance. *Antibiotics* 2022, *11*, 1724. https://doi.org/10.3390/antibiotics11121724.
5. Suster, K.; Cor, A. Induction of Viable but Non-Culturable State in Clinically Relevant Staphylococci and Their Detection with Bacteriophage K. *Antibiotics* 2023, *12*, 311. https://doi.org/10.3390/antibiotics12020311.
6. Habib, S.; Gibbon, M.; Couto, N.; Kakar, K.; Habib, S.; Samad, A.; Munir, A.; Fatima, F.; Mohsin, M.; Feil, E. The Diversity, Resistance Profiles and Plasmid Content of *Klebsiella* spp. Recovered from Dairy Farms Located around Three Cities in Pakistan. *Antibiotics* 2023, *12*, 539. https://doi.org/10.3390/antibiotics12030539.
7. Khan, M.; Azam, S.; Ahmad, S.; Ali, Q.; Liaqat, Z.; Rehman, N.; Khan, I.; Alharbi, M.; Alshammari, A. Molecular Characterization and Epidemiology of Antibiotic Resistance Genes of β-Lactamase Producing Bacterial Pathogens Causing Septicemia from Tertiary Care Hospitals. *Antibiotics* 2023, *12*, 617. https://doi.org/10.3390/antibiotics12030617.
8. Al Fadhli, A.; Mouftah, S.; Jamal, W.; Rotimi, V.; Ghazawi, A. Cracking the Code: Unveiling the Diversity of Carbapenem-Resistant Klebsiella pneumoniae Clones in the Arabian Peninsula through Genomic Surveillance. *Antibiotics* 2023, *12*, 1081. https://doi.org/10.3390/antibiotics12071081.
9. Sheck, E.; Romanov, A.; Shapovalova, V.; Shaidullina, E.; Martinovich, A.; Ivanchik, N.; Mikotina, A.; Skleenova, E.; Oloviannikov, V.; Azizov, I.; et al. Acinetobacter Non-baumannii Species: Occurrence in Infections in Hospitalized Patients, Identification, and Antibiotic Resistance. *Antibiotics* 2023, *12*, 1301. https://doi.org/10.3390/antibiotics12081301.
10. Ghazawi, A.; Strepis, N.; Anes, F.; Yaaqeib, D.; Ahmed, A.; AlHosani, A.; AlShehhi, M.; Manzoor, A.; Habib, I.; Wani, N.; et al. First Report of Colistin-Resistant Escherichia coli Carrying *mcr-1* IncI2(delta) and IncX4 Plasmids from Camels (*Camelus dromedarius*) in the Gulf Region. *Antibiotics* 2024, *13*, 227. https://doi.org/10.3390/antibiotics13030227.

# References

1. Rayan, R.A. Flare of the silent pandemic in the era of the COVID-19 pandemic: Obstacles and opportunities. *World J. Clin. Cases* 2023, *11*, 1267–1274. [CrossRef] [PubMed]
2. Antimicrobial Resistance Collaborators. Global burden of bacterial antimicrobial resistance in 2019: A systematic analysis. *Lancet* 2022, *399*, 629–655. [CrossRef] [PubMed]
3. Shelenkov, A.; Petrova, L.; Zamyatin, M.; Mikhaylova, Y.; Akimkin, V. Diversity of International High-Risk Clones of *Acinetobacter baumannii* Revealed in a Russian Multidisciplinary Medical Center during 2017–2019. *Antibiotics* 2021, *10*, 1009. [CrossRef] [PubMed]
4. Arcari, G.; Carattoli, A. Global spread and evolutionary convergence of multidrug-resistant and hypervirulent *Klebsiella pneumoniae* high-risk clones. *Pathog. Glob. Health* 2023, *117*, 328–341 [CrossRef] [PubMed]
5. Velazquez-Meza, M.E.; Galarde-Lopez, M.; Carrillo-Quiroz, B.; Alpuche-Aranda, C.M. Antimicrobial resistance: One Health approach. *Vet. World* 2022, *15*, 743–749. [CrossRef] [PubMed]
6. Djordjevic, S.P.; Jarocki, V.M.; Seemann, T.; Cummins, M.L.; Watt, A.E.; Drigo, B.; Wyrsch, E.R.; Reid, C.J.; Donner, E.; Howden, B.P. Genomic surveillance for antimicrobial resistance—A One Health perspective. *Nat. Rev. Genet.* 2024, *25*, 142–157. [CrossRef] [PubMed]
7. Lakicevic, B.; Jankovic, V.; Pietzka, A.; Ruppitsch, W. Wholegenome sequencing as the gold standard approach for control of Listeria monocytogenes in the food chain. *J. Food Prot.* 2023, *86*, 100003. [CrossRef] [PubMed]

8. Bogaerts, B.; Winand, R.; Van Braekel, J.; Hoffman, S.; Roosens, N.H.C.; De Keersmaecker, S.C.J.; Marchal, K.; Vanneste, K. Evaluation of WGS performance for bacterial pathogen characterization with the Illumina technology optimized for time-critical situations. *Microb. Genom.* **2021**, *7*, 699. [CrossRef] [PubMed]
9. Shaji, S.; Selvaraj, R.K.; Shanmugasundaram, R. *Salmonella* Infection in Poultry: A Review on the Pathogen and Control Strategies. *Microorganisms* **2023**, *11*, 2814. [CrossRef] [PubMed]
10. Okada, N.; Takahashi, M.; Yano, Y.; Sato, M.; Abe, A.; Ishizawa, K.; Azuma, M. Hospital outbreak of extended-spectrum beta-lactamase-producing *Escherichia coli* potentially caused by toilet and bath chair use. *Infect. Prev. Pract.* **2022**, *4*, 100239. [CrossRef] [PubMed]
11. Pazos-Rojas, L.A.; Cuellar-Sanchez, A.; Romero-Ceron, A.L.; Rivera-Urbalejo, A.; Van Dillewijn, P.; Luna-Vital, D.A.; Munoz-Rojas, J.; Morales-Garcia, Y.E.; Bustillos-Cristales, M.D.R. The Viable but Non-Culturable (VBNC) State, a Poorly Explored Aspect of Beneficial Bacteria. *Microorganisms* **2023**, *12*, 39. [CrossRef] [PubMed]

**Disclaimer/Publisher's Note:** The statements, opinions and data contained in all publications are solely those of the individual author(s) and contributor(s) and not of MDPI and/or the editor(s). MDPI and/or the editor(s) disclaim responsibility for any injury to people or property resulting from any ideas, methods, instructions or products referred to in the content.

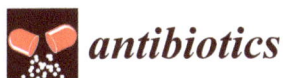

Article

# Induction of Viable but Non-Culturable State in Clinically Relevant Staphylococci and Their Detection with Bacteriophage K

Katja Šuster [1,*] and Andrej Cör [1,2]

1 Department of Research, Valdoltra Orthopaedic Hospital, 6280 Ankaran, Slovenia
2 Faculty of Education, University of Primorska, 6000 Koper, Slovenia
* Correspondence: katja.suster@ob-valdoltra.si

**Abstract:** Prosthetic joint infections are frequently associated with biofilm formation and the presence of viable but non-culturable (VBNC) bacteria. Conventional sample culturing remains the gold standard for microbiological diagnosis. However, VBNC bacteria lack the ability to grow on routine culture medium, leading to culture-negative results. Bacteriophages are viruses that specifically recognize and infect bacteria. In this study, we wanted to determine if bacteriophages could be used to detect VBNC bacteria. Four staphylococcal strains were cultured for biofilm formation and transferred to low-nutrient media with different gentamycin concentrations for VBNC state induction. VBNC bacteria were confirmed with the BacLight[TM] viability kit staining. Suspensions of live, dead, and VBNC bacteria were incubated with bacteriophage K and assessed in a qPCR for their detection. The VBNC state was successfully induced 8 to 19 days after incubation under stressful conditions. In total, 6.1 to 23.9% of bacteria were confirmed alive while not growing on conventional culturing media. During the qPCR assay, live bacterial suspensions showed a substantial increase in phage DNA. No detection was observed in dead bacteria or phage non-susceptible *E. coli* suspensions. However, a reduction in phage DNA in VBNC bacterial suspensions was observed, which confirmed the detection was successful based on the adsorption of phages.

**Keywords:** phage typing; molecular detection; bacteriophages; VBNC; pathogenic bacteria; PJI; biofilm

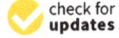

Citation: Šuster, K.; Cör, A. Induction of Viable but Non-Culturable State in Clinically Relevant Staphylococci and Their Detection with Bacteriophage K. *Antibiotics* 2023, 12, 311. https://doi.org/10.3390/antibiotics12020311

Academic Editor: Andrey Shelenkov

Received: 5 January 2023
Revised: 27 January 2023
Accepted: 1 February 2023
Published: 2 February 2023

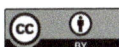

**Copyright:** © 2023 by the authors. Licensee MDPI, Basel, Switzerland. This article is an open access article distributed under the terms and conditions of the Creative Commons Attribution (CC BY) license (https://creativecommons.org/licenses/by/4.0/).

## 1. Introduction

In the last decade, research on bacteriophage use has increased for diagnostic and therapeutic purposes in human medicine [1]. Bacteriophages are viruses that specifically recognize and attach to their target host bacteria, inject their genetic material, reproduce inside the host, and release their progeny by lysing the bacterium. Due to the extraordinary specificity of phages for a particular genus, species, or even strain of bacteria, they could be a promising new tool for the rapid detection of bacteria in clinical samples. Bacteriophage K is a broad-spectrum staphylococcal bacteriophage [2–5]. Previous research work showed that combining bacteriophage K with qPCR technology enabled the detection of staphylococci in the sonicate fluid of infected prosthetic joints [6,7].

The replacement of joints with artificial joint prostheses is one of the most successful surgical procedures in orthopedic surgery as it has improved the life quality of millions of patients by saving them from chronic pain and improving their mobility. Due to technological advances, the number of prostheses that need to be replaced is decreasing; however, it is still necessary to replace approximately 10% of them [8]. The most serious complication leading to joint prosthesis revision is bacterial prosthetic joint infection (PJI), which is reported to occur in 0.8 to 1.9% of knee arthroplasties and 0.3 to 1.7% of hip arthroplasties [9]. The microbiological culturing of samples represents the gold standard for establishing the microbiological diagnosis (microbial typing) of PJI but does not always identify the pathogen. Culture-negative infections have been widely reported in the literature and account for about 7–42% [10–13] of PJI cases, occurring at a higher rate in late PJI. Culture-negative infections unable the selection of targeted antimicrobials; instead, broad-spectrum or multiple antibiotics are administered to cover the most common microorganisms, which can be less effective and lead to treatment failure. Failure to isolate the causative pathogen by culture is mostly due to antibiotic administration prior to sampling, infections with fastidious or uncommon microorganisms, improper sampling and lack of resuscitation in the laboratory, and biofilm formation on biomaterial. Biofilms are associated with the persistence and chronicity of infections and represent an important threat to human health, especially due to their increased virulence and tolerance to antimicrobials.

The inaccurate use of antibiotics due to misdiagnosis or the administration of inadequate doses importantly contributes to the emerging multidrug-resistant strains, and may induce persistence and a VBNC state in bacteria [14,15]. As for antibiotic pressure, other environmental conditions can also act as stressors on bacterial cells. Within layers of a biofilm, different stressful microenvironments form that are low in oxygen and nutrients and have a low pH due to higher waste concentrations. Such conditions promote phenotypic heterogeneity within bacterial populations in a biofilm, giving rise to persisters and VBNC bacteria [14,16,17]. As a response to stressors, bacteria activate a cascade of stress-related mechanisms followed by important morphological changes and lower metabolic activity. The transition of bacteria into those states is generally accepted as a bacterial mechanism of survival.

Due to all the changes that bacteria undergo while transitioning to the VBNC state, they also lose their ability to grow on routinely used bacteriological media [18–20]. Currently, there is no validated and specific method for the identification of all viable bacteria in clinical specimens. This leads to false negative results due to a lack of growth by conventional microbiological culturing methods or underestimation of the total bacterial number or species in a sample. Under continued stressful conditions, bacteria can remain in the VBNC state over long periods. However, during the process known as resuscitation, bacteria can revive into the culturable state, regaining full metabolic activity and virulence, and thus causing a recurrence of infection in patients weeks or months later [21]. Therefore, the underestimation or non-detection of bacteria due to biofilm formation on medical devices and the presence of VBNC bacteria pose a great risk to public health.

Identifying the causative pathogen is of the utmost importance for an optimal outcome in treating implant-related infections as it directly influences the choice of antimicrobial and surgical therapy. However, further studies for the detection of all viable bacteria in clinical samples are needed. In this study, we demonstrate that phage K combined with qPCR enables the detection of VBNC staphylococci within biofilms. The use of bacteriophages for bacterial typing could therefore represent an important alternative to conventional microbiological diagnostic procedures that will allow the specific detection of all viable bacteria in clinical specimens.

## 2. Results

### 2.1. Biofilm Formation and Induction of VBNC State

Minimal inhibitory concentrations (MIC) of gentamycin were determined to be 3.12 µg/mL for *S. aureus* ATCC 25923, *S. epidermidis* DSM 3269, and *S. lugdunensis* OBV 20/143, whereas for the *S. aureus* OBV 17/166 strain, the MIC was determined to be 12.5 µg/mL.

All strains successfully formed biofilms on filter paper membranes during the 48 h incubation on BHI agar plates supplemented with 1% glucose. The biofilms' morphology was observed macroscopically and differed between strains. *S. aureus* OBV 17/166 biofilms appeared thicker and retained a more intense yellow color than other bacterial biofilms. *S. aureus* ATCC 25923 formed thinner biofilms than other staphylococcal strains (Figure 1).

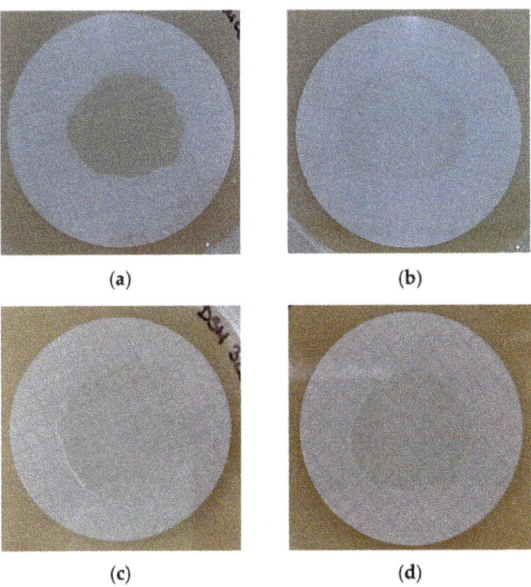

**Figure 1.** Biofilm formation on ø 47 mm membranes placed on BHI agar plates with 1% glucose: (**a**) *S. aureus* OBV 17/166; (**b**) *S. aureus* ATCC 25923; (**c**) *S. epidermidis* DSM 3269; (**d**) *S. lugdunensis* OBV 20/143.

The VBNC state in all tested staphylococcal strains was successfully induced in vitro by starvation on a low-nutrient M9 medium and antibiotic pressure using different concentrations of gentamycin. All control biofilms exposed only to starvation without gentamycin still retained their culturability after 30 days of exposure. Results are presented in Table 1.

**Table 1.** Results of VBNC state induction in four staphylococcal strains.

| Bacterial Strain | Conditions for VBNC Induction | Days under Stress Conditions Until Loss of Culturability (Mean ± SE) [1] | % of Viable Bacterial Cells after Culturability Loss (Mean ± SE) [1] |
|---|---|---|---|
| *S. aureus* ATCC 25923 | S | >30 | - |
|  | S + G 4 × MIC | 11.3 ± 1.3 | 11.9 ± 1.5 |
|  | S + G 8 × MIC | 8.0 ± 1.0 | 13.5 ± 0.4 |
|  | S + G 16 × MIC | 9.0 ± 1.0 | 14.0 ± 0.7 |
| *S. aureus* OBV 17/166 | S | >30 | - |
|  | S + G 4 × MIC | 19.3 ± 1.4 | 9.7 ± 0.1 |
|  | S + G 8 × MIC | 19.3 ± 1.4 | 14.2 ± 0.0 |
|  | S + G 16 × MIC | 13.7 ± 3.3 | 10.3 ± 0.9 |
| *S. epidermidis* DSM 3269 | S | >30 | - |
|  | S + G 4 × MIC | 16.0 ± 0.0 | 6.1 ± 0.4 |
|  | S + G 8 × MIC | 12.7 ± 1.3 | 10.7 ± 1.6 |
|  | S + G 16 × MIC | 8.0 ± 1.0 | 12.0 ± 0.7 |
| *S. lugdunensis* OBV 20/143 | S | >30 | - |
|  | S + G 4 × MIC | 15.3 ± 0.7 | 15.2 ± 3.5 |
|  | S + G 8 × MIC | 14.0 ± 0.0 | 23.7 ± 0.5 |
|  | S + G 16 × MIC | 10.0 ± 0.0 | 23.9 ± 0.5 |

S, starvation; G, gentamycin. [1] Values obtained from three independent parallel experiments and expressed as mean ± SE.

*S. aureus* ATCC 25923 was the first strain that stopped growing on a nutrient medium regardless of the antibiotic concentration used. The loss of culturability was first observed after $8.0 \pm 1.0$ days of starvation and exposure to gentamycin at an $8 \times$ MIC. No correlation was observed between the used concentrations and time to growth cessation in both tested *S. aureus* strains. In other tested strains, a correlation between antibiotic concentration and the exposure time until culturability loss has been found. There was a statistically significant difference between the use of $16 \times$ MIC and $8 \times$ MIC or $4 \times$ MIC in *S. epidermidis* ($p < 0.001$) and *S. lugdunensis* ($p = 0.014$ and $p = 0.003$, respectively), but not between the use of $4 \times$ MIC and $8 \times$ MIC ($p = 0.05$), analyzed with the Newman–Keuls method.

The presence of VBNC bacteria was confirmed after staining bacterial suspensions with the BacLight™ kit followed by visualization with fluorescence microscopy (Figure 2) and spectrophotometric measurements of emitted green and red fluorescence. The percentages of live bacteria present in samples are presented in Table 1.

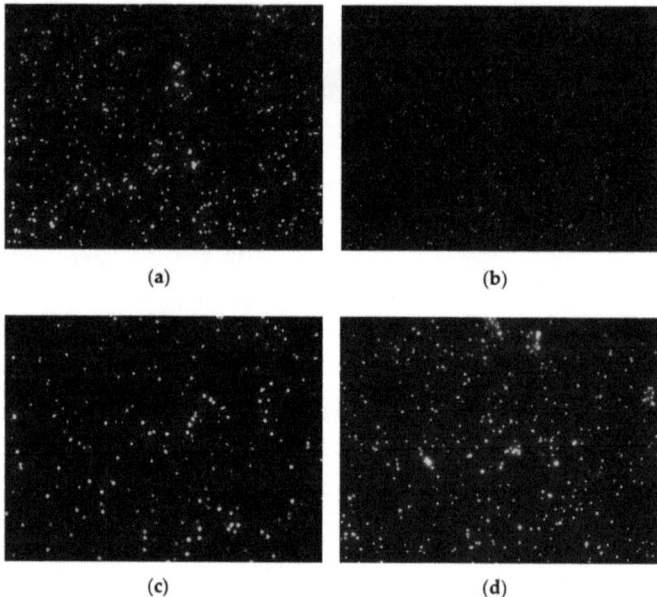

**Figure 2.** Examples of viable (green) and dead (red) bacteria (*S. epidermidis* DSM 3269) visualized using fluorescence microscopy: (**a**) suspension of live bacteria; (**b**) suspension of dead bacteria; (**c**) suspension of induced VBNC bacteria by gentamycin at $4 \times$ MIC; (**d**) suspension of induced VBNC bacteria by gentamycin at $16 \times$ MIC. Magnification, $600\times$.

The percentage of live bacteria in suspensions where the VBNC state was induced by exposure to gentamycin at $4 \times$ MIC ranged between $6.1 \pm 0.4\%$ and $15.2 \pm 3.5\%$, between $10.7 \pm 1.6\%$ and $23.7 \pm 0.5\%$ when biofilms were exposed to $8 \times$ MIC of gentamycin, and between $10.3 \pm 0.9\%$ and $23.9 \pm 0.5\%$ when exposed to $16 \times$ MIC of gentamycin. In *S. aureus* ATCC 25923 and *S. lugdunensis* OBV 20/143, no correlation between the percentage of viable bacteria and used gentamycin concentration has been found ($p = 0.069$ and $p = 0.059$, respectively). In *S. epidermidis* and *S. aureus* OBV 17/166 strains, there was a statistically significant difference in the percentage of viable bacteria in samples that were exposed to gentamycin $4 \times$ MIC and $8 \times$ MIC ($p = 0.02$). In *S. aureus* OBV 17/166, there was also a significant difference in the number of viable bacteria when comparing $8 \times$ MIC and $16 \times$ MIC results ($p = 0.002$), whereas in *S. epidermidis* the difference was significant, when comparing $4 \times$ MIC with $16 \times$ MIC ($p = 0.017$).

## 2.2. Detection of VBNC Bacteria with Bacteriophages and qPCR

To evaluate the possibility of the detection of VBNC staphylococci with our previously developed method for the detection of staphylococci from sonicate fluid samples of explanted prosthetic joints [6], suspensions of four different induced VBNC staphylococcal strains were inoculated with phage K and assayed for phage K DNA detection in the qPCR as described in the methods.

During the qPCR assay, a delay in amplification of a specific phage DNA sequence was observed in samples where phage K was added to VBNC bacterial suspensions compared to the reference sample, which contained only the initial amount of added phages. This was due to the phage adsorption on living cells, which did not allow phage multiplication because of their low metabolic state. Suspensions containing only dead bacteria, on the other hand, did not show any statistical difference compared to the reference sample. This indicated that the initial phage DNA was available for qPCR, whether or not the virions adsorbed onto dead cells or cell debris, with a particularity of dead *S. epidermidis*, which showed a statistically significant delay in the amplification of a specific phage sequence. However, the differences between the tested VBNC suspensions and dead bacterial suspensions were statistically different, showing an increased loss of phage DNA in samples where VBNC bacteria were present. For live bacterial suspensions, sequence amplification started 6–12 PCR cycles earlier than the reference control, due to phage proliferation, which was expected since the samples were incubated for 180 min at 37 °C. No difference was observed between the reference sample and live or dead *E. coli* suspensions, which represented the negative control strain, non-susceptible to phage K (Figure 3).

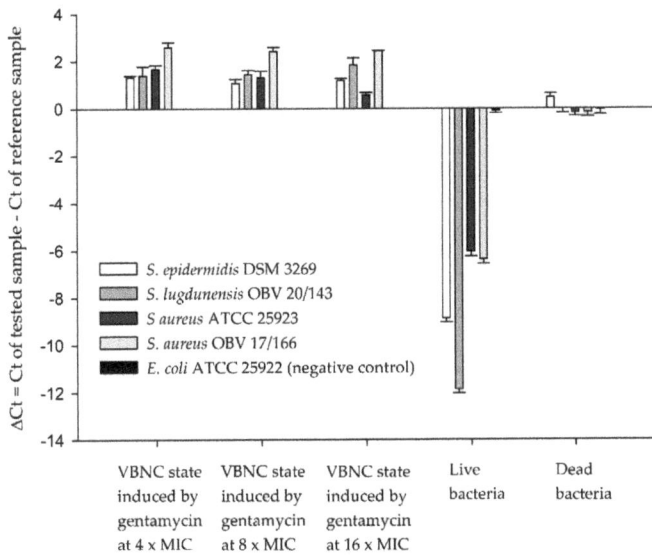

**Figure 3.** Detection of VBNC, live, and dead bacteria with bacteriophage K and qPCR. Values are expressed as mean ± SD.

## 3. Discussion

Lytic bacteriophages are virulent bacterial viruses that are gaining interest in modern medicine because of their extraordinary properties, which could be useful both for therapeutic and diagnostic purposes. They can specifically recognize their bacterial host, adsorb to their surface via specific cell receptors, and inject their genetic material into the cell. In that way, they take control of the bacterial metabolism by expressing their genes and assembling new phage particles. During this process, lysins accumulate in the bacterial cell, lysing the bacterium at a certain point, and releasing new progeny phages [22]. For that, more and more studies are focused on possibilities of phage use, not only for treatment but also for the diagnosis of bacterial infections [23]. In this study, we aimed to examine the induction and indirect detection of staphylococci in a low-metabolic state (the VBNC state) with a broad-spectrum staphylococcal bacteriophage (phage K) and qPCR. We demonstrated that phage K combined with qPCR enabled the detection of clinically relevant VBNC staphylococci within biofilms. The detection was based on the adsorption of added phages to VBNC bacteria, which was observed as a delay in phage DNA multiplication in the samples where phage K was added to VBNC bacterial suspensions. The method used in this study was previously developed for the detection of staphylococci in sonicate fluid samples of explanted prosthetic joints [6,7]. Now, we show that both actively growing and VBNC bacteria can be successfully and specifically detected with the bacteriophage-based method in 4 h. The main difference between detecting actively growing bacteria and bacteria in the VBNC state was in the phage adsorption to the bacteria and their reproduction. Bacteriophage K adsorbed and infected all viable bacteria; however, it was able to reproduce only in actively growing bacteria, which resulted in an increase in phage DNA. On the other hand, a decrease in phage DNA was observed in VBNC bacterial suspensions, as phage reproduction strongly depends on the bacterial physiological state [24]. Furthermore, dead bacterial cells were not detected with the method, whether or not the virions could adsorb onto dead cells or cell debris. This was probably due to the sample's chloroform treatment. Chloroform dissolves the bacterial outer membrane and has been long used for periplasmic protein extraction [25]. The treatment could therefore trigger the release of phages attached to dead bacteria or cell debris, making phage DNA available for qPCR. Chloroform treatment was previously determined to importantly improve the detection of live bacteria with the used method, as it induced the premature lysis of phage-infected bacteria [6]. By disrupting the cell membrane, chloroform provides phage endolysins with access to the peptidoglycan. This triggers the premature lysis of bacteria and the release of bacterial cell content including progeny bacteriophages and/or their components and DNA. However, the results indicate that chloroform did not induce the premature lysis of VBNC bacteria. This is probably because bacteriophages need a live and metabolically active host for their replication, and phage endolysins (or at least enough endolysins) do not form in VBNC bacteria for their lysis. In addition, VBNC bacteria are more resistant to harsh environmental conditions and chemicals, and this could also implicate a higher resistance to chloroform treatment.

Phage selectivity in specific strain recognition minimizes false-negative and false-positive results often associated with detection methods and offers the possibility for the detection of only live bacteria. Phage typing is used to identify bacteria, especially in the food industry, but also in water and environmental pollution. Although the diagnosis with the use of the phage is fast and sensitive, its use in clinical practice is not common [26]. Different already-developed phage-based diagnostic methods are focused on the detection of one bacterial species/strain with a specific bacteriophage. Available FDA-approved and clinically used diagnostic tests are used so far for the identification of *M. tuberculosis*, *Y. pestis*, *B. anthracis*, and *S. aureus* [9].

Culture-negative infections have been widely reported in the literature. Traditional microbiologic culturing does not yield any growth in about 7–42% [10–13] of PJI cases and occurs at a higher rate in late PJI. In a recent prospective cohort study [27], culture-negative PJI was determined in 19.7% of late PJI and 6.2% of early/delayed PJI cases. The microbiological assessment of device-related biofilm infections improved significantly by sonication fluid culture [28–32]. During sonication, biofilm is detached from the removed device by applying low-intensity ultrasound waves. The culture of sonicate fluid is now widely in use in combination with periprosthetic tissue/synovial fluid cultures to improve the detection of microorganisms in PJI. However, as bacteria in the VBNC state cannot be detected with conventional culturing methods, they contribute importantly to culture-negative results, representing an important clinical issue leading to inadequate antibiotic administration and inadequate patient treatment. For some, the infection goes undetected (silent infections) at first; for others, the prescribed antibiotics (if prescribed) are not needed; and in other cases, patients receive weak epidemiologically inadequate broad-spectrum antibiotics instead of specific ones. Not being able to detect and efficiently treat VBNC bacterial infections contributes to infection recurrence, increases in health care costs, patient dissatisfaction, and importantly to the emerging antimicrobial resistance, which is becoming more and more common today.

The detection of VBNC bacteria remains a challenge in clinical practice, and there is a need for a new specific and sensitive method for the quick detection of non-culturable bacteria. Existing research on their detection includes different staining and molecular methods [33], but so far, none of them is in use in clinical practice. Cerca et al. [34] suggested the use of SYBR green (a component of the existing commercially available BacLight™ LIVE/DEAD viability kit) as a fluorescent probe to assess the metabolic state of *S. epidermidis* bacteria by flow cytometry. Ou et al. [35] induced the VBNC state in MRSA strains with freezing at $-20\ ^\circ C$, and subsequently evaluated their detection from contaminated food samples with the use of propidium monoazide-crossing priming amplification. Li et al. [36] successfully applied a propidium monoazide-polymerase chain reaction assay to rapidly detect VBNC *S. aureus* in food. A few studies also demonstrated that the detection of bacteria in the VBNC state with phages is possible. Awais et al. [37] engineered a GFP-labeled phage for the detection of *E. coli* and showed that also the detection of VBNC *E. coli* was possible with the method. Fernandez et al. [38] immobilized phage PVP-SE1 on the gold surface in a biosensor for the quantitative detection of VBNC *S. enteriditis*. They were able to successfully distinguish viable and VBNC cells from dead cells with a detection rate of 3–4 cells per sensor. As far as we know, no research on the detection of VBNC bacteria in biofilms formed by clinical isolates from patients with PJI using bacteriophages has been made.

*Staphylococcus aureus* and coagulase-negative staphylococci account for more than half of the cases of PJI, and the prevalence of methicillin-resistant *S. aureus* PJI is increasing [39,40]. Therefore, four clinically relevant and biofilm-forming staphylococcal strains—*S. epidermidis*, *S. lugdunensis*, and two *S. aureus* strains—were selected for this study. Importantly, two of the tested strains (*S. aureus* OBV 17/166 and *S. lugdunensis* OBV 20/143) were PJI clinical isolates. Bacteria were cultured for biofilm formation and transferred to low-nutrient media with three different gentamycin concentrations ($4 \times$ MIC, $8 \times$ MIC, and $16 \times$ MIC) for their induction into the VBNC state. We demonstrated that all tested strains were able to enter the VBNC state as early as 8 days and up to 19 days of exposure to gentamycin, regardless of the concentration used. To date, several foodborne and clinical bacterial species have been reported to be able to transition into the VBNC state, among them *S. aureus* and *S. epidermidis*. In the literature, different environmental conditions were used for induction. Pasquaroli et al. [18,19] successfully induced the VBNC state in *S. aureus* 10,850 biofilms with different concentrations of antibiotic vancomycin, quinupristin/dalfopristin, daptomycin, and/or nutrient depletion. Yan et al. [41] demonstrated the induction of the VBNC state in *S. aureus* in a citric acid buffer at $-20\ ^\circ C$. Bacteria showed changes in biological characteristics and were able to resuscitate under many different conditions. Robben et al. [42] showed that non-ionic surfactants can induce the VBNC state in *S. aureus* in just about 5 min and up to 1 h of exposure. Cerca et al. [43] observed that pH and extracellular levels of calcium and magnesium induced the VBNC state in *S. epidermidis* biofilms. Most of the conducted research on VBNC bacteria is, however, still from the fields of the food industry and water monitoring. Furthermore, several human pathogens associated with medical device infection were also reported as being able to enter the VBNC state. Zandri et al. [44] analyzed 44 central venous catheters negative by the Maki technique (rolling the catheter segment across blood agar) for the presence of VBNC bacteria in the biofilm. An analysis of 39 culture-negative samples with fluorescent staining and a bacterial 16S rDNA analysis by qPCR confirmed the presence of VBNC bacteria in 77% of samples that did not grow on culture media, mostly from the *Staphylococci* spp. (*S.*

*epidermidis* and *S. aureus*). However, the standard microbiology blood culture was positive only in 18% of patients. In a recent study, Wilkins et al. [45] demonstrated the presence of VBNC *P. aeruginosa*, *P. mirabilis*, and *E. coli* bacteria in biofilms forming on different antimicrobial urinary catheters, explaining why antimicrobial materials do not show a significantly important clinical improvement in vivo. However, we did not find any studies reporting the VBNC state in *S. lugdunensis*. Additionally, *S. epidermidis* has been reported in the literature as the only coagulase-negative *staphylococcus* to enter the VBNC state so far [46].

The results obtained in our study improved a previously developed method. The sensitivity of the method has already been determined previously by testing 104 clinical samples (sonicate fluid) with the method, and results were compared with the results obtained from microbiological conventional culturing. The sensitivity was 94.12%, with only one false negative result. However, in that patient, only conventional tissue culture was positive, while the culture of SF remained sterile [7]. For an exact determination of the method's sensitivity in also detecting VBNC bacteria, a larger number of SF samples would need to be tested in an extended future research study, to sample patients with a confirmed PJI but negative microbiological results (cases suspicious for VBNC presence). The method could be additionally improved by the application of new bacteriophages, specific to other bacterial species, or even by the bacteriophages with a narrower host range, to distinguish between *S. aureus* and coagulase-negative staphylococci. Results could therefore contribute importantly to the development of a new fast and effective diagnostic tool for the detection of device-associated biofilm infections, and, more broadly, other difficult-to-diagnose infections.

## 4. Materials and Methods

### 4.1. Bacteria and Bacteriophages

*Staphylococcus aureus* subsp. *aureus* bacteriophage K ATCC 19685-B1™, *S. aureus* ATCC 25923, and *E. coli* ATCC 25922 were purchased from the American Type Culture Collection (ATCC, Manassas, Vancouver, BC, Canada). *E. coli* ATCC 25922 was used in the study only as a negative control in the detection with phage K and qPCR. *S. epidermidis* DSM 3269 was purchased from the German Collection of Microorganisms and Cell Cultures GmbH (DSMZ, Deutsche Sammlung von Mikroorganismen und Zellkulturen GmbH). Clinical isolates *S. lugdunensis* OBV 20/143 and *S. aureus* OBV 17/166 were from an »in-house«on-growing isolates library of Valdoltra Orthopaedic Hospital, and they were isolated from patients undergoing revision surgery at our institution due to PJI during routine microbiological diagnostic procedures. Species were determined by conventional microbiological culturing methods and confirmed by sequencing.

### 4.2. Biofilm Formation and Induction of VBNC State

For the preparation of M9 minimal nutrient agar, 200 mL of M9 salts solution, 20 mL of 20% glucose solution, 2 mL of 1 M $MgSO_4$ (Carl Roth GmbH, Karlsruhe, Germany), 100 µL of 1 M $CaCl_2$ (Fisher Scientific, Loughborough, UK), 14 g of Agar Bios Special LL (Biolife Italiana srl, Milan, Italy), and $dH_2O$ were combined for the preparation of 1 L media. The M9 salt solution was prepared by dissolving 56.8 g $Na_2HPO_4$ (Sigma-Aldrich, St. Louis, MO), 15 g $KH_2PO_4$ (Sigma-Aldrich, St. Louis, MO), 2.5 g NaCl (Carlo Erba, Milan, Italy), and 5 g $NH_4Cl$ (Honeywell Fluka, Seelze, Germany) into 1 L $dH_2O$ and sterilized by autoclaving. D-Glucose anhydrous (Fisher Scientific, Loughborough, UK) was used for the preparation of 1% and 20% glucose solutions, which were sterilized by filtration through 0.22 µm pore-size Minisart syringe filters (Sartorius Stedim Biotech GmbH, Goettingen, Germany).

For the selected bacteria, minimal inhibitory concentrations (MIC) for the antibiotic gentamycin were determined by the microdilution technique in 96-well microtiter plates according to the protocol described by Wiegand et al. [47]. Two-times dilutions of gentamycin (Sigma-Aldrich, St. Louis, MO) were prepared in BHI broth (Merck KGaA, Darmstadt,

Germany) so that tested concentrations ranged from 100 µg/mL to 0.1 µg/mL. After the overnight incubation of plates at 37 °C, PrestoBlue™ Cell Viability Reagent (Invitrogen Life Technologies, Carlsbad, CA) was added to wells according to the manufacturer's instructions, and fluorescence was measured with a Tecan Infinite 200 Pro MPlex plate reader (Tecan, Männedorf, Switzerland) to determine the proliferation of bacterial cells. Fluorescence values were plotted vs. antibiotic concentration, and MIC values were determined as the lowest concentrations of gentamycin, which prevented the visible growth of bacteria.

For biofilm development on a solid surface, the colony biofilm assay was performed [48,49]. A late logarithmic bacterial culture was diluted to match the 0.5 McFarland standard (Carl Roth GmbH, Karlsruhe, Germany), and a 100 µL of the diluted culture was spotted on a 0.22 µm sterile cellulose nitrate filter disc (Sartorius Stedim Biotech GmbH, Goettingen, Germany) placed on the BHI agar plate supplemented with 1% glucose. Plates were incubated at 37 °C for 48 h.

To induce the VBNC state in bacteria, each filter disc with biofilm was transferred to M9 minimal nutrient agar plates with gentamycin at $4 \times$ MIC, $8 \times$ MIC, and $16 \times$ MIC. As a control, M9 minimal nutrient agar plates without gentamycin were used. Three parallel independent experiments were conducted for each tested bacterial strain under the same conditions. Plates were incubated aerobically at 37 °C and were weekly transferred to fresh plates of the same composition. The loss of culturability was monitored by sampling biofilms every other day and culturing biofilm samples on BHI agar plates at 37 °C for 7 days. The loss of culturability was determined if no visible growth was obtained after 7 days of culturing.

After the loss of culturability, biofilms were detached from filter paper discs by sonication. The applied sonication protocol is routinely used at our hospital for the sonication of explanted prosthetic devices for the microbiological assessment of PJI. Briefly, filter papers were placed in 5 mL sterile 0.85% NaCl solution, vortexed for 30 s, and then subjected to sonication at a frequency of 40 kHz and power density of 0.22 W/cm$^2$ in a BactoSonicR ultrasonic bath (Bandelin GmbH, Berlin, Germany) filled with 4% Tickopur solution (TR3, Bandelin, Berlin, Germany) for 5 min, followed by additional vortexing for 30 s. The suspension was then transferred into a new 50 mL falcon tube (Isolab, Wertheim, Germany) and centrifuged for 15 min at $10,000 \times g$ using a Sigma 3–18 KS centrifuge (Sigma Laborzentrifugen GmbH, Osterode am Harz, Germany). Bacteria were resuspended in 5 mL of sterile 0.85% NaCl solution.

To determine the presence of VBNC bacteria in the detached biofilms, the LIVE/DEAD™ BacLight™ Bacterial Viability Kit (Invitrogen™, Molecular Probes Inc., OR, USA) was used according to the manufacturer's instructions. Fluorescence was measured in black flat-bottom microtiter plates using a Tecan Infinite 200 Pro MPlex plate reader for the determination of viable cells percentages. Viable (green) and dead (red) bacteria were also visualized using a Fluorescence microscope Nikon Eclipse 80i (Nikon Corporation, Tokyo, Japan). Suspensions of live and dead bacterial cells were used as controls and were prepared as described in the BacLight™ kit manufacturer's instructions. According to their protocol, 70% 2-propanol (Merck, Darmstadt, Germany) was used to kill bacteria by incubating at room temperature for 1 h and mixing every 15 min. Prepared suspensions were used also in subsequent qPCR experiments.

*4.3. Detection of VBNC Bacteria with Bacteriophages and qPCR*

Suspensions of VBNC, live, and dead bacterial cells were adjusted to OD$_{670nm}$ of 0.6 diluting samples with the sterile 0.85% NaCl solution. A 100 µL of bacterial dilutions was then combined with BHI and bacteriophage K in a total volume of 1 mL. The final bacteriophage K concentration was $1.8 \times 10^4$ PFU/mL. A reference control sample was assessed and consisted of BHI with phage K at the same concentration. As a negative control, live and dead *E. coli* ATCC 25922 suspensions were used. Samples were incubated at 37 °C with shaking for 180 min. After that, 30 µL of chloroform (Sigma-Aldrich, St.

Louis, MO) was added to each sample and vortexed for 2 min. Afterward, samples were centrifuged in a tabletop MiniSpin centrifuge (Eppendorf AG, Hamburg, Germany) at $3287\times g$ for 5 min, and 1 µL of each supernatant was assayed in the qPCR in triplicates.

During the qPCR, the phage's DNA was quantified using previously designed [6] phage K-specific primers (forward 5'-CGTAGGTCACTCTCGTTTCG-3' and reverse 5'-CGTCACCGTAGAATGAAGCC -3') at a final concentration of 450 nM. DNA isolation prior to qPCR was previously proven unnecessary [6]. Reactions were performed in a total volume of 20 µL containing 10 µL of 2× Syber Green PowerUp master mix (Applied Biosystems, Life Technologies, Burlington, ON, Canada), 0.9 µL of each primer, 7.2 µL nuclease-free water, and 1 µL of the sample. The thermal cycling conditions were as follows: 2 min at 50 °C for UDG activation, 2 min at 95 °C for polymerase activation, and 45 cycles of 1 s at 95 °C and 30 s at 60 °C. In each qPCR run, a non-template control (using 1 µL nuclease-free water) as well as a reference control, containing only the initial amount of added phages, were included. The suspensions of live and dead bacterial cells with added phages were assessed as experimental controls. The protocols used for the detection of bacteria with phage K and qPCR, as well as the concentrations, were as optimized and defined in previous studies [6,7].

*4.4. Statistical Analysis*

The data shown are values obtained from three independent parallel experiments and expressed as mean ± SE (standard error) or mean ± SD (standard deviation). The SigmaPlot 12.0 (Systat Software, Chicago, IL, USA) program was used for the statistical analysis. A statistical analysis was performed by an analysis of variance (ANOVA, followed by the Student–Newman–Keuls test for comparisons across multiple groups) and Student's t-test. Statistical significance was defined as $p < 0.05$.

## 5. Conclusions

We successfully induced the VBNC state in the biofilms of *S. epidermidis*, *S. lugdunensis*, and two *S. aureus* strains with starvation and antibiotic pressure. With the tested method, we were able to specifically detect both live and VBNC staphylococci in a 4 h assay, through the detection of the increase or decrease in phage K DNA in the real-time PCR. Additionally, here, we first report the induction of the VBNC state in *S. lugdunensis*. To the best of our knowledge, *S. epidermidis* has been the only coagulase-negative *Staphylococcus* reported to enter the VBNC state up to today.

**Author Contributions:** Conceptualization, K.Š. and A.C.; Data Curation, K.Š.; Formal Analysis, K.Š.; Funding Acquisition, K.Š.; Investigation, K.Š.; Methodology, K.Š.; Project Administration, K.Š.; Resources, K.Š.; Software, K.Š.; Supervision, A.C.; Validation, K.Š. and A.C.; Visualization, A.C.; Writing—Original Draft, K.Š.; Writing—Review and Editing, A.C. All authors have read and agreed to the published version of the manuscript.

**Funding:** This research and the APC were funded by the Slovenian Research Agency, grant number Z3-4506.

**Institutional Review Board Statement:** Not applicable.

**Informed Consent Statement:** Not applicable.

**Data Availability Statement:** The data presented in this study are available in the Results section of this article.

**Conflicts of Interest:** The authors declare no conflict of interest. The funders had no role in the design of the study; in the collection, analyses, or interpretation of data; in the writing of the manuscript; or in the decision to publish the results.

## References

1. Abdelsattar, A.; Dawoud, A.; Makky, S.; Nofal, R.; Aziz, R.; El-Shibiny, A. Bacteriophages: From Isolation to Application. *Curr. Pharm. Biotechnol.* **2022**, *23*, 337–360. [CrossRef] [PubMed]
2. O'Flaherty, S.; Ross, R.P.; Meaney, W.; Fitzgerald, G.F.; Elbreki, M.F.; Coffey, A. Potential of the Polyvalent Anti-Staphylococcus Bacteriophage K for Control of Antibiotic-Resistant Staphylococci from Hospitals. *Appl. Environ. Microbiol.* **2005**, *71*, 1836–1842. [CrossRef]
3. Estrella, L.A.; Quinones, J.; Henry, M.; Hannah, R.M.; Pope, R.K.; Hamilton, T.; Teneza-mora, N.; Hall, E.; Biswajit, B. Characterization of Novel *Staphylococcus aureus* Lytic Phage and Defining Their Combinatorial Virulence Using the OmniLog® System. *Bacteriophage* **2016**, *6*, e1219440. [CrossRef]
4. Šuster, K.; Podgornik, A.; Cör, A. Quick Bacteriophage-Mediated Bioluminescence Assay for Detecting *Staphylococcus* spp. in Sonicate Fluid of Orthopaedic Artificial Joints. *New Microbiol* **2017**, *40*, 190–196. [PubMed]
5. Plota, M.; Sazakli, E.; Giormezis, N.; Gkartziou, F.; Kolonitsiou, F.; Leotsinidis, M.; Antimisiaris, S.G.; Spiliopoulou, I. In Vitro Anti-Biofilm Activity of Bacteriophage K (ATCC 19685-B1) and Daptomycin against Staphylococci. *Microorganisms* **2021**, *9*, 1853. [CrossRef] [PubMed]
6. Šuster, K.; Podgornik, A.; Cör, A. An Alternative Molecular Approach for a Rapid and Specific Detection of Clinically Relevant Bacteria Causing Prosthetic Joint Infections with Bacteriophage K. *New Microbiol.* **2020**, *43*, 107–114.
7. Šuster, K.; Cör, A. Fast and Specific Detection of Staphylococcal PJI with Bacteriophage-based Methods within 104 Sonicate Fluid Samples. *J. Orthop. Res.* **2022**, *40*, 1358–1364. [CrossRef] [PubMed]
8. Goodman, S.B.; Gallo, J.; Gibon, E.; Takagi, M. Diagnosis and Management of Implant Debris-Associated Inflammation. *Expert Rev. Med. Devices* **2020**, *17*, 41–56. [CrossRef]
9. Esteban, J.; Pérez-Jorge, C.; Pérez-Tanoira, R.; Gómez-Barrena, E. Microbiological Diagnosis of Prosthetic Joint Infection. In *Infected Total Joint Arthroplasty: The Algorithmic Approach*; Trebše, R., Ed.; Springer: London, UK, 2012; pp. 165–179.
10. Berbari, E.F.; Marculescu, C.; Sia, I.; Lahr, B.D.; Hanssen, A.D.; Steckelberg, J.M.; Gullerud, R.; Osmon, D.R. Culture-Negative Prosthetic Joint Infection. *Clin. Infect. Dis.* **2007**, *45*, 1113–1119. [CrossRef]
11. Malekzadeh, D.; Osmon, D.R.; Lahr, B.D.; Hanssen, A.D.; Berbari, E.F. Prior Use of Antimicrobial Therapy Is a Risk Factor for Culture-Negative Prosthetic Joint Infection. *Clin. Orthop.* **2010**, *468*, 2039–2045. [CrossRef]
12. Kim, Y.-H.; Park, J.-W.; Kim, J.-S.; Kim, D.-J. The Outcome of Infected Total Knee Arthroplasty: Culture-Positive Versus Culture-Negative. *Arch. Orthop. Trauma Surg.* **2015**, *135*, 1459–1467. [CrossRef]
13. Kalbian, I.; Park, J.W.; Goswami, K.; Lee, Y.-K.; Parvizi, J.; Koo, K.-H. Culture-Negative Periprosthetic Joint Infection: Prevalence, Aetiology, Evaluation, Recommendations, and Treatment. *Int. Orthop.* **2020**, *44*, 1255–1261. [CrossRef]
14. Ayrapetyan, M.; Williams, T.; Oliver, J.D. Relationship between the Viable but Nonculturable State and Antibiotic Persister Cells. *J. Bacteriol.* **2018**, *200*, e00249-18. [CrossRef]
15. Charani, E.; McKee, M.; Ahmad, R.; Balasegaram, M.; Bonaconsa, C.; Merrett, G.B.; Busse, R.; Carter, V.; Castro-Sanchez, E.; Franklin, B.D.; et al. Optimising Antimicrobial Use in Humans—Review of Current Evidence and an Interdisciplinary Consensus on Key Priorities for Research. *Lancet Reg. Health Eur.* **2021**, *7*, 100161. [CrossRef]
16. Stewart, P.S.; Franklin, M.J. Physiological Heterogeneity in Biofilms. *Nat. Rev. Microbiol.* **2008**, *6*, 199–210. [CrossRef]
17. Ayrapetyan, M.; Williams, T.C.; Oliver, J.D. Bridging the Gap between Viable but Non-Culturable and Antibiotic Persistent Bacteria. *Trends Microbiol.* **2015**, *23*, 7–13. [CrossRef]
18. Pasquaroli, S.; Zandri, G.; Vignaroli, C.; Vuotto, C.; Donelli, G.; Biavasco, F. Antibiotic Pressure Can Induce the Viable but Non-Culturable State in Staphylococcus Aureus Growing in Biofilms. *J. Antimicrob. Chemother.* **2013**, *68*, 1812–1817. [CrossRef]
19. Pasquaroli, S.; Citterio, B.; Cesare, A.; Amiri, M.; Manti, A.; Vuotto, C.; Biavasco, F. Role of Daptomycin in the Induction and Persistence of the Viable but Non-Culturable State of Staphylococcus Aureus Biofilms. *Pathogens* **2014**, *3*, 759–768. [CrossRef]
20. Ramamurthy, T.; Ghosh, A.; Pazhani, G.P.; Shinoda, S. Current Perspectives on Viable but Non-Culturable (VBNC) Pathogenic Bacteria. *Front. Public Health* **2014**, *2*, 103. [CrossRef]
21. Dong, K.; Pan, H.; Yang, D.; Rao, L.; Zhao, L.; Wang, Y.; Liao, X. Induction, Detection, Formation, and Resuscitation of Viable but Non-Culturable State Microorganisms. *Compr. Rev. Food Sci. Food Saf.* **2020**, *19*, 149–183. [CrossRef]
22. Hyman, P.; Abedon, S.T. Practical Methods for Determining Phage Growth Parameters. In *Bacteriophages: Methods and Protocols, Volume 1: Isolation, Characterization, and Interactions*; Clokie, M.R.J., Kropinski, A.M., Eds.; Humana Press: Totowa, NJ, USA, 2009; pp. 175–202. ISBN 978-1-60327-164-6.
23. Meile, S.; Kilcher, S.; Loessner, M.J.; Dunne, M. Reporter Phage-Based Detection of Bacterial Pathogens: Design Guidelines and Recent Developments. *Viruses* **2020**, *12*, 944. [CrossRef]
24. Jurač, K.; Nabergoj, D.; Podgornik, A. Bacteriophage Production Processes. *Appl. Microbiol. Biotechnol.* **2019**, *103*, 685–694. [CrossRef] [PubMed]
25. Ames, G.F.; Prody, C.; Kustu, S. Simple, Rapid, and Quantitative Release of Periplasmic Proteins by Chloroform. *J. Bacteriol.* **1984**, *160*, 1181–1183. [CrossRef] [PubMed]
26. Schofield, D.; Sharp, N.J.; Westwater, C. Phage-Based Platforms for the Clinical Detection of Human Bacterial Pathogens. *Bacteriophage* **2012**, *2*, 105–121. [CrossRef]

27. Triffault-Fillit, C.; Ferry, T.; Laurent, F.; Pradat, P.; Dupieux, C.; Conrad, A.; Becker, A.; Lustig, S.; Fessy, M.H.; Chidiac, C.; et al. Microbiologic Epidemiology Depending on Time to Occurrence of Prosthetic Joint Infection: A Prospective Cohort Study. *Clin. Microbiol. Infect.* **2019**, *25*, 353–358. [CrossRef]
28. Sebastian, S.; Malhotra, R.; Sreenivas, V.; Kapil, A.; Chaudhry, R.; Dhawan, B. Sonication of Orthopaedic Implants: A Valuable Technique for Diagnosis of Prosthetic Joint Infections. *J. Microbiol. Methods* **2018**, *146*, 51–54. [CrossRef]
29. Erivan, R.; Villatte, G.; Eymond, G.; Mulliez, A.; Descamps, S.; Boisgard, S. Usefulness of Sonication for Diagnosing Infection in Explanted Orthopaedic Implants. *Orthop. Traumatol. Surg. Res.* **2018**, *104*, 433–438. [CrossRef] [PubMed]
30. Ueda, N.; Oe, K.; Nakamura, T.; Tsuta, K.; Iida, H.; Saito, T. Sonication of Extracted Implants Improves Microbial Detection in Patients with Orthopedic Implant-Associated Infections. *J. Arthroplasty* **2019**, *34*, 1189–1196. [CrossRef]
31. Inacio, R.C.; Klautau, G.B.; Murça, M.A.S.; da Silva, C.B.; Nigro, S.; Rivetti, L.A.; Pereira, W.L.; Salles, M.J.C. Microbial Diagnosis of Infection and Colonization of Cardiac Implantable Electronic Devices by Use of Sonication. *Int. J. Infect. Dis.* **2015**, *38*, 54–59. [CrossRef] [PubMed]
32. Jost, G.F.; Wasner, M.; Taub, E.; Walti, L.; Mariani, L.; Trampuz, A. Sonication of Catheter Tips for Improved Detection of Microorganisms on External Ventricular Drains and Ventriculo-Peritoneal Shunts. *J. Clin. Neurosci.* **2014**, *21*, 578–582. [CrossRef] [PubMed]
33. Fleischmann, S.; Robben, C.; Alter, T.; Rossmanith, P.; Mester, P. How to Evaluate Non-Growing Cells—Current Strategies for Determining Antimicrobial Resistance of VBNC Bacteria. *Antibiotics* **2021**, *10*, 115. [CrossRef] [PubMed]
34. Cerca, F.; Trigo, G.; Correia, A.; Cerca, N.; Azeredo, J.; Vilanova, M. SYBR Green as a Fluorescent Probe to Evaluate the Biofilm Physiological State of *Staphylococcus epidermidis*, Using Flow Cytometry. *Can. J. Microbiol.* **2011**, *57*, 850–856. [CrossRef] [PubMed]
35. Ou, A.; Wang, K.; Mao, Y.; Yuan, L.; Ye, Y.; Chen, L.; Zou, Y.; Huang, T. First Report on the Rapid Detection and Identification of Methicillin-Resistant Staphylococcus Aureus (MRSA) in Viable but Non-Culturable (VBNC) Under Food Storage Conditions. *Front. Microbiol.* **2021**, *11*, 615875. [CrossRef] [PubMed]
36. Li, Y.; Huang, T.-Y.; Mao, Y.; Chen, Y.; Shi, F.; Peng, R.; Chen, J.; Yuan, L.; Bai, C.; Chen, L.; et al. Study on the Viable but Non-Culturable (VBNC) State Formation of Staphylococcus Aureus and Its Control in Food System. *Front. Microbiol.* **2020**, *11*, 599739. [CrossRef] [PubMed]
37. Awais, R.; Fukudomi, H.; Miyanaga, K.; Unno, H.; Tanji, Y. A Recombinant Bacteriophage-Based Assay for the Discriminative Detection of Culturable and Viable but Nonculturable Escherichia Coli O157:H7. *Biotechnol. Prog.* **2006**, *22*, 853–859. [CrossRef]
38. Fernandes, E.; Martins, V.C.; Nóbrega, C.; Carvalho, C.M.; Cardoso, F.A.; Cardoso, S.; Dias, J.; Deng, D.; Kluskens, L.D.; Freitas, P.P.; et al. A Bacteriophage Detection Tool for Viability Assessment of Salmonella Cells. *Biosens. Bioelectron.* **2014**, *52*, 239–246. [CrossRef]
39. Zimmerli, W.; Trampuz, A.; Ochsner, P.E. Prosthetic-Joint Infections. *N. Engl. J. Med.* **2004**, *351*, 1645–1654. [CrossRef]
40. Peel, T.N.; Buising, K.L.; Choong, P.F.M. Prosthetic Joint Infection: Challenges of Diagnosis and Treatment: Prosthetic Joint Infection. *ANZ J. Surg.* **2011**, *81*, 32–39. [CrossRef]
41. Yan, H.; Li, M.; Meng, L.; Zhao, F. Formation of Viable but Nonculturable State of Staphylococcus Aureus under Frozen Condition and Its Characteristics. *Int. J. Food Microbiol.* **2021**, *357*, 109381. [CrossRef]
42. Robben, C.; Fister, S.; Witte, A.K.; Schoder, D.; Rossmanith, P.; Mester, P. Induction of the Viable but Non-Culturable State in Bacterial Pathogens by Household Cleaners and Inorganic Salts. *Sci. Rep.* **2018**, *8*, 15132. [CrossRef] [PubMed]
43. Cerca, F.; Andrade, F.; Franca, A.; Andrade, E.B.; Ribeiro, A.; Almeida, A.A.; Cerca, N.; Pier, G.; Azeredo, J.; Vilanova, M. Staphylococcus Epidermidis Biofilms with Higher Proportions of Dormant Bacteria Induce a Lower Activation of Murine Macrophages. *J. Med. Microbiol.* **2011**, *60*, 1717–1724. [CrossRef]
44. Zandri, G.; Pasquaroli, S.; Vignaroli, C.; Talevi, S.; Manso, E.; Donelli, G.; Biavasco, F. Detection of Viable but Non-Culturable Staphylococci in Biofilms from Central Venous Catheters Negative on Standard Microbiological Assays. *Clin. Microbiol. Infect.* **2012**, *18*, 259–261. [CrossRef] [PubMed]
45. Wilks, S.A.; Koerfer, V.V.; Prieto, J.A.; Fader, M.; Keevil, C.W. Biofilm Development on Urinary Catheters Promotes the Appearance of Viable but Nonculturable Bacteria. *Mbio* **2021**, *12*, e03584-20. [CrossRef] [PubMed]
46. França, A.; Gaio, V.; Lopes, N.; Melo, L.D.R. Virulence Factors in Coagulase-Negative Staphylococci. *Pathogens* **2021**, *10*, 170. [CrossRef] [PubMed]
47. Wiegand, I.; Hilpert, K.; Hancock, R.E.W. Agar and Broth Dilution Methods to Determine the Minimal Inhibitory Concentration (MIC) of Antimicrobial Substances. *Nat. Protoc.* **2008**, *3*, 163–175. [CrossRef] [PubMed]
48. Merritt, J.H.; Kadouri, D.E.; O'Toole, G.A. Growing and Analyzing Static Biofilms. In *Current Protocols in Microbiology*; Coico, R., Kowalik, T., Quarles, J., Stevenson, B., Taylor, R., Eds.; John Wiley & Sons, Inc.: Hoboken, NJ, USA, 2005; ISBN 978-0-471-72925-9.
49. De Kievit, T. 1.39—Biofilms. In *Comprehensive Biotechnology*, 3rd ed.; Moo-Young, M., Ed.; Pergamon: Oxford, UK, 2011; pp. 529–540. ISBN 978-0-444-64047-5.

**Disclaimer/Publisher's Note:** The statements, opinions and data contained in all publications are solely those of the individual author(s) and contributor(s) and not of MDPI and/or the editor(s). MDPI and/or the editor(s) disclaim responsibility for any injury to people or property resulting from any ideas, methods, instructions or products referred to in the content.

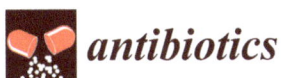 

Article

# The Detection of Potential Native Probiotics *Lactobacillus* spp. against *Salmonella* Enteritidis, *Salmonella* Infantis and *Salmonella* Kentucky ST198 of Lebanese Chicken Origin

Rima El Hage [1,2,*], Jeanne El Hage [3], Selma P. Snini [2], Imad Ammoun [4], Joseph Touma [1], Rami Rachid [1], Florence Mathieu [2], Jean-Marc Sabatier [5], Ziad Abi Khattar [6,*] and Youssef El Rayess [7]

1. Food Microbiology Laboratory, Lebanese Agricultural Research Institute (LARI), Fanar Station, Jdeideh El-Metn P.O. Box 901965, Lebanon
2. Laboratoire de Génie Chimique, UMR 5503 CNRS/INPT/UPS, INP-ENSAT, 1, Université de Toulouse, Avenue de l'Agrobiopôle, 31326 Castanet-Tolosan, France
3. Animal Health Laboratory, Lebanese Agricultural Research Institute (LARI), Fanar Station, Jdeideh El-Metn P.O. Box 901965, Lebanon
4. Milk and Milk Products Laboratory, Lebanese Agricultural Research Institute (LARI), Fanar Station, Jdeideh El-Metn P.O. Box 901965, Lebanon
5. CNRS UMR 7051, INP, Inst Neurophysiopathol, Aix-Marseille Université, 13385 Marseille, France
6. Microbiology/Tox-Ecotoxicology Team, Laboratory of Georesources, Geosciences and Environment (L2GE), Faculty of Sciences 2, Lebanese University, Campus Fanar, Jdeideh El-Metn P.O. Box 90656, Lebanon
7. Faculty of Agricultural and Food Sciences, Holy Spirit University of Kaslik, Jounieh P.O. Box 446, Lebanon
* Correspondence: relhage@lari.gov.lb (R.E.H.); ziad.abikhattar@ul.edu.lb (Z.A.K.)

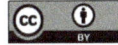

Citation: El Hage, R.E.; El Hage, J.E.; Snini, S.P.; Ammoun, I.; Touma, J.; Rachid, R.; Mathieu, F.; Sabatier, J.-M.; Abi Khattar, Z.; El Rayess, Y. The Detection of Potential Native Probiotics *Lactobacillus* spp. against *Salmonella* Enteritidis, *Salmonella* Infantis and *Salmonella* Kentucky ST198 of Lebanese Chicken Origin. *Antibiotics* **2022**, *11*, 1147. https://doi.org/10.3390/antibiotics11091147

Academic Editor: Andrey Shelenkov

Received: 26 July 2022
Accepted: 22 August 2022
Published: 24 August 2022

**Publisher's Note:** MDPI stays neutral with regard to jurisdictional claims in published maps and institutional affiliations.

Copyright: © 2022 by the authors. Licensee MDPI, Basel, Switzerland. This article is an open access article distributed under the terms and conditions of the Creative Commons Attribution (CC BY) license (https://creativecommons.org/licenses/by/4.0/).

**Abstract:** *Salmonella* continues to be a major threat to public health, especially with respect to strains from a poultry origin. In recent years, an increasing trend of antimicrobial resistance (AMR) in *Salmonella* spp. was observed due to the misuse of antibiotics. Among the approaches advised for overcoming AMR, probiotics from the *Lactobacillus* genus have increasingly been considered for use as effective prophylactic and therapeutic agents belonging to the indigenous microbiota. In this study, we isolated lactobacilli from the ilea and ceca of hens and broilers in order to evaluate their potential probiotic properties. Four species were identified as *Limosilactobacillus reuteri* (n = 22, 45.8%), *Ligilactobacillus salivarius* (n = 20, 41.6%), *Limosilactobacillus fermentum* (n = 2, 4.2%) and *Lactobacillus crispatus* (n = 1, 2%), while three other isolates (n = 3, 6.25%) were non-typable. Eight isolates, including *Ligilactobacillus salivarius* (n = 4), *Limosilactobacillus reuteri* (n = 2), *L. crispatus* (n = 1) and *Lactobacillus* spp. (n = 1) were chosen on the basis of their cell surface hydrophobicity and auto/co-aggregation ability for further adhesion assays using the adenocarcinoma cell line Caco-2. The adhesion rate of these strains varied from 0.53 to 10.78%. *Ligilactobacillus salivarius* A30/i26 and 16/c6 and *Limosilactobacillus reuteri* 1/c24 showed the highest adhesion capacity, and were assessed for their ability to compete in and exclude the adhesion of *Salmonella* to the Caco-2 cells. Interestingly, *Ligilactobacillus salivarius* 16/c6 was shown to significantly exclude the adhesion of the three *Salmonella* serotypes, *S.* Enteritidis, *S.* Infantis and *S.* Kentucky ST 198, to Caco-2 cells. The results of the liquid co-culture assays revealed a complete inhibition of the growth of *Salmonella* after 24 h. Consequently, the indigenous *Ligilactobacillus salivarius* 16/c6 strain shows promising potential for use as a preventive probiotic added directly to the diet for the control of the colonization of *Salmonella* spp. in poultry.

**Keywords:** *Salmonella* spp.; poultry; probiotic; *Ligilactobacillus salivarius*; inhibition; adhesion

## 1. Introduction

Non-typhoidal *Salmonella* strains are the leading cause of foodborne gastroenteritis [1]. Poultry products are primarily consumed worldwide and are commonly known to be reservoirs for a variety of microorganisms. *Salmonella* is the most frequently encountered pathogen in poultry products, as well as the most prominent inhabitant of avian gastrointestinal tracts (GIT) [2]. In developing countries, a high prevalence of *Salmonella* has been recorded, ranging from 13% to 39% in South America, estimated at 35% in Africa, and ranging from 35% to 50% in Asia [3]. In Lebanon, according to our recent study, the percentage of contamination of poultry meat at the retail level (supermarkets and restaurants) was estimated at 22.4% [4].

Several control strategies have been adopted to reduce or eliminate *Salmonella* at the farm level. It is well known that the use of antibiotic growth promoters (AGPs) and other prophylactic treatments improve animal health and productivity rates in livestock farming [5]. However, the mass use of antibiotics as feed additives has led to the emergence and spread of antimicrobial resistant pathogens and epidemic multi-drug-resistant clones and/or resistance genes in poultry reservoirs [6]. Recently, resistance to critical antibiotics, namely fluoroquinolones and expanded-spectrum β-lactam antibiotics, has spread worldwide and reached humans through the food chain [7]. Consequently, since 2006, AGP use in the animal industry has been completely banned in the EU [8] and reduced in many other countries [9]. However, in Lebanon, there are no current regulations concerning the use of AGPs in animal husbandry (personal communication with the ministry of agriculture).

Many countries have also implemented control programs to tackle *Salmonella* in poultry farms. Such was the case in the USA (National Poultry Improvement Plan (NPIP) for the eradication of *Salmonella* in eggs (1989) and meats (1994)) and the EU (Commission Regulation (EC), No. 2160/2003). These measurements ultimately led to the successful reduction of targeted *Salmonella* spp., but unfortunately cleared the way for the emergence of more resistant, less common serotypes, such as *S.* Heidelberg and *S.* Kentucky [10].

A promising alternative strategy against enteropathogens is the use of lactic acid bacteria (LAB) as probiotics. Probiotics are non-pathogenic live microorganisms which confer health benefits on their host when ingested in adequate quantities [11]. The use of (direct-fed microbial) probiotics as broiler growth promoters [12,13] could improve livestock health and might reduce the emergence of antimicrobial resistance (AMR) [14]. Strains of *Lactobacillus* spp. and *Bifidobacterium* spp. are the most widely studied probiotics acting against gastrointestinal microbial pathogens [15], especially against *Salmonella* infections in the broiler gastrointestinal tract [16,17]. Two fundamental mechanisms of inhibition of pathogenic microorganisms have been described, namely the direct cell competitive exclusion and the production of inhibitory compounds, including lactic and acetic acids, hydrogen peroxide, bacteriocin or bacteriocin-like inhibitors, and fatty and amino acid metabolites [18].

Intestinal adhesion and colonization are the first steps of the *Salmonella* infection process in poultry. Therefore, the adhesion ability is an essential prerequisite of, and one of the main criteria for selecting, potential probiotic strains [11]. The probiotic ability prevents the selected strains from undergoing direct elimination by peristalsis and inhibits the colonization of enteric pathogens in chickens by competitive exclusion [19]. Methods of evaluating the capacity of LAB to adhere to poultry epithelia may include in vitro analysis of, for example, cell aggregation, cell wall hydrophobicity, and adhesion to the human colorectal adenocarcinoma cell line (Caco-2) and chicken hepatocellular carcinoma cell line (LMH) [12]. Since bacterial populations of GIT are specific to their animal hosts, poultry-derived probiotics could be more effective than non-specific microbial agents [20].

This study aims to develop an effective probiotic derived from broiler and chicken GITs. In this regard, in vitro experiments were conducted to reveal the probiotic activity of native poultry-derived lactobacilli strains against the most relevant and drug-resistant *Salmonella* spp. (*S.* Enteritidis, *S.* Infantis and *S.* Kentucky ST198) in Lebanese poultry farms. The screening of lactobacilli strains for their anti-*Salmonella* activity, safety and surface probiotic properties was also carried out. Finally, the lactobacilli showing a great probiotic potential were selected for the further in vitro characterization of their adhesion ability and kinetics in co-culture. In fact, their adhesion and abilities to exclude and compete with *Salmonella* serotypes in epithelial tissues, using the Caco-2 cell line as an experimental model, were evaluated, as well as their capacity to inhibit pathogen growth in a mixed co-culture model.

## 2. Results

### 2.1. Screening of Lactobacilli and Their Anti-Salmonella Activity

In total, 210 stains (155 from the 16 trials and 55 from commercial birds) which presented as gram-positive bacilli/coccobacilli with no catalase activity were collected from broiler ceca and ileum samples. All lactobacilli were found to produce inhibition zones against the three serotypes of *Salmonella* based on the agar spot-on-lawn assay. The radii of their inhibition zones ranged from 1.2 to 4.4 cm (data not shown). However, the cell-free supernatants (CFSs) of all lactobacilli, neutralized to pH 6.8, did not display any antimicrobial effects against the *Salmonella* serotypes studied.

### 2.2. Genotypic Identification of Lactobacilli Isolates with Phylogenetic Relations

Lactobacilli strains ($n$ = 48) were chosen according to their high anti-*Salmonella* activity in the spot-on-lawn test. The 16S rRNA gene sequence analysis identified four species: *Limosilactobacillus reuteri* (formerly *Lactobacillus reuteri*) ($n$ = 22, 45.83%), *Ligilactobacillus salivarius* (formerly *Lactobacillus salivarius*) ($n$ = 20, 41.66%), *Limosilactobacillus fermentum* (formerly *Lactobacillus fermentum*) ($n$ = 2, 4.16%) and *Lactobacillus crispatus* ($n$ = 1, 2%) (Figure 1). The three remaining isolates (16/i10, 14/i15, A30/c2, 6.25%) were non-typable. The most common species were *Limosilactobacillus reuteri* and *Ligilactobacillus salivarius*. The phylogenetic tree demonstrated a close relation among the same species. However, we could not obtain a better strain resolution at the subspecies level among *Limosilactobacillus reuteri*. To gain further insight into the genetic dissimilarities and evolutionary relationships among the lineages isolated here would require profound core-gene-based phylogenetic analyses. These analyses are not considered here, since the focus of our study is the probiotic potential of lactobacilli strains.

### 2.3. Analysis of Surface Properties

The visual screening of the forty-eight chosen lactobacilli isolates showed that most of the strains were Agg+/Agg− (75%), while Agg+ and Agg− represented 14,6% and 10.4%, respectively (data not shown). These results were confirmed by auto-aggregation assays at 4 h. As shown in Figure 2, category I demonstrated a significant auto-aggregation percentage ($\geq$65%) compared to category II ($\leq$10%), while category III ranged from 10 to 65% except for three strains: one > 65% and two $\leq$ 10%. Auto-aggregation was determined in all the lactobacilli tested ($n$ = 45, 90%) at 24 h.

The co-aggregation properties of the lactobacilli strains with *Salmonella* serotypes differed among the strains and ranged from 0 to 94.6% (data not shown). They co-aggregated with *S.* Kentucky ST198, *S.* Enteritidis and *S.* Infantis at 52%, 58% and 63%, respectively. Otherwise, a high affinity for xylene was shown (65%) compared to non-hydrophobic isolates (31%).

### 2.4. Hydrophobicity and Auto/co-Aggregation Correlation

The results obtained from the analysis of the lactobacilli surfaces were subjected to principal component analysis (PCA) (Figure 3). The first PC1 and second PC2 principal components could explain 47.1% and 28.13% of the total variance, respectively. Based on the cell surface properties, eight lactobacilli strains were chosen for further adhesion assays, whose characteristics are summarized in Table 1. *Ligilactobacillus salivarius* A30/126 was shown to be highly hydrophobic (98.84% ± 1.34), possessing an aggregation phenotype (Agg+) and an ability to aggregate rapidly at 4 h (76.15% ± 3.93). The most co-aggregative strains were *L. crispatus* 16/c2, *Limosilactobacillus reuteri* 12/c8 and *Ligilactobacillus salivarius* (16/c4, 16/c6 and 14/i8). In addition to these properties, *Ligilactobacillus salivarius* 16/c6 did not exhibit auto-aggregation at 4 h but only at 24 h (9.89% ± 3.63 and 95.91% ± 2.58, respectively). However, *Ligilactobacillus salivarius* 16/c4 displayed an aggregation phenotype

(Agg+) and rapidly auto-aggregated at 4 h (76.23% ± 3.38). Both *Lactobacillus* spp. 16/i10 and *Limosilactobacillus reuteri* 1/c24 displayed high hydrophobicity levels (98.36% ± 3.63 and 91.81% ± 7.78, respectively); however, they either did not show an auto-aggregation capacity at 4 h, or only did so to a moderate degree (6.16% ± 5.53 and 13.76% ± 1.87, respectively) (Table 1).

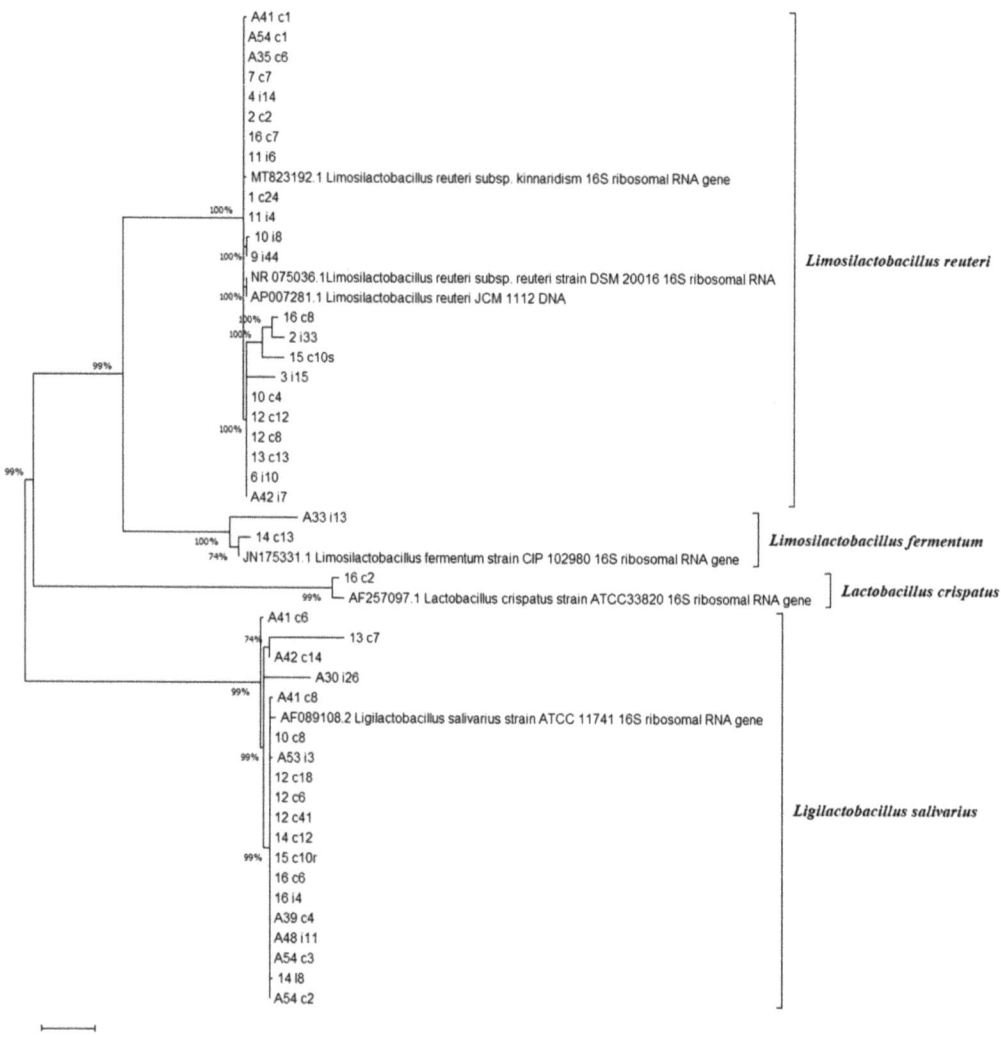

**Figure 1.** A maximum-likelihood phylogenetic tree reconstructed using 16S rRNA gene sequences. The percentage of replicate trees in which the associated species clustered together in the bootstrap test (1000 replicates) are shown next to the branches [21]. Evolutionary analyses were conducted in MEGA X. *Limosilactobacillus fermentum* comb. nov. CIP 102980 (JN175331), *Lactobacillus crispatus* ATCC 33820T (AF257097), *Ligilactobacillus salivarius* comb. nov. ATCC 11741T (AF089108), *Limosilactobacillus reuteri* comb. nov. JCM 1112 (AP007281), *Limosilactobacillus reuteri* subsp.*kinnaridis* (MT823192), and *Limosilactobacillus reuteri* subsp. *reuteri* DSM20016 (NR075036) were selected as type strains. The 16S rRNA gene accession numbers are provided in parentheses.

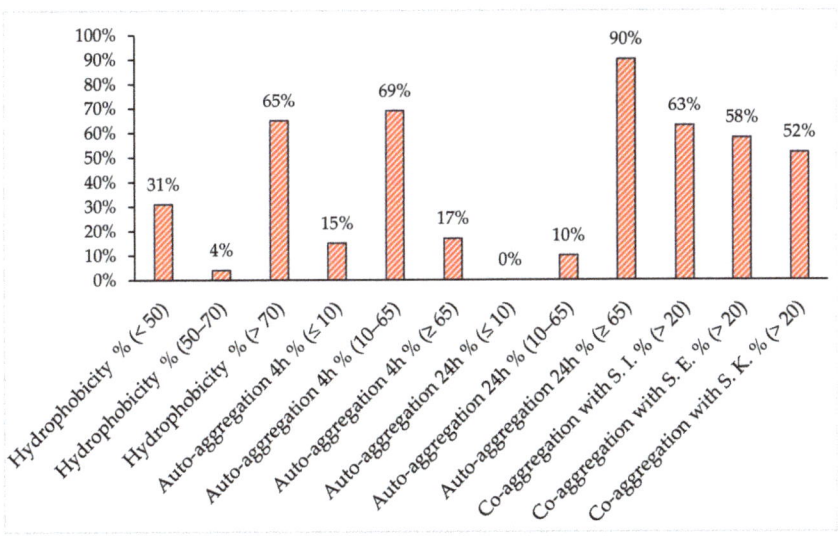

**Figure 2.** Isolate distribution in defined ranges of percentage of hydrophobicity, auto-aggregation and co-aggregation with the three *Salmonella* spp. (*S.* Enteritidis (S.E.), *S.* Kentucky ST198 (S.K.) and *S.* Infantis (S.I.).

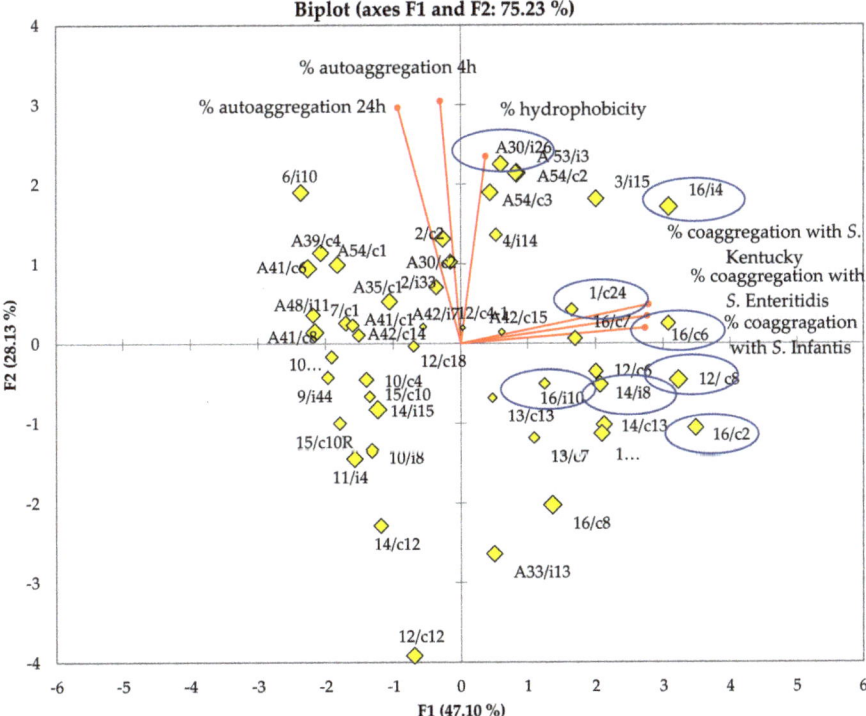

**Figure 3.** Graphic representation of the principal component analysis (PCA) of surface proprieties, including hydrophobicity and auto/co-aggregation, for the 48 lactobacilli isolated stains. The selected stains are encircled.

Table 1. Cell surface properties of the eight selected strains of lactobacilli.

| Isolates | Visual Aggregation | Auto-Aggregation 4 h (%) | Auto-Aggregation 24 h (%) | % Co-Aggregation with | | | Hydrophobicity (%) |
|---|---|---|---|---|---|---|---|
| | | | | S. Enteritidis | S. Infantis | S. Kentucky ST198 | |
| L. crispatus 16/c2 | Agg+/Agg− | 14.46 ± 2.78 | 58.67 ± 7.62 | 89.36 | 75.06 | 69.66 | 84.58 ± 1.92 |
| Ligilactobacillus salivarius 16/c6 | Agg− | 9.89 ± 3.63 | 95.91 ± 2.58 | 71.07 | 69.55 | 94.55 | 90.26 ± 3.91 |
| Ligilactobacillus salivarius 16/i4 | Agg+ | 76.23 ± 3.38 | 92.95 ± 10.5 | 82.49 | 80.45 | 79.94 | 82.25 ± 5.84 |
| Lactobacillus sp. 16/i10 | Agg+/Agg− | 6.16 ± 5.53 | 79.46 ± 1.18 | 45.60 | 34.32 | 63.51 | 98.36 ± 0.75 |
| Ligilactobacillus salivarius 14/i8 | Agg+/Agg− | 23.14 ± 5.29 | 73.47 ± 3.67 | 62.30 | 70.35 | 47.54 | 81.63 ± 1.2 |
| Limosilactobacillus reuteri 12/c8 | Agg+/Agg− | 33.93 ± 6.44 | 71.86 ± 1.89 | 83.47 | 73.87 | 80.00 | 52.66 ± 2.98 |
| Limosilactobacillus reuteri 1/c24 | Agg+/Agg− | 13.76 ± 1.87 | 91.81 ± 7.78 | 50.43 | 62.47 | 58.93 | 97.53 ± 0.96 |
| Ligilactobacillus salivarius A30/i26 | Agg+ | 76.15 ± 3.93 | 99.63 ± 0.26 | 49.54 | 25.71 | 60.00 | 98.84 ± 1.34 |

Values of auto-aggregation and hydrophobicity are the means of triplicate assays with their standard deviations.

There was no significant correlation between hydrophobicity, auto-aggregation, and co-aggregation among the forty-eight strains tested (Table 2). On the contrary, a significant correlation was detected ($p < 0.05$) between the co-aggregation results of the three *Salmonella* serotypes with lactobacilli isolates, since the correlation coefficient value reached up to 0.890.

Table 2. Correlation of Pearson coefficients between hydrophobicity, auto-aggregation and co-aggregation of the 48 lactobacilli isolates. The index of Pearson was used to evaluate the correlation between the six assays, hydrophobicity, auto-aggregation and co-aggregation between the lactobacilli strains and *S.* Enteritidis, *S.* Infantis and *S.* Kentucky stains.

| Variables | Hydrophobicity (%) | Auto-Aggregation 4 h (%) | Auto-Aggregation 24 h (%) | Co-Aggregation with S. Infantis (%) | Co-Aggregation with S. Enteritidis (%) | Co-Aggregation with S. Kentucky (%) |
|---|---|---|---|---|---|---|
| Hydrophobicity (%) | 1 | | | | | |
| Auto-aggregation 4 h (%) | 0.2264 | 1 | | | | |
| Auto-aggregation 24 h (%) | 0.2665 | 0.5302 | 1 | | | |
| Co-aggregation with S. Infantis (%) | 0.0595 | −0.0537 | −0.1878 | 1 | | |
| Co-aggregation with S. Enteritidis (%) | 0.1524 | 0.0202 | −0.1880 | 0.8782 | 1 | |
| Co-aggregation with S. Kentucky (%) | 0.1496 | −0.0208 | −0.2181 | 0.8439 | 0.8887 | 1 |

*2.5. Assays for Tolerance to Simulated Gastrointestinal Conditions of Chickens*

The eight chosen lactobacilli were further evaluated for their survival capacity in a medium simulating the GIT conditions of chickens (Figure 4). All strains were able to tolerate acidity and 0.1% (*w/v*) bile salts. However, at 0.3% bile salts, the survival rate was reduced for *Ligilactobacillus salivarius* 16/i4 and A33/i26 to 0% and 37%, respectively.

*2.6. Adhesion Assays*

The attachment of the lactobacilli isolates varied from 0.53 to 10.78% (Figure 5). *Ligilactobacillus salivarius* (A30/i26, 16/c6 and 16/i4) and *Limosilactobacillus reuteri* 1/c24 showed the highest adhesion abilities ($p < 0.05$) of 10.78% ± 4.2, 6.5% ± 1.82, 5% ± 0.99 and 6.43% ± 2.26, respectively. The remaining *Lactobacillus* spp. 16/i10, *Ligilactobacillus salivarius* 14/i8, *Limosilactobacillus reuteri* 12/c8 and *L. crispatus* 16/c2 strains showed no significant differences, with low adhesion capacities of 3.61% ± 1.14, 2.35% ± 0.86, 1.99% ± 0.66 and 0.53% ± 0.21, respectively.

*S.* Infantis, *S.* Enteritidis and *S.* Kentucky ST198 attached to the Caco-2 cells at a percentage of 8.81% ± 0.87, 7.81% ± 1.41 and 6.77% ± 0.89, respectively. No significant difference was found between the different serotypes (Figure 5).

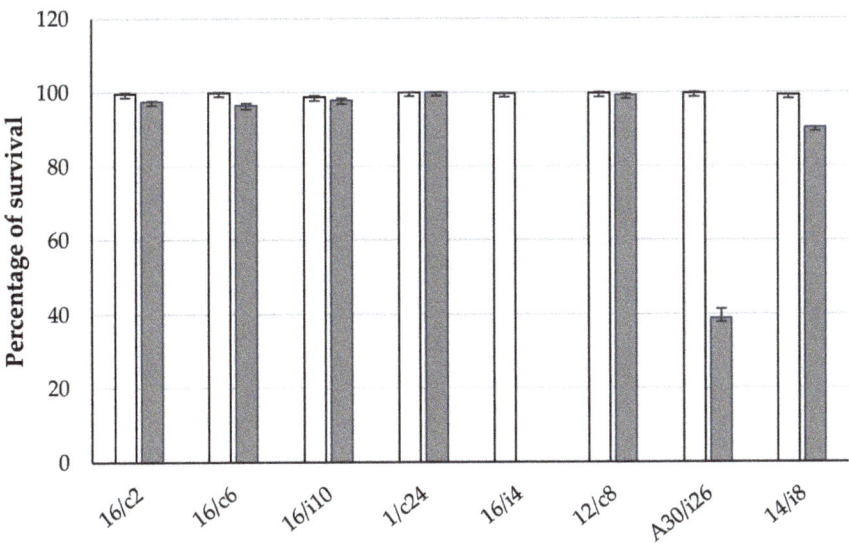

**Figure 4.** Effects of simulated gastrointestinal conditions on lactobacilli viability. White and grey columns correspond to lactobacilli subjected to 0.15% and 0.3% bile salts, respectively. *L. crispatus* 16/c2, *Ligilactobacillus salivarius* (16/c6, 16/i4, A30/i26, 14/i8), *Lactobacillus sp.* 16/i10 and *Limosilactobacillus reuteri* (1/c24 and 12/c8).

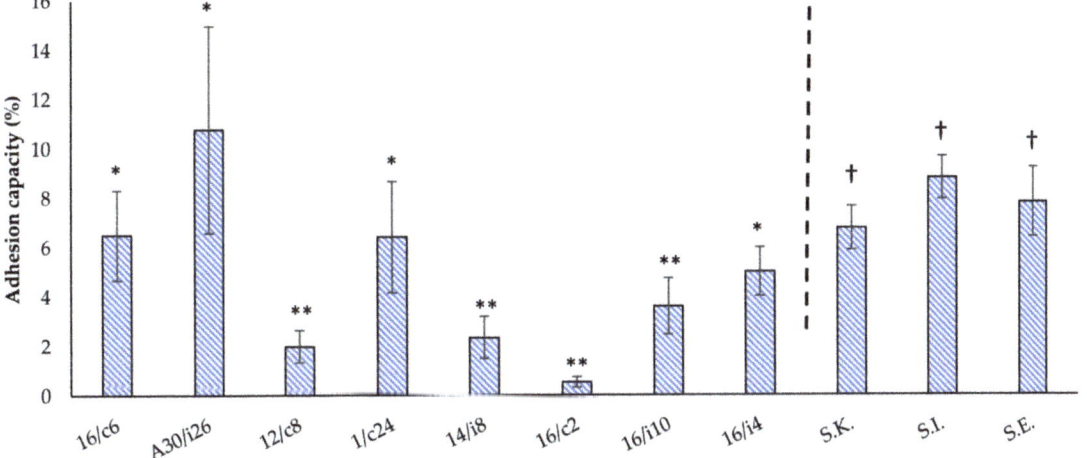

**Figure 5.** Adhesion capacities of the eight-native poultry-derived lactobacilli strains and the three *Salmonella* serotypes (*S.* Kentucky ST 198 (S.K.), *S.* Infantis (S.I.) and *S.* Enteritidis (S.E.)) to Caco-2 monolayers. The means and standard deviations of the two independent experiments are shown, each with three replicates. The differences between the levels of strain adhesion were evaluated separately for the lactobacilli strains and *Salmonella* serotypes. *Ligilactobacillus salivarius* 16/c6, 16/i4 and A30/i26 and *Limosilactobacillus reuteri* 1/c24 revealed no significant differences (*) in their adhesion capacity, a finding which was dissimilar from the four remaining tested strains (**). The differences in the adhesion capacities of *S.* Enteritidis, *S.* Infantis and *S.* Kentucky ST198 were also not significant among the three serotypes (†).

## 2.7. Competition/Exclusion Assays

Three lactobacilli strains that showed the highest adhesion capacity, namely, *Ligilactobacillus salivarius* A30/i26 and 16/c6 and *Limosilactobacillus reuteri* 1/c24, were assessed for their ability to compete with the pathogen for the adhesion site on the Caco-2 monolayers (Figure 6). The results showed that none of these strains displayed an effect on the pathogen adhesion to the Caco-2 cells. In the exclusion assays, *Ligilactobacillus salivarius* 16/c6 excluded the pathogens to a better degree than *Ligilactobacillus salivarius* A30/i26 and *Limosilactobacillus reuteri* 1/c24. The percentages of anti-adhesion to the Caco-2 cells of *S.* Enteritidis, *S.* Infantis and *S.* Kentucky ST198 were 70.30% ± 6.22, 86.57% ± 9.22 and 79.54% ± 9.26, respectively ($p < 0.05$).

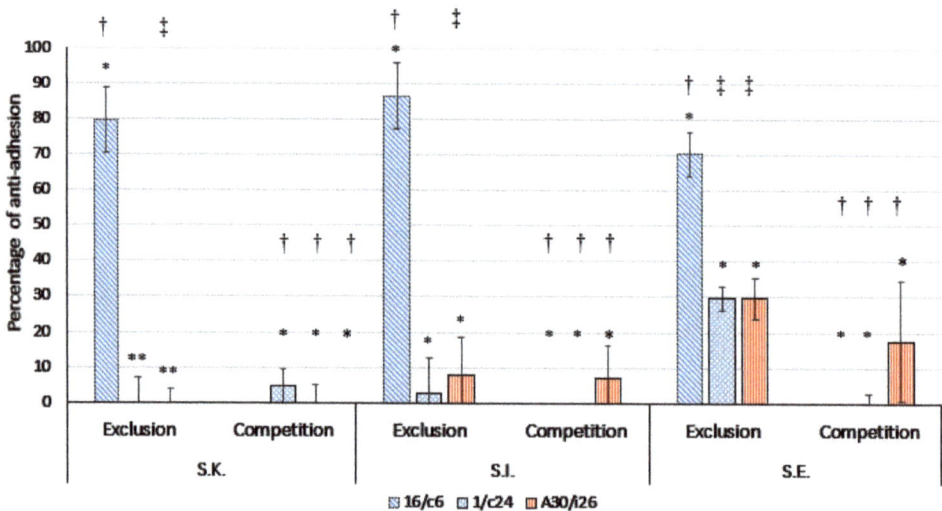

**Figure 6.** Inhibition of the adherence of *S.* Kentucky ST 198 (S.K.), *S.* Infantis (S.I.) and *S.* Enteritidis (S.E.) to Caco-2 cells by *Ligilactobacillus salivarius* 16/c6 and A30/i26 and *Limosilactobacillus reuteri* 1/c24 in competition and exclusion assays. The means and standard deviations of three independent experiments are shown, each with three replicates. (*) *Lactobacillus* strains were fixed and the differences in inhibition were calculated between the three serotypes in the same assay. (*) $p > 0.05$, (**) $p \leq 0.05$. (†) *Salmonella* serotypes were fixed, and the differences in inhibition were calculated between the three lactobacilli strains in the same assay. (†) $p > 0.05$, (‡) $p \leq 0.05$.

## 2.8. Co-Culture Growth Kinetics

Since *Ligilactobacillus salivarius* 16/c6 was able to inhibit the adhesion of *Salmonella* to the Caco-2 monolayers, its ability to inhibit the growth of *Salmonella* serotypes was assessed in a broth co-culture assay. Pure cultures of the lactobacilli and *Salmonella* serotypes (S.E., S.K., and S.I.) grew very well in the chosen Laptg medium (Figure 7).

In both experiments, without (Figure 7 A) or with (Figure 7 B) vortexing, differences in the CFUs between the control cultures of *Salmonella* (S.E., S.K., and S.I.) and co-cultures (S.E./LAB, S.K./LAB and S.I./LAB) were observed from the early incubation hours. However, the numbers of CFUs estimated from the co-cultures without vortexing were lower than those determined from the vortexed co-cultures and those of the control cultures at 8 h. In fact, the *Salmonella* in the co-cultures increased from $10^5$ to $10^6$ CFU /mL in the first 4 h and then sharply decreased to $10^2$ and $10^1$ CFU/mL, until a negligible cell viability was obtained between 8 h and 24 h. Simultaneously, the *Ligilactobacillus salivarius* count decreased from $10^7$ to $10^6$ at 8 h, then was reduced to almost $10^4$ at 24 h in the monoculture (16/c6) and co-cultures (LAB/S.E., LAB/S.K and LAB/S.I.).

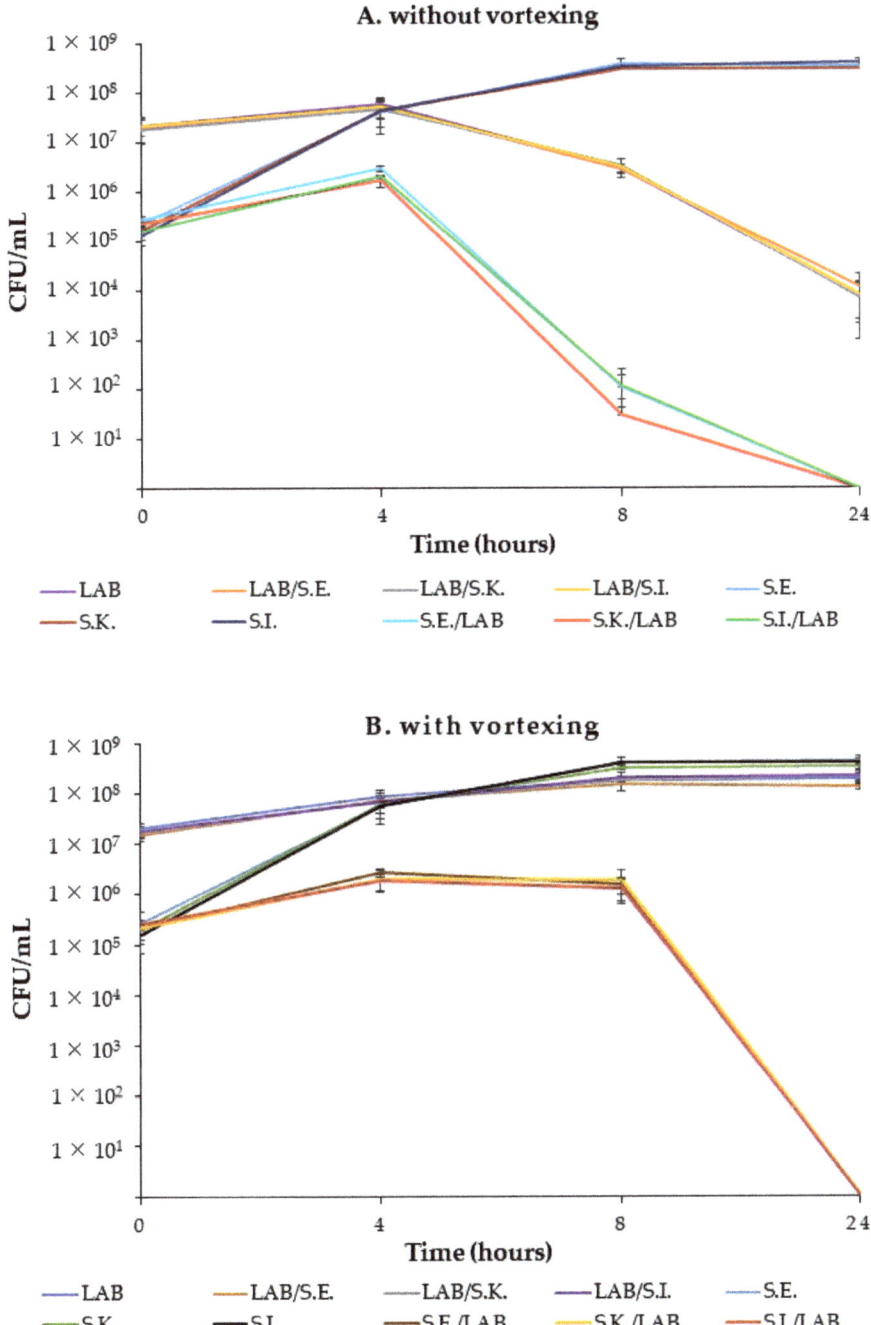

**Figure 7.** Kinetic growths of the pure cultures and co-cultures of *Ligilactobacillus salivarius* 16/c6 and *S.* Enteritidis, *S.* Infantis and *S.* Kentucky ST198 without (**A**) or with (**B**) vortexing. The means and standard deviations of the three independent experiments are shown, each with three replicates.

In the second set of experiments, *Salmonella* counts from the co-cultures (S.E./LAB, S.K./LAB and S.I./LAB) slightly increased in 4 h and remained constant until 8 h, then decreased to an undetectable level (<10 CFU/mL) at 24 h. However, the pure cultures of *Salmonella* slightly increased at 8 h and remained constant until the end of the experiments. The lactobacilli counts in the LAB–*Salmonella* mix (LAB/S.E., LAB/S.K and LAB/S.I.) were similar to those of the control monoculture. The pH value in both the mono- and co-cultures dropped from approximately 6.97 to 3.9 at 24 h.

## 3. Discussion

LAB are considered the principal residents of the GIT, where they provide the host with protection against enteric pathogen colonization (competition for nutrients and secretion of inhibitory substances). These LAB were the focus of many works, substituting the use of probiotics as growth promotors and/or subtherapeutic additives in animal feeds [22]. Numerous factors affect the microbial biodiversity of the poultry GIT, such as the GIT section (ileum or caeca) and the breed, diet and age of the chicken. The microbiota change significantly in the first 2–3 weeks until their stabilization at 5–6 weeks of age. It was found that, when broilers were fed with antibiotic and an additive-free corn-soy diet, 70% of their ileum population was comprised of *Lactobacillus* spp. The use of antibiotics in broilers was shown to induce changes in the composition of the intestinal bacterial community, namely *Ligilactobacillus salivarius* [23]. In this regard, our experiments did not detect an important species diversity among the lactobacilli isolates identified. Strains of *Lactobacillus acidophilus*, *Ligilactobacillus salivarius* and *Limosilactobacillus fermentum* were permanently found in all birds aged from two days old to market age. Babot and colleagues showed that the most common *Lactobacillus* species were *L. crispatus*, *Limosilactobacillus reuteri* and *Ligilactobacillus salivarius*, which was also the case in our findings [24].

In vitro tests have been used to assess the probiotic potential of lactobacilli. The production of hydrogen peroxide, organic acids and bacteriocins are the main strategies of *Lactobacillus* in inhibiting *Salmonella* growth [18]. However, in the present study, hydrogen peroxide production was unlikely to be the cause of this inhibition in the agar diffusion test due to the anaerobic growth conditions of the lactobacilli [25]. The well-diffusion antagonism method did not show any inhibition, thereby excluding the hypothesis of secreted bacteriocins or bacteriocin-like as *Salmonella* inhibitors. Decreasing the pH by organic acid production was likely to be the cause of such an effect [26]. Although the bacteriocin or bacteriocin-like activity produced by LAB is commonly more effective against Gram-positive bacteria, such as *Listeria monocytogenes* [27], the inhibition of the Gram-negative *Salmonella* has also been reported [28].

The adhesion behavior of bacteria is a complex multistep process which includes specific and non-specific ligand–receptor mechanisms [29]. The latter are controlled by physicochemical reactions of the cell wall, including electrostatic and Van der Waals interactions, as well as hydrophobic properties. These are the most reliable long-range non-covalent interactions (Lewis acid–base) due to the surface proteins and lipoteichoic acids covering the peptidoglycan, and conferring a net negative bacterial surface charge in physiological conditions [24]. According to the authors, this feature is strain-specific and may vary depending on the medium, age and surface structures of bacteria. Indeed, considerable variability in the hydrophobicity capacity has been observed in our study, with 65% of the isolates showing high hydrophobicity (70%).

Auto-aggregation properties, together with the co-aggregation ability, of a probiotic strain are necessary for adhering to the intestinal tract by forming a defensive barrier against the colonization of foodborne pathogens [30]. Moreover, the LAB co-aggregating ability might regulate the pathogen microenvironment and stimulate the excretion of antimicrobial substances [31]. *Lactobacillus* spp. also favors many aggregation-promoting factors (APFs) involved in auto-aggregation and/or adhesion in a strain-specific manner [32]. Furthermore, exopolysaccharides (EPS) are believed to play an essential role in cell aggregation, biofilm formation and adhesion. Polak-Berecka and colleagues concluded that the adherence and/or co-aggregation ability of *Lactobacillus rhamnosus* are strongly related to specific interactions based on surface proteins and specific fatty acids, whereas polysaccharides (hydrophilic nature) hinder the adhesion and aggregation by masking protein receptors [33].

Aggregation values have been shown to increase over time, typically at 20 h of incubation, in a strain-dependent manner [34], which is in accordance with our results. All isolates with the (Agg+) phenotype were identified as *Ligilactobacillus salivarius*, thus corroborating the findings of Ait Seddik and colleagues, who demonstrated the high auto-aggregation ability of this strain [35]. According to Solieri and colleagues, co-aggregation values below 20% are indicative of a weak co-aggregation ability [36]. Our isolates differed in their co-aggregation abilities (0 to 94.6%), highlighting once again these strain-specific characteristics.

Another probiotic protective mechanism involves the competition for adhesion sites [37]. *Ligilactobacillus salivarius* (16/c6, 16/i4, 14/i8 and A30/i26), *Limosilactobacillus reuteri* (1/c24), *L. crispatus* (16/c2) and *Limosilactobacillus fermentum* (12/c8 and 16/i10) were selected according to their cell hydrophobicity and auto/co-aggregation abilities. The adherence capacity differed significantly between the lactobacilli strains isolated, which is consistent with other studies, showing that this ability is species and strain-dependent [38]. The highest adhesion ability was shown in four isolates of lactobacilli: *Ligilactobacillus salivarius* A30/i26 and 16/i4, being highly auto-aggregative and hydrophobic, as well as in *Ligilactobacillus salivarius* 16/c6 and *Limosilactobacillus reuteri* 1/c24, showing great co-aggregation and hydrophobicity abilities. *L. crispatus* 16/c2, *Limosilactobacillus reuteri* 12/c8 and *Ligilactobacillus salivarius* 14/i8 had the lowest adhesion percentages, despite their high co-aggregation capacities. Interestingly, *Limosilactobacillus* sp.16/i10, a high hydrophobic strain, also exhibited a low adhesion percentage.

The studied parameters, i.e., hydrophobicity, aggregation / co-aggregation and adhesion, illustrated no interrelation. However, some studies mentioned that the cell surface hydrophobicity is related to the attachment to epithelial cells [39,40], while others have excluded this relationship in their analyses [27]. García-Cayuela and colleagues revealed a correlation between auto-aggregation and co-aggregation [29], which disagrees with our results. Del Re and colleagues proposed that auto-aggregation and hydrophobicity are independent characteristics, but both are necessary for adhesion [41]. Multitude interrelated surface factors (fatty acids, surface proteins, LPS and EPS) may have unpredictable effects on adherence, co-aggregation and cell-to-cell interactions [38].

Survival in the GIT is a critical probiotic property. Bile tolerance is strain-specific and related to the hydrolase activity [42]. By mimicking the GIT conditions, all the eight lactobacilli strains were capable of growing at 0.1% (w/v) bile salts, but two *Ligilactobacillus salivarius* strains, namely, A30/i26 and 16/i4, were affected by 0.3%. This concentration is considered critical for screening for resistant probiotic strains [27]. Genes involved in bile salt hydrolysis, *bsh-1* and *bsh-2*, were found to be responsible for the acid and bile tolerance in *Ligilactobacillus salivarius* UCC118 [26]. In favor of our findings, a significantly decreasing cell count in most of the *Ligilactobacillus salivarius* isolates has been observed when the strains were incubated with a high concentration of bile salts (0.5%), whereas most of the *Limosilactobacillus reuteri* isolates showed a high tolerance [43].

*Ligilactobacillus salivarius* A30/i26 and 16/c6 and *Limosilactobacillus reuteri* 1/c24 were selected for their high adhesion abilities and were further evaluated for their potential to compete with the three *Salmonella* serotypes in, or exclude them from, epithelial adhesion using the Caco2 cells as an experimental model. The inhibition of the pathogen adhesion by the three probiotic strains indicated a high variability in a strain-dependent manner. *Ligilactobacillus salivarius* 16/c6 significantly inhibited the adhesion of the three *Salmonella* serotypes to the Caco-2 cell monolayers only by exclusion assays, which is in accordance with findings of Campana, Van Hemert and Baffone [38]. The authors suggested that *Ligilactobacillus salivarius* W24 could significantly inhibit the adhesion of pathogens to Caco-2 cells only by exclusion. Jankowska and colleagues showed that *L. paracasei* reduced *Salmonella's* adhesion to Caco-2 cells by 4- and 7-fold in competition and exclusion experiments, respectively [44]. However, the inhibition of *Salmonella*'s attachment to Caco-2 cells by exclusion, as well as by competition, has been frequently reported [37,45,46].

The inhibition of the *Salmonella* serotypes by *Ligilactobacillus salivarius* 16/c6 was similarly demonstrated by a mixed co-culture assay. When the co-cultures were tested without vortexing, the kinetic growth results of the lactobacilli and the pathogens confirmed what was previously distinguished by the auto-aggregation and co-aggregation assays and emphasized the ability for these features over time. Indeed, both co-cultures and the *Ligilactobacillus salivarius* monoculture revealed a clear supernatant after 8 h of incubation. Additionally, it has been demonstrated that the efficient aggregation and proper settling of flocs are essential for the management of effluent in the activated sludge process [47]. In this regard, such a feature of our strain might be promising in regard to the purification and decontamination of wastewater of slaughterhouses, which is mainly polluted by pathogens and organic materials.

When *Ligilactobacillus salivarius* 16/c6 and the *Salmonella* serotypes were subjected to the same co-culture assay but with vortexing, the reduction in the *Salmonella* counts in the mixed cultures co-occurred with a decrease in the pH, which is in accordance with findings of other studies [43]. Some bacterial strains have acid-adaptation systems that enable them to survive at pH < 2 [2]. Other non-negligible antimicrobial factors are involved in the *Salmonella* inhibition, such as competition for nutrients [43] and the contact-dependent inhibition (CDI) mechanism [48]. The latter case, where cell-to-cell contact is required, could be explained by the exchange of and interactions between bacteria mediated by conjugation, secretion systems, contact-dependent inhibition, allolysis and nanotubes. In fact, in our study, the low count was observed at 4 h among the *Salmonella* monocultures and mixed co-cultures.

## 4. Materials and Methods

### 4.1. Isolation and Phenotypic Characterization of Lactobacillus spp.

The different lactobacilli were isolated from the digestive tracts (ileum and cecum) of 16 antibiotic-free healthy broiler groups of different ages (four levels), breeds (four species) and diet formulas (four levels), as well as from 10 antibiotic-treated commercial broilers (Table 3). Experiments coded from 1 to 16 corresponded to the antibiotic-free broiler group, the "A"-coded experiment represents the group of antibiotic-treated commercial broilers, and the sample origin was designated as "i" for ileum and "c" for cecum. Samples of the ileum or cecum content of each category were homogenized at a ratio of 1:10 (10 g of ileum or cecum content in 90 mL of buffered peptone water (Scharlau-Chemie, Barcelona, Spain)). The homogenate was diluted $10^7$-fold and 0.1 mL was plated onto de Man, Rogosa and Sharpe (MRS) agar (Sigma-Aldrich, Burlington, MA, USA). The plates were incubated anaerobically for 3 to 4 days at 37 °C. In total, 210 randomly selected strains were first characterized by Gram staining, motility and the detection of catalase activity. Gram-positive, catalase-negative bacilli were presumptively considered as *Lactobacillus* for further identification. Isolates were preserved in MRS broth with 20% glycerol at −70 °C until further use. All strains were revivified by successive streaking on MRS agar prior to performing any assay.

### 4.2. Salmonella Isolates

The antagonistic activity and co-aggregation ability of the lactobacilli strains were tested on three native avian *Salmonella* strains isolated from our previous study [4,49]. *S.* Enteritidis is the most predominant avian pulsotype causing human illness, whereas *S.* Kentucky ST198 and *S.* Infantis were chosen for their MDR pattern and their high prevalence in Lebanese poultry production. Strains were inoculated into 15 mL tryptic soy broth (TSB) (Sigma-Aldrich) and incubated at 37 °C for 18 h for further analyses.

Table 3. List of coded experiments numbered according to age, breed and diet formula of the broilers and hens deprived of any antibiotics and feed additives. The A-coded sample refers to non-antibiotic-free commercial broilers.

| Experiment Number | Category, Age | Breed | Diet Formula |
|---|---|---|---|
| 1 | Broiler, 35 days | Cobb | High starch diet: corn 60%, soya 20%, wheat 20% |
| 2 | Broiler, 35 days | Cobb | High protein diet: soya 40%, corn 40%, wheat 20% |
| 3 | Broiler, 35 days | Cobb | High gluten diet: wheat 60%, soya 20%, corn 20% |
| 4 | Broiler, 35 days | Ross | High starch diet: corn 60%, soya 20%, wheat 20% |
| 5 | Broiler, 35 days | Ross | High protein diet: soya 40%, corn 40%, wheat 20% |
| 6 | Broiler, 35 days | Ross | High gluten diet: wheat 60%, soya 20%, corn 20% |
| 7 | Broiler, one day | Cobb | High starch diet: corn 60%, soya 20%, wheat 20% |
| 8 | Broiler, one day | Cobb | High protein diet: soya 40%, corn 40%, wheat 20% |
| 9 | Broiler, one day | Cobb | High gluten diet: wheat 60%, soya 20%, corn 20% |
| 10 | Broiler, one day | Ross | High starch diet: corn 60%, soya 20%, wheat 20% |
| 11 | Broiler, one day | Ross | High protein diet: soya 40%, corn 40%, wheat 20% |
| 12 | Broiler, one day | Ross | High gluten diet: wheat 60%, soya 20%, corn 20% |
| 13 | Layer, 69 weeks | Isa Brown | Normal feed: corn 40%, soya 32%, wheat 20% |
| 14 | Layer, 69 weeks | Isa White | Normal feed: corn 40%, soya 32%, wheat 20% |
| 15 | Layer, 27 weeks | Isa Brown | Normal feed: corn 40%, soya 32%, wheat 20% |
| 16 | Layer, 27 weeks | Isa White | Normal feed: corn 40%, soya 32%, wheat 20% |
| A | Broiler, 35 weeks | Ross | Normal feed: corn 40%, soya 32%, wheat 20% |

### 4.3. Assessment of the Lactobacilli Antagonism

The anti-*Salmonella* activities of 210 presumptive lactobacilli were preliminarily screened using the simple spot-on-lawn antimicrobial assay and the agar well-diffusion method [25], with minor modifications. In brief, 10 µL of overnight lactobacilli cultures were spotted onto the surfaces of MRS agar plates and then incubated anaerobically for 18 h at 37 °C. In parallel, an overnight culture of each selected *Salmonella* serotype was inoculated at $10^5$ CFU/mL into 7 mL of TSB soft agar (0.7% agar) and then poured onto the agar plates previously cultured with a strain of lactobacilli. After solidification, the plates were incubated for an additional 18 h at 37 °C under anaerobic conditions. The anti-*Salmonella* activity was evaluated by observing the inhibition zones around lactobacilli spots.

The agar well-diffusion assay was performed to identify the inhibitory substances secreted in the culture supernatants. The lactobacilli isolates showing antagonism were grown overnight at 37 °C in 15 mL of MRS broth. The cell-free supernatants (CFSs) were obtained by centrifugation ($4000\times g$, 20 min, 4 °C) and filtration using 0.22 µm-pore Hi-MED syringe filters. The pH of the CFSs was then adjusted to 6.5 by 1 N NaOH. The *Salmonella* isolates were added at $10^6$ CFU/mL to 20 mL of TSB supplemented with 0.75% agar-agar (semi-solid) and then poured into an empty Petri dish. After solidification, 6 mm wells were punched and 50 µL of the CFS was added to each well. The plates were left to settle at 8 °C for 24 h to enable the diffusion of the secreted antimicrobial substances, then incubated at 37 °C for 24 h. The absence or presence of any inhibitory zones was recorded after 24 h of incubation at 37 °C. The two assays were performed in triplicate.

### 4.4. Selection of Strains Based on Their Phenotypic Aggregation

A preliminary visual aggregation screening was performed according to Del Re et al. [41], with minor modifications. In brief, the lactobacilli cultured in the MRS broth were classified into three categories: category I for strains with an aggregation phenotype (Agg+) showing visible aggregates even after vigorous vortexing, category II for strains with constant turbidity and without precipitate (Agg−), and category III for strains with a mixed phenotype forming a precipitate and a clear or small turbid supernatant (Agg+/Agg−).

### 4.5. Species Identification and Phylogenetic Relationships

The 48 selected lactobacilli isolates were identified by 16S rRNA gene sequence analysis. The DNA extraction was achieved with a Qiamp DNA Mini Kit (Qiagen, Hilden, Germany). The amplification of the 16S rRNA gene sequence was performed in a Veriti thermal cycler (Applied Biosystem, CA, USA) under the following cycling conditions:: denaturation at 95 °C for 15 min, 30 cycles of denaturation at 94 °C for 1 min, annealing at 52 °C for 1 min and extension at 72 °C for 2 min, followed by another extension at 72 °C for 7 min. Reaction mixtures (50 µL) were prepared as follows: reaction buffer 10 × (5 µL), 10 mM dNTPs mix (1 µL), 0.5 mM of primer (27F (5′-GTGCTGCAGAGAGTTTGATCCTGGCTCAG-3′) and 1492R (5′-CACGGATCCTACGGGTACCTTGTTACGACTT-3′), bacterial DNA (5 µL) and 2.5 U of HotStarTaq DNA polymerase (Qiagen, Hilden, Germany). Th amplicon separation was completed by electrophoresis at 100 V on 1% (w/v) agarose, stained with ethidium bromide in 1 × TBE buffer and purified using the GenElute TM PCR Clean-Up Kit (Sigma-Aldrich) according to the manufacturer's instructions. The DNA sequencing was carried out on a SeqStudio Genetic Analyzer (Applied Biosystem, USA). The editing was performed with Bioedit (version 7.2.5, 2013), and the 16S rDNA sequences were compared with other sequences using NCBI BLAST (http://blast.ncbi.nlm.nih.gov/Blast.cgi, accessed on 25 April 2022). A phylogenetic tree was assembled using the neighboring methods [50], with the tree builder function of MEGA X [51].

*4.6. Cell Surface Properties*

4.6.1. Auto-Aggregation and Co-Aggregation Assays

Auto-aggregation and co-aggregation capacities of the selected lactobacilli strains, according to their auto-aggregation visual features, were further assessed by spectrophotometric analysis at 4 h and 24 h, as described by Collado and colleagues [34], with minor modifications. An overnight lactobacilli culture ($10^8$ CFU/mL) was centrifuged (4000× g, 20 min, 4 °C) and the pellet was washed with phosphate-buffered saline (PBS) at pH 7.1 and then resuspended in the same buffer. The cell suspension (4 mL) was placed into glass bijou bottles and incubated at room temperature for 24 h. The absorbances at 600 nm ($A_{600\,nm}$) were measured at different times of incubation (t0, t4 and t24).

The auto-aggregation percentage was calculated using the following formula: $1 - (A_t/A_0) \times 100$, where $A_t$ represents the absorbance at different times (4 and 24 h) and $A_0$ the absorbance at time = 0 ($t_0$). The aggregation ability was classified according to Del Re and colleagues [41], with minor modifications. Results with values $\geq 65\%$ and $\leq 10\%$ were considered as highly auto-aggregative and non-auto-aggregative, respectively.

For the co-aggregation assay, mixed cultures with equal volumes (2 mL) of lactobacilli and *Salmonella* strains, as well as monocultures (4 mL), were prepared and incubated at room temperature without agitation. $A_{600\,nm}$ were measured at 24 h of incubation.

The percentage of co-aggregation was calculated according to Handley and colleagues [39], as follows: $(1 - A_{mix}/(A_{Sal} + A_{Lac})/2) \times 100$, where $A_{Sal}$ and $A_{Lac}$ represent the absorbances of the monocultures, *Salmonella* and lactobacilli, respectively, while $A_{mix}$ represents the absorbance of the mixed culture at 24 h. Values below 20% are indicative of a weak co-aggregation capability [36].

4.6.2. Hydrophobicity Assays

The microbial adhesion to the hydrocarbons (MATH) test was evaluated as defined by Rosenberg and colleagues [52], with slight changes. Lactobacilli cultures were centrifuged, and the pellet was washed with PBS buffer pH = 7.1 and suspended in the same buffer to adjust the concentration to $10^8$ CFU/mL. An equal volume of 2 mL cell culture and xylene (nonpolar solvent) were mixed and vigorously vortexed for 5 min before measuring the $A_{600\,nm}$ ($A_0$). After incubation at room temperature for 1 h, the aqueous phase was cautiously removed, and its $A_{600\,nm}$ ($A_1$) was measured.

The cell surface hydrophobicity (H) was calculated as follows: H% = $(1 - A_1/A_0) \times 100$. Isolates with (H) values > 70%, between 50–70% and < 50% were classified as highly, moderately and low-hydrophobic, respectively [53].

## 4.7. In Vitro Cell Tolerance to Gastrointestinal Conditions

The tolerance to gastrointestinal conditions of the eight lactobacilli strains, which were chosen according to their hydrophobicity and auto/ co-aggregation capacities, was assessed according to Babot and colleagues [24], with minor modifications. Overnight lactobacilli cultures were centrifuged (4000× $g$, 4 °C, 20 min) and adjusted to approximately $10^8$ CFU/mL in PBS buffer. A volume of 1.75 mL was inoculated in 2.25 mL of a simulated gastric juice (125 mM NaCl, 7 mM KCl, 45 mM $NaHCO_3$, 3 g/L pepsin pH 2.0). After incubation at 41.5 °C (poultry corporal temperature) for 1 h (mean retention time in the proventriculus and gizzard), the suspension was centrifuged and washed twice with PBS buffer. The pellet was then suspended in 3 mL of simulated intestinal juice (NaCl 22 mM, KCl 3.2 mM, $NaHCO_3$ 7.6 mM, pancreatin 0.1% $w/v$, bile salts 0.15% or 0.3% $w/v$, pH = 8.00) and incubated at 41.5 °C for 2 h (mean retention time in the small intestine). The concentrations of bile salts were selected to simulate the 0.1 to 1% bile concentration range of the poultry GIT, with approximately 0.25% in the ileum and 0.1% in the cecum [12]. After the serial dilutions, 0.1 mL of the suspensions was plated onto the MRS agar and incubated anaerobically for three days at 37 °C.

Tolerance to the GIT conditions was evaluated as follows: % survival = ($Log_{10} N_1$/ $Log_{10} N_0$) × 100, where $Log_{10} N_0$ is the number of bacterial cells in the PBS, and $Log_{10} N_1$ represents the number of viable cells after exposure to gastrointestinal conditions.

## 4.8. Cell Culture

### 4.8.1. Cell Line and Growth Conditions

The human colorectal adenocarcinoma Caco-2 cell line was used to perform the adhesion assays. Cells were grown in a 75 $cm^2$ flask containing Dulbecco's modified Eagle's medium (DMEM) (1× DMEM, 1M-1Glutamax, Gibco), supplemented with 10% ($v/v$) heat-inactivated fetal bovine serum (FBS) (Eurobio), 1× non-essential amino acids (NEAA), 100 U/mL penicillin and 10 mg/mL streptomycin (Sigma-Aldrich). Cells were incubated at 37 °C in a humidified atmosphere containing 5% $CO_2$ until 80% confluence was reached. Prior to the adhesion assay, $5 \times 10^4$ cells were seeded in 24-well tissue culture plates and incubated in the same conditions as mentioned above for 16 days (full differentiation). At the end of the incubation time, the cell line monolayers were washed twice with Dubelcco's PBS (Eurobio) to remove antibiotics before adding the bacterial suspension.

### 4.8.2. Adhesion to Caco-2 Cells

Overnight cultures of the selected lactobacilli strains (16/c6, 16/c2, 16/i10, 16/c4, 14/i8, 12/c8, 1/c24 and A30/i26) and *Salmonella* serotypes were centrifuged, washed twice in Dulbecco's PBS (Eurobio) and suspended in an antibiotic-free DMEM medium at a concentration of $10^8$ CFU/mL. Then, 1 mL of bacterial culture was added to each cell well and incubated for 1 h at 37 °C in a humidified atmosphere containing 5% $CO_2$. After that, the supernatant was removed and the wells were gently washed three times with Dulbecco's PBS buffer to eliminate non-adherent bacteria. Finally, the Caco-2 monolayers were trypsinized with 0.25% trypsin-EDTA solution (Eurobio), and the adherent bacteria were enumerated by plating serial dilutions onto MRS agar medium for *Lactobacillus* and TSA agar medium for *Salmonella*. The adhesion ability was calculated as ($N_1/N_0$) × 100, where $N_1$ and $N_0$ represent the CFUs of the total adhered and added bacteria, respectively. Two independent experiments were conducted in triplicate for each condition.

### 4.8.3. Inhibition of the Adhesion of *Salmonella* to Caco-2 Cells

Two different protocols were followed to evaluate the ability of the selected lactobacilli strains to inhibit *Salmonella*'s adhesion to the Caco-2 cells. The *Ligilactobacillus salivarius* (16/c6 and A30/i26) and *Limosilactobacillus reuteri* (1/c24) strains were selected based on their adhesion properties. The competition adhesion assay was performed by seeding Caco-2 cell monolayers with a mixed culture of each of the selected lactobacilli ($10^8$ CFU/mL) with each of the *Salmonella* strains ($10^7$ CFU/mL) in complete DMEM. The *Salmonella* monocultures were used as controls. After an incubation period of 2 h at 37 °C in a humidified atmosphere containing 5% $CO_2$, the supernatants with the non-adherent bacteria were removed, and then the Caco-2 cells were trypsinized. The adherent bacterial cells were serially diluted and plated onto TSA agar medium and MRS agar medium to enumerate the *Salmonella* and *Lactobacillus*, respectively.

The ability of the *Salmonella* strains to adhere to the Caco-2 cells in the absence ($N_{Sal}$) and the presence ($N_{Mix}$) of lactobacilli was calculated as follows:

Anti-adhesion ability% = $1 - (N_{Mix}/N_{Sal})$% [54].

For the exclusion assays, the Caco-2 cell monolayers were pre-exposed to lactobacilli strains ($10^8$ CFU/mL) for 1 h [37]. Then, the Caco-2 cell monolayers were gently washed three times with Dulbecco's PBS prior to the addition of the *Salmonella* strains ($10^7$ CFU/mL) and incubation for 2 h. At the end of incubation time, supernatants with the non-adherent bacteria were removed, and the Caco-2 cells were then trypsinized. The adherent bacterial cells were serially diluted and plated onto TSA and MRS agar media to enumerate the *Salmonella* and *Lactobacillus*, respectively. Two independent experiments for each strain were conducted in triplicate for each condition.

*4.9. Co-Culture Growth Kinetic Study*

Two series of experiments were carried out to evaluate the effects of *Ligilactobacillus salivarius* 16 / c6 on the growth of the *Salmonella* strains in a co-culture model. In the first co-culture experiment, an 18 h-old culture of the 16 /c6 strain ($10^7$ CFU/mL) was co-inoculated with each culture of the three *Salmonella* strains (approximately $10^5$ CFU/mL) into 100 mL of Laptg medium (peptone 15 g/L, tryptone 10 g/L, yeast extract 10 g/L, glucose 10 g/L, tween 80 0.1%; all media/chemicals were purchased from Sigma-Aldrich) at pH 6.9 and then incubated in a shaker incubator at 100 rpm at 37 °C for 24 h. Pure cultures of each of the strains served as controls. Before enumeration, the culture was left for 10 min without vortexing to evaluate the auto/co-aggregation capacity of *Ligilactobacillus salivarius*. Then, 0.1 mL of supernatant was plated out at different times (0, 4, 8 and 24 h) in triplicate onto the selective media (XLD agar for *Salmonella* and MRS agar for *Lactobacillus*) for counting. The pH of the culture medium was checked regularly. In the second experiment, the bacterial cultures were prepared as described above. Before enumeration, the culture was vigorously vortexed.

*4.10. Statistical Analyses*

Statistical analyses were performed using XLSTAT version 2021.4 (Addinsoft Inc. Paris, France). The surface properties of the forty-eight lactobacilli ($n$ = 3) strains were assessed by principal component analysis (PCA). The index of Pearson was used to evaluate the correlation between the six assays, hydrophobicity, auto-aggregation and co-aggregation between a given lactobacilli strain and each of the *S.* Enteritidis, *S.* Infantis and *S.* Kentucky strains. Differences between the results for the adhesion and inhibition by competitive/exclusion were performed by one-way ANOVA, and $p$-values $\leq 0.05$ were considered statistically significant.

## 5. Conclusions

This work was the first national tentative attempt to isolate potential candidates from the lactobacilli of Lebanese poultry to act as probiotics. The *Ligilactobacillus. salivarius* 16/c6 isolate that we highlighted here could be used as a potent probiotic dietary supplement in order to reinforce the intestinal microbiota of newly hatched chickens due to its high viability and long persistence in the poultry intestinal tract, as well as its ability to block the adhesion sites against *Salmonella* spp. The adhesion of lactobacilli strains to epithelial cells should also be investigated using the chicken LMH cell line to evaluate its probiotic potential in poultry. The study of these parameters is a crucial step in disseminating such native probiotic strains. However, further in vivo studies are required in order to ultimately better our understanding of how lactobacilli strains interact with and affect the fitness of *Salmonella* in the GITs of chicken hosts.

**Author Contributions:** Conceptualization, R.E.H. and Y.E.R.; methodology, R.E.H., S.P.S., F.M. and Y.E.R.; software, R.E.H., Z.A.K. and Y.E.R.; validation, R.E.H., F.M., J.-M.S., Z.A.K. and Y.E.R.; formal analysis, R.E.H. and Z.A.K.; investigation, R.E.H., J.E.H., S.P.S., J.T. and R.R.; resources, R.E.H., J.E.H., F.M. and J.-M.S.; data curation, R.E.H. and Z.A.K.; writing—original draft preparation, R.E.H. and I.A.; writing—review and editing, S.P.S., F.M., J.-M.S., Z.A.K. and Y.E.R.; visualization, R.E.H., J.E.H., Z.A.K. and Y.E.R.; supervision, F.M. and Y.E.R.; project administration, F.M. and Y.E.R. All authors have read and agreed to the published version of the manuscript.

**Funding:** This research received no external funding.

**Acknowledgments:** The authors would like to thank the general director of the LARI, Michel Afram, and INP-ENSAT in Toulouse for their full support. The authors also thank Chantal Ghanem for her help in plotting the principal component analysis (PCA).

**Conflicts of Interest:** The authors declare no conflict of interest. The funders had no role in the design of the study; in the collection, analyses, or interpretation of data; in the writing of the manuscript; or in the decision to publish the results.

## References

1. European Food Safety Authority/European Centre for Disease Prevention and Control. The European Union Summary Report on Trends and Sources of Zoonoses, Zoonotic Agents and Food-Borne Outbreaks in 2016. *EFSA J.* **2017**, *15*, e04676. [CrossRef]
2. Tan, S.M.; Lee, S.M.; Dykes, G.A. Buffering Effect of Chicken Skin and Meat Protects *Salmonella* Enterica Strains against Hydrochloric Acid but Not Organic Acid Treatment. *Food Control* **2014**, *42*, 329–334. [CrossRef]
3. Antunes, P.; Mourão, J.; Campos, J.; Peixe, L. Salmonellosis: The Role of Poultry Meat. *Clin. Microbiol. Infect.* **2016**, *22*, 110–121. [CrossRef] [PubMed]
4. El Hage, R.; El Rayess, Y.; Bonifait, L.; El Hafi, B.; Baugé, L.; Viscogliosi, E.; Hamze, M.; Mathieu, F.; Matar, G.M.; Chemaly, M. A National Study through a 'Farm-to-Fork' Approach to Determine *Salmonella* Dissemination along with the Lebanese Poultry Production Chain. *Zoonoses Public Health* **2022**, *69*, 499–513. [CrossRef] [PubMed]
5. Pan, D.; Yu, Z. Intestinal Microbiome of Poultry and Its Interaction with Host and Diet. *Gut Microbes* **2014**, *5*, 108–119. [CrossRef] [PubMed]
6. Ferri, M.; Ranucci, E.; Romagnoli, P.; Giaccone, V. Antimicrobial Resistance: A Global Emerging Threat to Public Health Systems. *Crit. Rev. Food Sci. Nutr.* **2017**, *53*, 2857–2876. [CrossRef]
7. Franco, A.; Leekitcharoenphon, P.; Feltrin, F.; Alba, P.; Cordaro, G.; Iurescia, M.; Tolli, R.; D'Incau, M.; Staffolani, M.; Di Giannatale, E.; et al. Emergence of a Clonal Lineage of Multidrug-Resistant ESBL-Producing *Salmonella* Infantis Transmitted from Broilers and Broiler Meat to Humans in Italy between 2011 and 2014. *PLoS ONE* **2015**, *10*, e144802. [CrossRef]
8. Regulation (EC) No 1831/2003. Regulation (EC) No 1831/2003 of the European Parliament and of the Council of 22 September 2003 on Additives for Use in Animal Nutrition. *Off. J. Eur. Communities* **2003**, *L268*, 15.
9. Krysiak, K.; Konkol, D.; Korczyński, M. Review Overview of the Use of Probiotics in Poultry Production. *Animals* **2021**, *11*, 1620. [CrossRef]
10. Foley, S.L.; Nayak, R.; Hanning, I.B.; Johnson, T.J.; Han, J.; Ricke, S.C. Population Dynamics of *Salmonella* Enterica Serotypes in Commercial Egg and Poultry Production. *Appl. Environ. Microbiol.* **2011**, *77*, 4273–4279. [CrossRef]
11. FAO; WHO. *Guidelines for the Evaluation of Probiotics in Food*; FAO: Rome, Italy; WHO: Geneva, Switzerland, 2002.
12. Spivey, M.A.; Dunn-Horrocks, S.L.; Duong, T. Epithelial Cell Adhesion and Gastrointestinal Colonization of *Lactobacillus* in Poultry. *Poult. Sci.* **2014**, *93*, 2910–2919. [CrossRef] [PubMed]
13. Saint-Cyr, M.J.; Guyard-Nicodème, M.; Messaoudi, S.; Chemaly, M.; Cappelier, J.M.; Dousset, X.; Haddad, N. Recent Advances in Screening of Anti-Campylobacter Activity in Probiotics for Use in Poultry. *Front. Microbiol.* **2016**, *7*, 553. [CrossRef]
14. Ouwehand, A.C.; Forssten, S.; Hibberd, A.A.; Lyra, A.; Stahl, B. Probiotic Approach to Prevent Antibiotic Resistance. *Ann. Med.* **2016**, *48*, 246–255. [CrossRef] [PubMed]
15. Muñoz-Quezada, S.; Gomez-Llorente, C.; Plaza-Diaz, J.; Chenoll, E.; Ramón, D.; Matencio, E.; Bermudez-Brito, M.; Genovés, S.; Romero, F.; Gil, A.; et al. Competitive Inhibition of Three Novel Bacteria Isolated from Faeces of Breast Milk-Fed Infants against Selected Enteropathogens. *Br. J. Nutr.* **2013**, *109* (Suppl. 2), S63–S69. [CrossRef] [PubMed]
16. Feng, J.; Wang, L.; Zhou, L.; Yang, X.; Zhao, X. Using in Vitro Immunomodulatory Properties of Lactic Acid Bacteria for Selection of Probiotics against *Salmonella* Infection in Broiler Chicks. *PLoS ONE* **2016**, *11*, e0147630. [CrossRef] [PubMed]
17. Rantala, M.; Nurmi, E. Prevention of the Growth of *Salmonella* Infantis in Chicks by the Flora of the Alimentary Tract of Chickens. *Br. Poult. Sci.* **1973**, *14*, 627–630. [CrossRef]
18. Ayeni, A.O.; Ruppitsch, W.; Ayeni, F.A. Characterization of Bacteria in Nigerian Yogurt as Promising Alternative to Antibiotics in Gastrointestinal Infections. *J. Diet. Suppl.* **2018**, *211*, 1–11. [CrossRef]
19. Yadav, A.K.; Tyagi, A.; Kumar, A.; Panwar, S.; Grover, S.; Saklani, A.C.; Hemalatha, R.; Batish, V.K. Adhesion of Lactobacilli and Their Anti-Infectivity Potential. *Crit. Rev. Food Sci. Nutr.* **2017**, *57*, 2042–2056. [CrossRef]

20. Vineetha, P.G.; Tomar, S.; Saxena, V.K.; Susan, C.; Sandeep, S.; Adil, K.; Mukesh, K. Screening of *Lactobacillus* Isolates from Gastrointestinal Tract of Guinea Fowl for Probiotic Qualities Using in vitro Tests to Select Species-Specific Probiotic Candidates. *Br. Poult. Sci.* **2016**, *57*, 474–482. [CrossRef]
21. Felsenstein, J. Confidence Limits on Phylogenies: An Approach Using the Bootstrap; Confidence Limits on Phylogenies: An Approach Using the Bootstrap. *Evolution* **1985**, *39*, 783–791. [CrossRef]
22. Chen, X.; Xu, J.; Shuai, J.; Chen, J.; Zhang, Z.; Fang, W. The S-Layer Proteins of *Lactobacillus Crispatus* Strain ZJ001 Is Responsible for Competitive Exclusion against *Escherichia coli* O157:H7 and *Salmonella* Typhimurium. *Int. J. Food Microbiol.* **2007**, *115*, 307–312. [CrossRef] [PubMed]
23. Albazaz, R.I.; Byukunal Bal, E.B. Microflora of Digestive Tract in Poultry. *Kahramanmaraş Sütçü İmam Üniversitesi Doğa Bilim. Derg.* **2014**, *17*, 39–42. [CrossRef]
24. Babot, J.D.; Argañaraz-Martínez, E.; Saavedra, L.; Apella, M.C.; Perez Chaia, A. Selection of Indigenous Lactic Acid Bacteria to Reinforce the Intestinal Microbiota of Newly Hatched Chicken—Relevance of in Vitro and Ex Vivo Methods for Strains Characterization. *Res. Vet. Sci.* **2014**, *97*, 8–17. [CrossRef] [PubMed]
25. Schillinger, U.; Lucke, F.K. Antimicrobial Activity of *Lactobacillus* Sake Isolated from Meat. *Appl. Environ. Microbiol.* **1989**, *55*, 1901–1906. [CrossRef]
26. Adetoye, A.; Pinloche, E.; Adeniyi, B.A.; Ayeni, F.A. Characterization and Anti-*Salmonella* Activities of Lactic Acid Bacteria Isolated from Cattle Faeces. *BMC Microbiol.* **2018**, *18*, 96. [CrossRef] [PubMed]
27. Ramos, C.L.; Thorsen, L.; Schwan, R.F.; Jespersen, L. Strain-Specific Probiotics Properties of *Lactobacillus fermentum*, *Lactobacillus plantarum* and *Lactobacillus crevis* Isolates from Brazilian Food Products. *Food Microbiol.* **2013**, *36*, 22–29. [CrossRef]
28. Gupta, A.; Tiwari, S.K. Plantaricin LD1: A Bacteriocin Produced by Food Isolate of *Lactobacillus plantarum* LD1. *Appl. Biochem. Biotechnol.* **2014**, *172*, 3354–3362. [CrossRef]
29. García-Cayuela, T.; Korany, A.M.; Bustos, I.; Gómez de Cadiñanos, L.P.; Requena, T.; Peláez, C.; Martínez-Cuesta, M.C. Adhesion Abilities of Dairy *Lactobacillus plantarum* Strains Showing an Aggregation Phenotype. *Food Res. Int.* **2014**, *57*, 44–50. [CrossRef]
30. Kos, B.; Šušković, J.; Vuković, S.; Šimpraga, M.; Frece, J.; Matošić, S. Adhesion and Aggregation Ability of Probiotic Strain *Lactobacillus acidophilus* M92. *J. Appl. Microbiol.* **2003**, *94*, 981–987. [CrossRef]
31. Potočnjak, M.; Pušić, P.; Frece, J.; Abram, M.; Janković, T.; Gobin, I. Three New *Lactobacillus plantarum* Strains in the Probiotic Toolbox against Gut Pathogen *Salmonella enterica* Serotype Typhimurium. *Food Technol. Biotechnol.* **2017**, *55*, 48–54. [CrossRef]
32. Nishiyama, K.; Sugiyama, M.; Mukai, T. Adhesion Properties of Lactic Acid Bacteria on Intestinal Mucin. *Microorganisms* **2016**, *4*, 34. [CrossRef]
33. Polak-Berecka, M.; Waśko, A.; Paduch, R.; Skrzypek, T.; Sroka-Bartnicka, A. The Effect of Cell Surface Components on Adhesion Ability of *Lactobacillus rhamnosus*. *Antonie Van Leeuwenhoek Int. J. Gen. Mol. Microbiol.* **2014**, *106*, 751–762. [CrossRef]
34. Collado, M.C.; Surono, I.; Meriluoto, J.; Salminen, S. Indigenous Dadih Lactic Acid Bacteria: Cell-Surface Properties and Interactions with Pathogens. *J. Food Sci.* **2007**, *72*, 89–93. [CrossRef] [PubMed]
35. Ait Seddik, H.; Bendali, F.; Cudennec, B.; Drider, D. Anti-Pathogenic and Probiotic Attributes of *Lactobacillus salivarius* and *Lactobacillus plantarum* Strains Isolated from Feces of Algerian Infants and Adults. *Res. Microbiol.* **2017**, *168*, 244–254. [CrossRef] [PubMed]
36. Solieri, L.; Bianchi, A.; Mottolese, G.; Lemmetti, F.; Giudici, P. Tailoring the Probiotic Potential of Non-Starter *Lactobacillus* Strains from Ripened Parmigiano Reggiano Cheese by in Vitro Screening and Principal Component Analysis. *Food Microbiol.* **2014**, *38*, 240–249. [CrossRef] [PubMed]
37. Singh, T.P.; Kaur, G.; Kapila, S.; Malik, R.K. Antagonistic Activity of *Lactobacillus reuteri* Strains on the Adhesion Characteristics of Selected Pathogens. *Front. Microbiol.* **2017**, *8*, 486. [CrossRef]
38. Campana, R.; Van Hemert, S.; Baffone, W. Strain-Specific Probiotic Properties of Lactic Acid Bacteria and Their Interference with Human Intestinal Pathogens Invasion. *Gut Pathog.* **2017**, *9*, 12. [CrossRef] [PubMed]
39. Handley, P.S.; Harty, D.W.; Wyatt, J.E.; Brown, C.R.; Doran, J.P.; Gibbs, A.C. A Comparison of the Adhesion, Coaggregation and Cell-Surface Hydrophobicity Properties of Fibrillar and Fimbriate Strains of *Streptococcus salivarius*. *J. Gen. Microbiol.* **1987**, *133*, 3207–3217. [CrossRef]
40. De Souza, B.M.S.; Borgonovi, T.F.; Casarotti, S.N.; Todorov, S.D.; Penna, A.L.B. *Lactobacillus casei* and *Lactobacillus fermentum* Strains Isolated from Mozzarella Cheese: Probiotic Potential, Safety, Acidifying Kinetic Parameters and Viability under Gastrointestinal Tract Conditions. *Probiotics Antimicrob. Proteins* **2018**, *11*, 382–396. [CrossRef]
41. Del Re, B.; Sgorbati, B.; Miglioli, M.; Palenzona, D. Adhesion, Autoaggregation and Hydrophobicity of 13 Strains of *Bifidobacterium longum*. *Lett. Appl. Microbiol.* **2000**, *31*, 438–442. [CrossRef]
42. Zommiti, M.; Connil, N.; Hamida, J.B.; Ferchichi, M. Probiotic Characteristics of *Lactobacillus curvatus* DN317, a Strain Isolated from Chicken Ceca. *Probiotics Antimicrob. Proteins* **2017**, *9*, 415–424. [CrossRef] [PubMed]
43. Abhisingha, M.; Dumnil, J.; Pitaksutheepong, C. Selection of Potential Probiotic *Lactobacillus* with Inhibitory Activity Against *Salmonella* and Fecal Coliform Bacteria. *Probiotics Antimicrob. Proteins* **2018**, *10*, 218–227. [CrossRef] [PubMed]
44. Jankowska, A.; Laubitz, D.; Antushevich, H.; Zabielski, R.; Grzesiuk, E. Competition of *Lactobacillus paracasei* with *Salmonella* Enterica for Adhesion to Caco-2 Cells. *J. Biomed. Biotechnol.* **2008**, *2008*, 357964. [CrossRef] [PubMed]
45. Jessie Lau, L.Y.; Chye, F.Y. Antagonistic Effects of *Lactobacillus plantarum* 0612 on the Adhesion of Selected Foodborne Enteropathogens in Various Colonic Environments. *Food Control* **2018**, *91*, 237–247. [CrossRef]

46. Hai, D.; Lu, Z.; Huang, X.; Lv, F.; Bie, X. In Vitro Screening of Chicken-Derived Lactobacillus Strains That Effectively Inhibit *Salmonella* Colonization and Adhesion. *Foods* **2021**, *10*, 569. [CrossRef] [PubMed]
47. Malik, A.; Sakamoto, M.; Hanazaki, S.; Osawa, M.; Suzuki, T.; Tochigi, M.; Kakii, K. Coaggregation among Nonflocculating Bacteria Isolated from Activated Sludge. *Appl. Environ. Microbiol.* **2003**, *69*, 6056–6063. [CrossRef]
48. Bian, X.; Evivie, S.E.; Muhammad, Z.; Luo, G.W.; Liang, H.Z.; Wang, N.N.; Huo, G.C. In Vitro Assessment of the Antimicrobial Potentials of *Lactobacillus helveticus* Strains Isolated from Traditional Cheese in Sinkiang China against Food-Borne Pathogens. *Food Funct.* **2016**, *7*, 789–797. [CrossRef]
49. El Hage, R.; Losasso, C.; Longo, A.; Petrin, S.; Ricci, A.; Mathieu, F.; Abi Khattar, Z.; El Rayess, Y. Whole-Genome Characterisation of TEM-1 and CMY-2 β-Lactamase-Producing *Salmonella* Kentucky ST198 in Lebanese Broiler Chain. *J. Glob. Antimicrob. Resist.* **2020**, *23*, 408–416. [CrossRef]
50. Saitou, N.N.M.; Nei, M. The Neighbor-Joining Method: A New Method for Reconstructing Phylogenetic Trees'. *Mol. Biol. Evol.* **1987**, *4*, 406–425.
51. Kumar, S.; Stecher, G.; Li, M.; Knyaz, C.; Tamura, K. MEGA X: Molecular Evolutionary Genetics Analysis across Computing Platforms. *Mol. Biol. Evol.* **2018**, *35*, 1547–1549. [CrossRef]
52. Rosenberg, M.; Gutnick, D.; Rosenberg, E. Adherence of Bacteria to Hydrocarbons: A Simple Method for Measuring Cell-Surface Hydrophobicity. *FEMS Microbiol. Lett.* **1980**, *9*, 29–33. [CrossRef]
53. Buahom, J.; Siripornadulsil, S.; Siripornadulsil, W. Feeding with Single Strains Versus Mixed Cultures of Lactic Acid Bacteria and *Bacillus subtilis* KKU213 Affects the Bacterial Community and Growth Performance of Broiler Chickens. *Arab. J. Sci. Eng.* **2018**, *43*, 3417–3427. [CrossRef]
54. Son, S.H.; Jeon, H.L.; Yang, S.J.; Lee, N.K.; Paik, H.D. In Vitro Characterization of *Lactobacillus brevis* KU15006, an Isolate from Kimchi, Reveals Anti-Adhesion Activity against Foodborne Pathogens and Antidiabetic Properties. *Microb. Pathog.* **2017**, *112*, 135–141. [CrossRef] [PubMed]

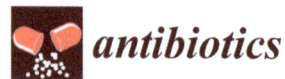 

*Article*

# *Acinetobacter* Non-*baumannii* Species: Occurrence in Infections in Hospitalized Patients, Identification, and Antibiotic Resistance

Eugene Sheck [1], Andrey Romanov [1], Valeria Shapovalova [1], Elvira Shaidullina [1], Alexey Martinovich [1], Natali Ivanchik [1], Anna Mikotina [1], Elena Skleenova [1], Vladimir Oloviannikov [1], Ilya Azizov [1], Vera Vityazeva [2], Alyona Lavrinenko [3], Roman Kozlov [1] and Mikhail Edelstein [1,*]

[1] Institute of Antimicrobial Chemotherapy, Smolensk State Medical University, 214019 Smolensk, Russia; evgeniy.sheck@antibiotic.ru (E.S.); ilya.azizov@antibiotic.ru (I.A.)
[2] Republican Children's Hospital, 185000 Petrozavodsk, Republic of Karelia, Russia
[3] Shared Resource Laboratory, Karaganda Medical University, 100008 Karaganda, Kazakhstan
* Correspondence: mikhail.edelstein@antibiotic.ru

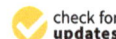

Citation: Sheck, E.; Romanov, A.; Shapovalova, V.; Shaidullina, E.; Martinovich, A.; Ivanchik, N.; Mikotina, A.; Skleenova, E.; Oloviannikov, V.; Azizov, I.; et al. *Acinetobacter* Non-*baumannii* Species: Occurrence in Infections in Hospitalized Patients, Identification, and Antibiotic Resistance. *Antibiotics* **2023**, *12*, 1301. https://doi.org/10.3390/antibiotics12081301

Academic Editor: Ilias Karaiskos

Received: 17 July 2023
Revised: 5 August 2023
Accepted: 7 August 2023
Published: 9 August 2023

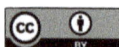

Copyright: © 2023 by the authors. Licensee MDPI, Basel, Switzerland. This article is an open access article distributed under the terms and conditions of the Creative Commons Attribution (CC BY) license (https://creativecommons.org/licenses/by/4.0/).

**Abstract:** Background: *Acinetobacter* species other than *A. baumannii* are becoming increasingly more important as opportunistic pathogens for humans. The primary aim of this study was to assess the prevalence, species distribution, antimicrobial resistance patterns, and carbapenemase gene content of clinical *Acinetobacter* non-*baumannii* (*Anb*) isolates that were collected as part of a sentinel surveillance program of bacterial infections in hospitalized patients. The secondary aim was to evaluate the performance of MALDI-TOF MS systems for the species-level identification of *Anb* isolates. Methods: Clinical bacterial isolates were collected from multiple sites across Russia and Kazakhstan in 2016–2022. Species identification was performed by means of MALDI-TOF MS, with the Autobio and Bruker systems used in parallel. The PCR detection of the species-specific $bla_{OXA-51-like}$ gene was used as a means of differentiating *A. baumannii* from *Anb* species, and the partial sequencing of the *rpoB* gene was used as a reference method for *Anb* species identification. The susceptibility of isolates to antibiotics (amikacin, cefepime, ciprofloxacin, colistin, gentamicin, imipenem, meropenem, sulbactam, tigecycline, tobramycin, and trimethoprim–sulfamethoxazole) was determined using the broth microdilution method. The presence of the most common in *Acinetobacter*-acquired carbapenemase genes ($bla_{OXA-23-like}$, $bla_{OXA-24/40-like}$, $bla_{OXA-58-like}$, $bla_{NDM}$, $bla_{IMP}$, and $bla_{VIM}$) was assessed using real-time PCR. Results: In total, 234 isolates were identified as belonging to 14 *Anb* species. These comprised 6.2% of *Acinetobacter* spp. and 0.7% of all bacterial isolates from the observations. Among the *Anb* species, the most abundant were *A. pittii* (42.7%), *A. nosocomialis* (13.7%), the *A. calcoaceticus/oleivorans* group (9.0%), *A. bereziniae* (7.7%), and *A. geminorum* (6.0%). Notably, two environmental species, *A. oleivorans* and *A. courvalinii*, were found for the first time in the clinical samples of patients with urinary tract infections. The prevalence of resistance to different antibiotics in *Anb* species varied from <4% (meropenem and colistin) to 11.2% (gentamicin). Most isolates were susceptible to all antibiotics; however, sporadic isolates of *A. bereziniae*, *A. johnsonii*, *A. nosocomialis*, *A. oleivorans*, *A. pittii*, and *A. ursingii* were resistant to carbapenems. *A. bereziniae* was more frequently resistant to sulbactam, aminoglycosides, trimethoprim–sulfamethoxazole, and tigecycline than the other species. Four (1.7%) isolates of *A. bereziniae*, *A. johnsonii*, *A. pittii* were found to carry carbapenemase genes ($bla_{OXA-58-like}$ and $bla_{NDM}$, either alone or in combination). The overall accuracy rates of the species-level identification of *Anb* isolates with the Autobio and Bruker systems were 80.8% and 88.5%, with misidentifications occurring in 5 and 3 species, respectively. Conclusions: This study provides important new insights into the methods of identification, occurrence, species distribution, and antibiotic resistance traits of clinical *Anb* isolates.

**Keywords:** *Acinetobacter* non-*baumannii*; MALDI-TOF MS; *rpoB* gene sequencing; antibiotic resistance; carbapenemases

## 1. Introduction

The genus *Acinetobacter* belongs to the family *Moraxellaceae*, class γ-proteobacteria, and comprises coccobacillary-shaped Gram-negative, aerobic, non-lactose fermenting, saprophytic bacteria. This genus has undergone substantial taxonomic modification and currently comprises 82 species with valid published names and 24 species with non-verified published or provisionally assigned names (https://lpsn.dsmz.de/genus/acinetobacter, accessed on 16 July 2023) [1]. Most *Acinetobacter* species are ubiquitous in the environment (soil, water, plants, and animals), and some have evolved as important opportunistic pathogens for humans and animals and have adapted to cause various infections, especially in compromised hosts [2]. *A. baumannii* is a primary human pathogen and is one of the main causes of nosocomial infections with the highest mortality rates [3,4]. Its intrinsic resistance to many antibiotics and its remarkable ability to acquire resistance to all available therapeutic agents, including carbapenems, have secured it a place in the group of ESKAPE pathogens (*E*nterococcus faecium, *S*taphylococcus aureus, *K*lebsiella pneumoniae, *A*cinetobacter baumannii, *P*seudomonas aeruginosa, and *E*nterobacter spp.) [5] and a top place in the WHO's global priority list of antibiotic-resistant bacteria [6]. *A. baumannii* and seven other closely related species (*A. calcoaceticus*, *A. geminorum* (the most recently described species), *A. lactucae* (formerly also known as *A. dijkshoorniae*), *A. nosocomialis*, *A. oleivorans* (effectively but not validly published named species), *A. pittii*, and *A. seifertii*) together form the *Acinetobacter calcoaceticus-baumannii* (*Acb*) complex [7–10]. Species within the *Acb* complex are almost indistinguishable phenotypically but differ significantly in terms of their ecology, pathogenicity, epidemiology, and susceptibility to antibiotics [11]. As an example, while all *Acb* species are capable of causing infections in humans, *A. calcoaceticus* and *A. oleivorans* are primarily environmental species and are less frequently isolated from human clinical specimens [9,12]. In contrast, *A. pittii* and *A. nosocomialis* are more often associated with hospital-acquired infections [11]. As well as *Acb*, 20 more species of the genus *Acinetobacter* were included in the recently updated list of bacteria cultured from humans [13]; among them, *A. bereziniae*, *A. johnsonii*, *A. junii*, *A. lwoffii*, *A. soli*, and *A. ursingii* have commonly been reported in human infections. Although significantly less prevalent than *A. baumannii* and typically less resistant to antibiotics, *Acinetobacter* non-*baumannii* (*Anb*) species are becoming increasingly more important as nosocomial pathogens [14–20].

The accurate identification of *Anb* species is therefore crucial but remains challenging, especially within the *Acb* complex [21]. In the last two decades, molecular methods have been introduced to enable the more efficient differentiation of *Acinetobacter* species as compared to conventional phenotypic identification by manual biochemical tests or automated systems. The sequencing of certain protein-encoding genes (*rpoB* for RNA polymerase subunit B, which is used the most often, *gyrB* for DNA gyrase subunit B, or *recA* for DNA repair recombinase) and/or multilocus sequence analysis (MLSA) have proven the most accurate methods and thus constitute the current reference standard for the identification of *Acinetobacter* species [8,21–23]. The PCR detection of *A. baumannii* species-specific genes for class D β-lactamase ($bla_{OXA-51-like}$) has also been used as a quick and effective means of differentiating *A. baumannii* from *Anb* species [24]. The use of matrix-assisted laser desorption/ionization time-of-flight mass spectrometry (MALDI-TOF MS) for the identification of bacterial species has been a major breakthrough in clinical microbiology. It has proven to be a rapid, cost-effective, and accurate method of differentiating even closely related bacterial species that are otherwise indistinguishable by conventional phenotypic methods [25]. Several studies have assessed the performance of MALDI-TOF MS systems for the identification of *Acinetobacter* species, and, notably, the results from these studies have demonstrated the crucial importance of the size and quality of reference spectra databases (libraries) for accurate species-level identification [21,26,27].

The epidemiology and mechanisms of antibiotic resistance have been most extensively studied for *A. baumannii*. In particular, numerous publications have addressed the problem of the global spread of carbapenem-resistant strains and acquired carbapenemase-producing strains of this species, which pose the most significant health threat [3,4,28].

Other *Acinetobacter* species have been less well studied, although there have been many reports from many parts of the world of isolates of different *Anb* species producing different carbapenemases [29–42]. A recent analysis of publicly available genome sequences showed that *Anb* species represent a reservoir of many transferrable resistance genes to different classes of antibiotics, other than carbapenems [43].

Therefore, this study specifically focused on clinical *Anb* isolates that were collected as part of a large sentinel surveillance program in 2016–2022. We aimed to assess: (i) the prevalence of *Anb* in infections in hospitalized patients; (ii) the performance of MALDI-TOF MS systems for the species-level identification of *Anb* in comparison with the reference *rpoB* sequencing method; and (iii) the prevalence of antibiotic resistance and acquired carbapenemases in *Anb* species.

## 2. Results

*2.1. Species Distribution of Acinetobacter Isolates*

A total of 3754 (10.9%) of the bacterial isolates collected in 2016–2022 within the frame of AMR sentinel surveillance program in Russia and Kazakhstan were identified as members of the *Acinetobacter* genus. *A. baumannii* was the most prevalent species, comprising 3520 (10.2%) isolates, while the other *Acinetobacter* species jointly comprised 234 (0.7%) bacterial isolates. The *Anb* isolates were collected from 41 hospitals in 27 cities across Russia and Kazakhstan. Using the phylogenetic clustering of *rpoB* gene sequence data, they were assigned to 14 different species (Figure 1). The clinical isolates clustered well with the corresponding reference strains and the clusters of different species were clearly separated on the tree. The only exception was *A. geminorum*, a species recently separated from *A. pittii* [7]. Fourteen isolates formed a monophyletic clade and had complete nucleotide sequence identity with the *A. geminorum* type strain J00019, which, however, was poorly discriminated from *A. pittii* (nucleotide distance 0.003; bootstrap value 67%). The two species *A. oleivorans* (https://lpsn.dsmz.de/species/acinetobacter-oleivorans, accessed on 16 July 2023) and *A. septicus* (https://lpsn.dsmz.de/species/acinetobacter-septicus, accessed on 16 July 2023), which have the nomenclatural status "not validly published", were considered the same species, respectively, as *A. calcoaceticus* (*A. calcoaceticus/oleivorans*) and *A. ursingii* (*A. ursingii/septicus*). The latter two species/groups, as well as *A. johnsonii* and *A. lwoffii*, showed the highest intraspecies variability in *rpoB* gene sequences, with a maximum nucleotide divergence between strains of the same species of 0.049, 0.029, 0.027, and 0.033, respectively (Supplementary Table S1: Pairwise nucleotide distance matrix of partial *rpoB* sequences of the studied clinical isolates and reference strains).

*A. pittii* was the major *Anb* species, with 100 isolates that were geographically scattered. Three other species of the *Acb* complex (*A. nosocomialis*, *A. calcoaceticus/oleivorans*, and *A. geminorum*) and one species (*A. bereziniae*) that does not belong to the *Acb* complex each included more than 10 isolates from diverse geographic sites. The nine remaining *Anb* species (*A. junii*, *A. soli*, *A. seifertii*, *A. johnsonii*, *A. lwoffii*, *A. ursingii/septicus*, *A. haemolyticus*, *A. radioresistens*, and *A. courvalinii*) comprised one to nine isolates each. Curiously, one isolate, M19-2435, showed the highest nucleotide sequence identity (>99.4%) with the reference strains of *A. courvalinii*, a soil-dwelling species that had not previously been isolated from humans [13,44,45]. This isolate was recovered from a urine sample of an eight-year-old male patient with a neurogenic bladder after he was operated at the Children's Hospital of Petrozavodsk, Russia, in April 2019.

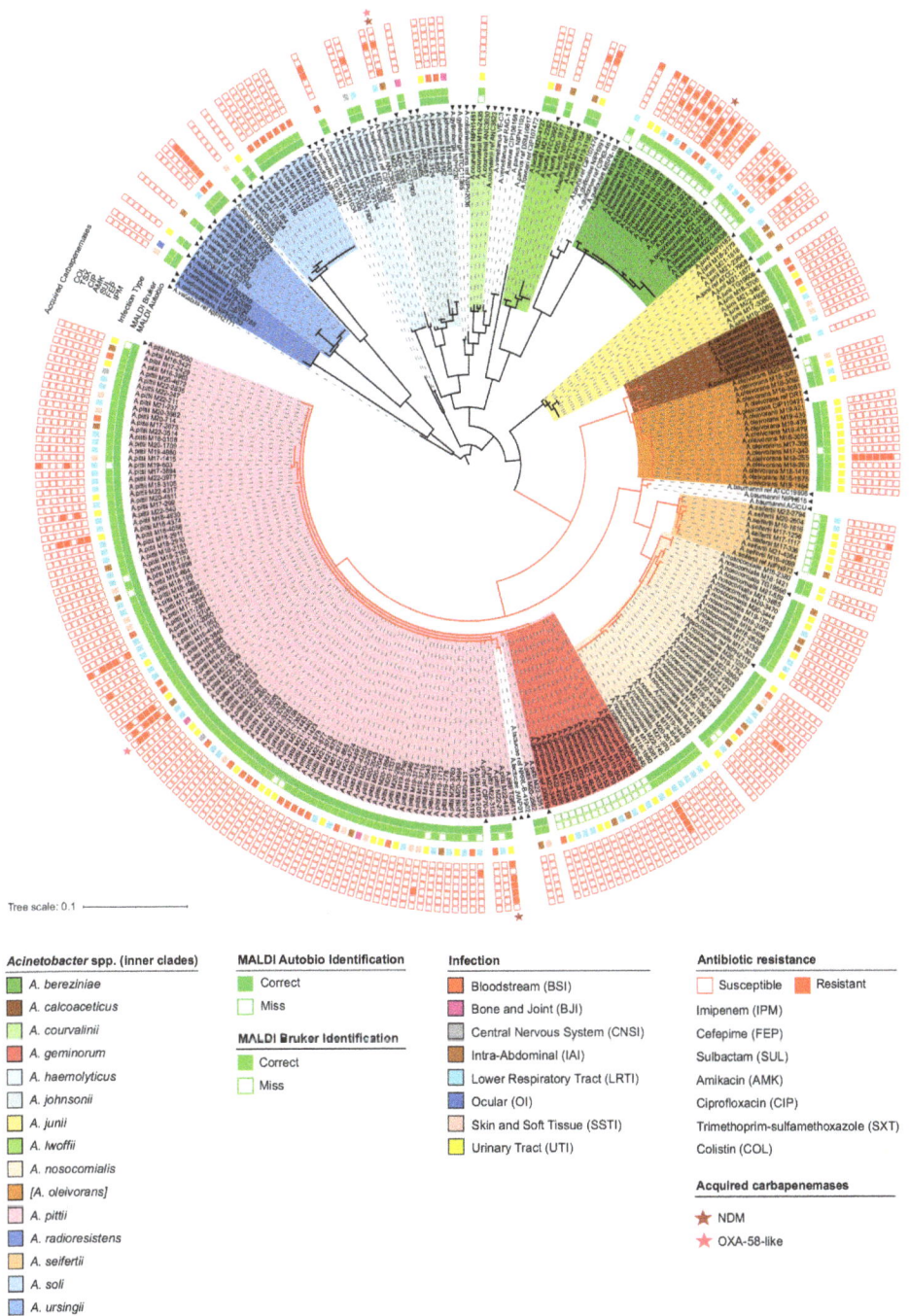

**Figure 1.** Midpoint-rooted maximum-likelihood distance tree of partial *rpoB* sequences from clinical isolates and reference strains of *Anb* species. The various species identified in this study are shown with the colored inner clades, according to the legend. Reference strains are marked with black triangles.

Species of the *A. calcoaceticus-baumannii* complex are shown with red branches. Concentric rings show (from the center to the outside): (i) the accuracy of the species identification with the Autobio and Bruker MALDI-TOF MS systems; (ii) the infection type; (iii) the antibiotic resistance profiles; and (iv) the presence of acquired carbapenemase genes (see legends).

*2.2. Accuracy of Anb Species Identification Using MALDI-TOF MS Systems*

Table 1 summarizes the results of the *Anb* species identification using two MALDI-TOF MS systems, the Autobio Autof and the Bruker Biotyper, compared to the reference method of *rpoB* gene sequencing. Figure 1 details the results for the individual isolates. Since *A. oleivorans* [9] has the nomenclatural status "not validly published", it was considered the same species as *A. calcoaceticus* (*A. calcoaceticus/oleivorans*), and the identification of *A. oleivorans* as *A. calcoaceticus* was not considered incorrect. The overall rates of correct species identification were 189/234 (80.8%) for Autobio and 207/234 (88.5%) for Bruker. Both systems provided confident species-level identification of all isolates of *A. haemolyticus*, *A. johnsonii*, *A. junii*, *A. lwoffii*, *A. radioresistens*, *A. soli*, and *A. ursingii*. In addition, Autobio correctly identified all isolates of *A. nosocomialis* and *A. pittii*, two and eleven of which were misidentified by Bruker, respectively, as *A. baumannii* (log scores: 2.15–2.3) and *A. lactucae* (log scores: 1.99–2.26). On the other hand, Bruker correctly identified all isolates of *A. bereziniae*, *A. calcoaceticus/oleivorans* (as *A. calcoaceticus*), *A. courvalinii*, and *A. seifertii*, while Autobio misidentified all isolates of *A. bereziniae* as *A. guillouiae* (scores: 9.416–9.705), *A. seifertii* as *A. pittii* (scores: 8.990–9.348), a single isolate of *A. courvalinii* as *A. haemolyticus* (score 9.181); additionally, it provided no confident identification for four isolates of *A. calcoaceticus/oleivorans* (scores: 4.437–5.688). Finally, both the Autobio and Bruker systems misidentified all isolates of *A. geminorum*, respectively, as *A. pittii* (scores: 7.445–9.607) and *A. lactucae* (log scores: 2.1–2.23). In order to improve the accuracy of the identification, we generated reference mass spectra of representative *Anb* isolates and added them to the user libraries. Subsequently, all *Anb* isolates from our collection were correctly identified to the species level when tested against both the proprietary and our custom spectra libraries (data not shown).

**Table 1.** Accuracy of the species identification of *Anb* isolates using MALDI-TOF MS systems.

| *Anb* Species [1] | No. of Isolates | No. (Percent) Correctly Identified | |
|---|---|---|---|
| | | Autobio Autof | Bruker Biotyper |
| *A. bereziniae* | 18 | 0 (0%) | 18 (100%) |
| *A. calcoaceticus/oleivorans* | 21 | 17 (81%) | 21 (100%) |
| *A. courvalinii* | 1 | 0 (0%) | 1 (100%) |
| *A. geminorum* | 14 | 0 (0%) | 0 (0%) |
| *A. haemolyticus* | 3 | 3 (100%) | 3 (100%) |
| *A. johnsonii* | 7 | 7 (100%) | 7 (100%) |
| *A. junii* | 9 | 9 (100%) | 9 (100%) |
| *A. lwoffii* | 5 | 5 (100%) | 5 (100%) |
| *A. nosocomialis* | 32 | 32 (100%) | 30 (93.8%) |
| *A. pittii* | 100 | 100 (100%) | 89 (89%) |
| *A. radioresistens* | 2 | 2 (100%) | 2 (100%) |
| *A. seifertii* | 8 | 0 (0%) | 8 (100%) |
| *A. soli* | 9 | 9 (100%) | 9 (100%) |
| *A. ursingii/septicus* | 5 | 5 (100%) | 5 (100%) |

[1] as determined by *rpoB* gene sequence analysis.

*2.3. Infections Caused by Anb Species*

The *Anb* isolates were most often isolated from clinical samples of hospitalized patients with lower respiratory tract infections (75/234 (32.1%)) and urinary tract infections (UTIs) (65/234 (27.8%)). Other primary sites of infection included, in order of decreasing abundance: heart and blood vessels, 43/234 (18.4%), the abdominal cavity, 25/234 (10.7%), skin and soft tissues, 18/234 (7.7%), bones and joints, 4/234 (1.7%), the central nervous system, 3/284 (1.3%), and eye appendages, 1/234 (0.4%). Overall, we did not find any association between particular *Anb* species and the site of infection. All species represented by more than one isolate were isolated from diverse infections (Figure 1). Only two species were statistically significantly more abundant in specific loci: 14/16 (87.5%) *A. oleivorans* isolates were recovered from UTIs (the proportion of UTI isolates among other species was 51/218 (23.4%), $p = 0.0001$, Fisher's exact test with the Holm correction), and 7/9 (77.8%) *A. soli* isolates were recovered from primary bloodstream infections (the proportion of bloodstream isolates among other species was 36/225 (16.0%), $p = 0.0001$). It should be noted, however, that all UTI isolates of *A. oleivorans* were isolated in the same pediatric hospital in Petrozavodsk city between October 2016 and February 2019. Likewise, all bloodstream isolates of *A. soli* were isolated in the same neonatal care unit in Kazan city between January 2019 and July 2019. Therefore, a common source of infection could not be excluded in the case of both *A. oleivorans* UTI and *A. soli* bloodstream isolates.

In addition to these two examples of potentially clonal expansions of *A. oleivorans* and *A. soli*, we observed a few more "in-hospital clusters" of isolates of the same species. These included five clusters of 7 to 15 isolates of *A. pittii* in different hospitals and one cluster of 11 isolates of *A. nosocomialis*. Records indicated that 171/234 (73.1%) infections due to *Anb* species were considered nosocomial as they occurred more than 48 h after patient admission to the hospital or were thought to be acquired during previous hospital admissions.

### 2.4. Susceptibility to Antibiotics and the Presence of Acquired Carbapenemase Genes

Table 2 provides a statistical summary of the susceptibility of *Anb* isolates to 11 antibiotics, and Figure 1 additionally shows the resistance profiles of the individual isolates to key agents representing major antibiotic classes. Most *Anb* isolates were susceptible to all antibiotics tested. The resistance rates to all β-lactam antibiotics and sulbactam were below 6%, and resistance to β-lactams was not confined to any particular species. Importantly, resistance to carbapenems (imipenem or meropenem) was detected in 11 sporadic isolates: 5 *A. pittii*, 2 *A. bereziniae*, and 1 isolate each of *A. johnsonii*, *A. nosocomialis*, *A. oleivorans*, and *A. ursingii*, all of which, except *A. johnsonii*, were additionally resistant to antibiotics of at least two other classes. Thirteen (5.6%) isolates, including five *A. pittii*, four *A. bereziniae*, and one isolate each of *A. nosocomialis*, *A. oleivorans*, *A. seifertii*, and *A. ursingii*, were resistant to sulbactam at an MIC breakpoint of $\geq 16$ mg/L. The overall resistance rates to non-β-lactam agents were: 8.7% to tobramycin, 9.9% to amikacin, 11.2% to gentamicin, 7.4% to ciprofloxacin, 8.7% to trimethoprim–sulfamethoxazole, and 3.0% to colistin. The seven colistin-resistant isolates belonged to three species: four *A. bereziniae*, two *A. pittii*, and one *A. seifertii*. Notably, *A. bereziniae* displayed significantly higher resistance rates than other *Anb* species to colistin (22.2% vs. 1.4%, $p = 0.0008$, Fisher's exact test with the Holm correction), sulbactam (22.2% vs. 4.21%, $p = 0.0118$), aminoglycosides (66.7% vs. 7.9%, $p = 0.0001$), and trimethoprim–sulfamethoxazole (66.7% vs. 3.8%, $p = 0.0001$); it also showed higher resistance levels to tigecycline ($MIC_{90\%}$: >16 mg/L vs. 1 mg/L).

Acquired carbapenemase genes were detected in 4/234 (1.7%) isolates collected at geographically distant sites. One isolate each of *A. bereziniae* and *A. pittii* carried the $bla_{NDM}$ gene, another isolate of *A. pittii* carried the $bla_{OXA\text{-}58\text{-like}}$ gene, and one isolate of *A. johnsonii* harbored the $bla_{NDM}$ and $bla_{OXA\text{-}58\text{-like}}$ genes simultaneously. The carbapenemase-positive isolates of *A. bereziniae* and *A. pittii* displayed high-level resistance to imipenem and meropenem, with MICs of $\geq 16$ mg/L. Curiously, however, the double-carbapenemase-positive isolate of *A. johnsonii* showed borderline resistance to imipenem, with an MIC of 8 mg/L, and susceptibility to meropenem with an MIC of 1 mg/L. Finally, as expected, the isolates of *A. radioresistens*, which were susceptible to carbapenems, tested positive by PCR for the $bla_{OXA\text{-}23\text{-like}}$ gene, which is known to be intrinsic chromosomally-encoded and usually weakly expressed in this species [46].

Table 2. Minimum inhibitory concentration (MIC) range, MIC50, MIC90, and proportion of Anb isolates by category of susceptibility to 11 antibiotics.

| Antibiotic | MIC, mg/L | | | Percent by Category [1] | | |
|---|---|---|---|---|---|---|
| | Range | 50% | 90% | S | I | R |
| Amikacin | ≤0.5–≥256 | 1 | 8 | 90.1 | - | 9.9 |
| Cefepime [2] | ≤0.5–≥256 | 2 | 16 | 88.7 | 5.7 | 5.7 |
| Ciprofloxacin | ≤0.06–≥128 | 0.125 | 0.5 | - | 92.6 | 7.4 |
| Colistin | ≤0.06–≥64 | 0.5 | 2 | 97.0 | - | 3.0 |
| Gentamicin | ≤0.25–≥256 | 0.5 | 8 | 88.8 | - | 11.2 |
| Imipenem | ≤0.06–≥128 | 0.125 | 0.5 | 95.7 | - | 4.3 |
| Meropenem | ≤0.06–≥128 | 0.25 | 0.5 | 95.2 | 0.9 | 3.9 |
| Sulbactam [3] | ≤0.25–≥256 | 1 | 4 | 92.2 | 2.2 | 5.6 |
| Tigecycline [4] | ≤0.03–≥16 | 0.25 | 1 | - | - | - |
| Tobramycin | ≤0.25–≥256 | 0.25 | 2 | 91.3 | - | 8.7 |
| Trimethoprim–sulfamethoxazole (1:19) [5] | ≤0.125–≥256 | 0.125 | 4 | 89.6 | 1.7 | 8.7 |

[1] S, susceptible; I, susceptible, increased exposure (EUCAST), or intermediate resistant (CLSI); R, resistant. EUCAST v13.0 MIC clinical breakpoints were used unless otherwise stated. [2] For cefepime, CLSI M100 ED33 MIC breakpoints were used. [3] For sulbactam, the MIC breakpoints (S ≤ 4 mg/L, I 8 mg/L, R ≥ 16 mg/L) were based on CLSI M100 ED33 ampicillin–sulbactam (2:1) MIC breakpoints (S ≤ 8/4 mg/L, I 16/8 mg/L, R ≥ 32/16 mg/L), where sulbactam comprises the active component of the combination against Acinetobacter. [4] For tigecycline, no MIC breakpoints were established by either EUCAST or CLSI. [5] MIC values refer to trimethoprim.

## 3. Discussion

This study characterized 234 clinical Anb isolates collected from hospitalized patients in multiple centers across Russia and Kazakhstan over the last seven years. These isolates belonged to 14 different species, as was determined by *rpoB* gene sequencing, and jointly comprised 6.2% of *Acinetobacter* spp. (the remaining isolates were *A. baumannii*) and 0.7% of all bacterial isolates collected as part of the sentinel surveillance program [47]. Among the Anb species, the most abundant was *A. pittii* (42.7%), followed by *A. nosocomialis* (13.7%), *A. calcoaceticus/oleivorans* (9.0%), *A. bereziniae* (7.7%), and *A. geminorum* (6.0%). *A. pittii* and *A. nosocomialis* are both known to be the next most common *Acinetobacter* spp. after *A. baumannii* to cause nosocomial infections [20]. *A. geminorum*, which has recently been separated from *A. pittii* [7], has a highly similar *rpoB* gene sequence. On the contrary, *A. oleivorans*, which has not been assigned the nomenclatural status of a validly published named species, and which was therefore regarded in our analysis as one species with *A. calcoaceticus*, has a more divergent *rpoB* gene sequence. It is worth mentioning that the *rpoB* sequences of 16 isolates of the *A. calcoaceticus/oleivorans* group clustered closely with those of the reference strains of *A. oleivorans*, while only 5 isolates clustered with the reference strains of *A. calcoaceticus*. This is an unexpected finding given that *A. oleivorans* has commonly been described as a soil-dwelling carbohydrate-hydrolyzing bacterium and has not been associated with humans [9,48–50]. Another interesting finding was the isolation of *A. courvalinii* [44,45] from a urine clinical sample of an eight-year-old male patient with cystitis, which, to our knowledge, represents the first documented case of human infection with this species.

The studied Anb isolates were recovered from different primary sites of infection, mostly the lower respiratory tract, urinary system, and blood stream, with no particular association between the infection locus and the species. It is worth noting that *A. oleivorans* and *A. soli* were isolated significantly more often, respectively, from urine and blood. However, all the urine isolates of *A. oleivorans* were collected in the same hospital and could therefore have a common origin, as were all the blood isolates of *A. soli*. In addition to these two examples, we observed several in-hospital clusters of infections due to *A. pittii* and *A. nosocomialis*, indicating their likely nosocomial transmission.

One of the most important tasks of this study was to assess the performance of two MALDI-TOF MS systems for the identification of Anb species. The Autobio and Bruker systems demonstrated the overall rates of correct species-level identification, respectively, of

80.8% and 88.5% for our collection of *Anb* isolates. These rates are lower than those reported from the study of the routine collection of bacterial isolates of any species (>97%) [51]. However, our results correspond well with the findings of many studies that focus specifically on the MALDI-TOF MS identification of *Acinetobacter* spp. [21,26,27]. In line with these studies, we found that most cases of misidentification were likely due to the absence or insufficient number of mass spectra of new species in the reference libraries, as was the case for *A. geminorum* in the Autobio and Bruker libraries and *A. courvalinii* in the Autobio library; the misidentifications could also be due to the potentially inconsistent species identification of the reference strains present in the library, as was the case for *A. bereziniae* and *A. seifertii* being identified with high scores as *A. guillouiae* and *A. pittii*, respectively, by Autobio. The low-score identification results of single isolates of *A. calcoaceticus/oleivorans*, *A. nosocomialis*, and *A. pittii* were also likely due to the small number of mass spectra of these species in the reference libraries. Importantly, however, we found that all identification errors could be eliminated by adding the spectra of "difficult" strains, correctly identified using the reference method, to the custom user libraries. These findings once again highlight the importance of maintaining the reference spectra libraries in accordance with current taxonomy and nomenclature of *Acinetobacter* spp. and the need to include strains of newly described species in the libraries.

The studied *Anb* isolates were mostly susceptible to antibiotics. The resistance rates to all agents did not exceed 10% (except for gentamicin, at 11.2%). These rates are significantly lower than those reported for *A. baumannii* isolates from the same surveillance program [47,52,53]. For example, the prevalence of resistance to trimethoprim–sulfamethoxazole, aminoglycosides, ciprofloxacin, and carbapenems was 6 to 20 times lower in *Anb* than in *A. baumannii* (https://amrmap.net/?id=BWSMM21DC29DC11, accessed on 16 July 2023) [47]. The exception was resistance to colistin, which was more than three times higher in *Anb* than in *A. baumannii* (3.0% vs. 0.8%), with most colistin-resistant isolates being identified as *A. bereziniae*. The latter species was also more resistant to sulbactam, aminoglycosides, trimethoprim–sulfamethoxazole, and tigecycline than other *Anb* species. The acquired resistance to colistin in *A. bereziniae* has previously been found to be associated with mutations in the *pmrB* gene involved in lipopolysaccharide modification [54]. Resistance to most aminoglycosides, including amikacin, has been attributed to plasmid-carried genes for aminoglycoside-modifying enzymes (*aphA6*, *aac(6′)-31* and *aadA1*) [36,55,56].

The primary mechanisms of resistance to carbapenems in *Acinetobacter* spp. include the overexpression of naturally occurring species-specific carbapenemases of molecular class D (OXA) [57] and the production of acquired carbapenemases of class D (mainly OXA-23-, OXA-24/40-, and OXA-58-like enzymes) and class B (mainly NDM and IMP) [4]. Our study revealed the low prevalence of acquired carbapenemases in *Anb* isolates (1.7%) as compared to *A. baumannii* (81.9%) (https://amrmap.net/?id=AN0Fl54mX14mX14, accessed on 16 July 2023). Moreover, only OXA-58-like and NDM carbapenemases were found alone or in combination in sporadic isolates of *A. bereziniae*, *A. johnsonii*, and *A. pittii*, whereas, in *A. baumannii* in Russia, these carbapenemases were rare, and the OXA-23- and OXA-24/40-types were the predominant carbapenemases detected [47,53]. Likewise, studies from many other countries have found the same differences in the frequency of various acquired carbapenemases in *A. baumannii* and *Anb*. OXA-58 has been detected in the early carbapenem-resistant isolates of *A. baumannii* in Europe, Asia, and South America [58,59] and, recently, mostly in *Anb* species, including *A. bereziniae*, *A. colistiniresistens*, *A. johnsonii*, *A. junii*, *A. nosocomialis*, *A. pittii*, *A. radioresistens*, *A. seifertii*, *A. towneri*, and *A. ursingii*, from all over the world [37,60–69]. Similarly, metallo-β-lactamases, mostly NDM-1 and IMP variants, have been found in global *Anb* isolates, often in combination with OXA-58 [62–64,70–78].

While our study covered a large geographic area and a long time period, it did not identify and include some of the *Anb* species that have been previously cultured from humans. This is an obvious limitation of the study, which demonstrates the importance of ongoing surveillance and research. Our further study will utilize whole-genome sequencing data to infer the phylogenetic relationships between closely related *Acinetobacter* spp., such as *A. pittii* and *A. geminorum*, and to explore in greater depth the mechanisms of antibiotic resistance in *Anb* isolates. Further studies will also be needed to continuously evaluate the performance of MALDI-TOF MS platforms with updated spectra libraries for identification of *Acinetobacter* spp.

## 4. Materials and Methods

### 4.1. Bacterial Isolates

All the studied isolates and accompanying metadata were collected as part of the national sentinel surveillance program of antimicrobial resistance (AMR) in bacterial pathogens isolated from hospitalized patients [47]. Between 1 January 2016 and 31 December 2022, 94 participating hospitals from 42 cities across Russia and 1 hospital in Karaganda, Kazakhstan, contributed a total of 34,524 non-duplicate (one per patient/case of infection) clinical bacterial isolates, of which 3754 (10.9%) were confirmed in the central surveillance laboratory as *Acinetobacter* species. The isolates were recovered from representative clinical specimens (blood, tissue biopsies, cerebrospinal fluid, bronchoalveolar lavage, sputum, urine, etc.) of patients with clinical symptoms of infections; isolates from surface swabs, screenings, and environmental samples were excluded. All isolates with accompanying clinical and epidemiological information were referred to the central surveillance laboratory of the Institute of Antimicrobial Chemotherapy (IAC), where species identification, antibiotic susceptibility testing, and molecular genetic characterizations of the isolates were performed.

### 4.2. Species Identification with MALDI-TOF MS

The bacterial isolates were identified with MALDI-TOF MS, using both the Microflex LT-MALDI Biotyper System with the Biotyper spectral database ver.11 (Bruker Daltonics, Bremen, Germany) and the Autof MS2000 System with the current online spectral library (Autobio Diagnostics, Zhengzhou, China). The standard methods of direct colony transfer and rapid (on-target) extraction with formic acid were used for sample preparation prior to the acquisition of mass spectra, as described previously [79,80]. The criteria for "confident species-level identification" were as follows: log scores $\geq 2.0$ for the Bruker Biotyper System and scores $\geq 9.0$ for the Autobio Autof System. Only the highest-match score values (1st of the 10 best hits) of the clinical isolates against the corresponding reference libraries were reported in the Results section. To generate the reference spectra of the selected *Acinetobacter* strains for the Autobio library, the full (in-tube) extraction method was used; the extracts from each culture were spotted four times onto a ground steel target and each spot was measured and processed three times according to the manufacturer's instruction.

### 4.3. Additional Tests to Distinguish A. baumannii

*A. baumannii* isolates were additionally distinguished by the detection of species-specific $bla_{\text{OXA-51-like}}$ genes using real-time PCR [24] and by multilocus sequencing typing (MLST) using the University of Oxford and the Institute Pasteur typing schemes [81,82].

### 4.4. Sequencing of the rpoB Gene and Analysis of the Sequence Data

All isolates preliminarily identified as *Anb* species were subjected to *rpoB* gene sequencing, which was used a reference identification method [21]. Briefly, a 397 bp internal fragment of the *rpoB* gene was amplified by PCR using the primers Ac696F, 5′-TAYCGYAAAGAYTTGAAAGAAG-3′, and Ac1093R, 5′-CMACACCYTTGTTMCCRTGA-3′, as described elsewhere [83]. The PCR products were purified with exonuclease I and a shrimp alkaline phosphatase treatment and were sequenced on both strands using the same primers and a BigDye Terminator v3.1 Cycle Sequencing Kit (Thermo Fisher Scientific, Waltham, MA, USA). The sequencing products were analyzed using a Applied Biosystems 3500 Genetic Analyzer (Life Technologies, Carlsbad, CA, USA). Quality assessments and the assembly of sequences were performed using a QIAGEN CLC Genomics Workbench 21.0 (QIAGEN, Aarhus, Denmark).

The *rpoB* gene sequences of the reference and type strains (one to three per species) of 27 *Acinetobacter* spp. (*A. baumannii*, *A. baylyi*, *A. beijerinckii*, *A. bereziniae*, *A. calcoaceticus*, *A. colistiniresistens*, *A. courvalinii*, *A. geminorum*, *A. guillouiae*, *A. haemolyticus*, *A. johnsonii*, *A. junii*, *A. lactucae*, *A. lwoffii*, *A. nosocomialis*, *A. oleivorans*, *A. parvus*, *A. pittii*, *A. radioresistens*, *A. schindleri*, *A. seifertii*, *A. septicus*, *A. soli*, *A. towneri*, *A. ursingii*, *A. variabilis*, and *A. venetianus*) were obtained from the NCBI GenBank (https://www.ncbi.nlm.nih.gov/genbank/, accessed on 16 July 2023) and the ATCC Genome Portal (https://genomes.atcc.org/, accessed on 16 July 2023). The *rpoB* gene sequences of the studied clinical isolates and reference strains were aligned together (after trimming the primer sites) and the resulting alignment was used to produce a maximum-likelihood tree with the Tamura–Nei model and 1000 bootstraps using MEGA v.11.0.13 [84]. The visualization and annotation of the phylogenetic tree were performed using iTOL v.6.7.6 [85].

*4.5. Antimicrobial Susceptibility Testing*

Antimicrobial susceptibility testing (AST) was conducted for the following agents: amikacin, cefepime, ciprofloxacin, colistin, gentamicin, imipenem, meropenem, sulbactam, tigecycline, tobramycin, and trimethoprim–sulfamethoxazole (1:19). This was accomplished by using a reference broth microdilution method according to ISO 20776-2:2021 [86] and the methodology of the European committee on antimicrobial susceptibility testing (EUCAST) [87]. *Escherichia coli* ATCC 25922, *E. coli* NCTC 13846, and *Pseudomonas aeruginosa* ATCC 27853 were used as quality control strains for AST. The AST results were interpreted according to the EUCAST v.13.0 Clinical Breakpoints [88] for all agents except for cefepime and sulbactam, for which the results were interpreted using the CLSI M100 ED33 breakpoints [89], and for tigecycline, for which only the $MIC_{50}$ and $MIC_{90}$ values were reported due to lack of EUCAST and CLSI interpretive criteria.

*4.6. Real-Time PCR Detection of Carbapenemase Genes*

The detection of genes encoding the most common *Acinetobacter*-spp.-acquired carbapenemases of molecular class D (OXA-23-, OXA-24/40-, and OXA-58-like) and class B (metallo-β-lactamases: NDM, IMP and VIM) was performed using commercial real-time PCR assays: AmpliSens MDR Acinetobacter-OXA-FL and AmpliSens MDR MBL-FL (Central research institute of epidemiology, Moscow, Russia), according to manufacturer's instructions. Amplification reactions were carried out using the DTPrime 5X1 Real-Time PCR System (DNA Technology, Moscow, Russia). Strains of *A. baumannii*, *A. pittii*, and *P. aeruginosa* carrying the genes of the known carbapenemases from the IAC collection [47] were used as positive controls.

*4.7. Data Availability*

The DNA sequences obtained in this study were deposited in the European Nucleotide Archive under the project accession number PRJEB61953. The clinical, epidemiological, geospatial, and temporal characteristics of the studied *Anb* isolates, the quantitative (MIC) and qualitative (categorical) AST data, the carbepenemase gene status, and the *rpoB* phylogenetic clustering data were made available as an open-access project at Microreact [90]: https://microreact.org/project/fKrejDn6vqcervyWwMAs8W-acinetobacter-non-baumannii-species (accessed on 16 July 2023).

## 5. Conclusions

This study represents one of the largest surveys of *Anb* isolates collected from infections in hospitalized patients. It provides new insights into the methods of identification, as well as the occurrence, species distribution, and antibiotic resistance traits of *Anb* isolates. It also reports for the first time the isolation of *A. oleivorans* and *A. courvalinii* from clinical samples of patients with urinary tract infections.

**Supplementary Materials:** The following supporting information can be downloaded at: https://www.mdpi.com/article/10.3390/antibiotics12081301/s1, Table S1: Pairwise nucleotide distance matrix of partial *rpoB* sequences of the studied clinical isolates and reference strains.

**Author Contributions:** Conceptualization, E.S. (Eugene Sheckand) and M.E.; methodology and experimental work, E.S. (Eugene Sheckand), A.R., E.S. (Elvira Shaidullinaand), A.M. (Alexey Martinovichand), N.I., A.M. (Anna Mikotina), E.S. (Elena Skleenova), V.O., I.A., V.V., and A.L.; data validation and analysis, V.S. and M.E.; writing—original draft preparation, E.S. (Eugene Sheckand); writing—review and editing, M.E.; supervision and project administration, R.K. and M.E. All authors have read and agreed to the published version of the manuscript.

**Funding:** The national sentinel surveillance program of antimicrobial resistance (AMR) in bacterial pathogens isolated from hospitalized patients is funded by the Ministry of Health of the Russian Federation (Grant no. 056-00050-21-03).

**Institutional Review Board Statement:** The studied bacterial isolates (ENA project accession no. PRJEB61953) from the national AMR surveillance program were recovered at local clinical hospitals in Russia as part of routine diagnostic sampling. The national AMR surveillance program was approved by the Review Board of the FSBEI HE "Smolensk State Medical University" of the Ministry of Health of the Russian Federation. Ethical approval was granted by the institutional Independent Ethics Committee, on 4 September 2015.

**Informed Consent Statement:** The informed consent was waived for this study because it did not involve any additional interventions; no personal patient data were collected and the data regarding the sources of the isolates were collected anonymously.

**Data Availability Statement:** The DNA sequences obtained in this study were deposited in the European Nucleotide Archive under the project accession number PRJEB61953. The clinical, epidemiological, geospatial, and temporal characteristics of studied Anb isolates, the quantitative (MIC) and qualitative (categorical) AST data, the carbapenemase gene status, and the *rpoB* phylogenetic clustering data were made available as an open-access project at Microreact (https://microreact.org/project/fKrejDn6vqcervyWwMAs8W-acinetobacter-non-baumannii-species, accessed on 16 July 2023).

**Acknowledgments:** We thank all the participants of the sentinel surveillance program for the collection of the clinical bacterial isolates used in this study. We also thank the entire IAC laboratory staff for maintaining the collection and undertaking susceptibility testing of isolates.

**Conflicts of Interest:** The authors declare no conflict of interest.

## References

1. Meier-Kolthoff, J.P.; Carbasse, J.S.; Peinado-Olarte, R.L.; Göker, M. TYGS and LPSN: A Database Tandem for Fast and Reliable Genome-Based Classification and Nomenclature of Prokaryotes. *Nucleic Acids Res.* **2022**, *50*, D801–D807. [CrossRef]
2. Wong, D.; Nielsen, T.B.; Bonomo, R.A.; Pantapalangkoor, P.; Luna, B.; Spellberg, B. Clinical and Pathophysiological Overview of *Acinetobacter* Infections: A Century of Challenges. *Clin. Microbiol. Rev.* **2017**, *30*, 409. [CrossRef] [PubMed]
3. Antunes, L.C.S.; Visca, P.; Towner, K.J. *Acinetobacter baumannii*: Evolution of a Global Pathogen. *Pathog. Dis.* **2014**, *71*, 292–301. [CrossRef]
4. Ramirez, M.S.; Bonomo, R.A.; Tolmasky, M.E. Carbapenemases: Transforming *Acinetobacter baumannii* into a Yet More Dangerous Menace. *Biomolecules* **2020**, *10*, 720. [CrossRef] [PubMed]
5. Boucher, H.W.; Talbot, G.H.; Bradley, J.S.; Edwards, J.E.; Gilbert, D.; Rice, L.B.; Scheld, M.; Spellberg, B.; Bartlett, J. Bad Bugs, No Drugs: No ESKAPE! An Update from the Infectious Diseases Society of America. *Clin. Infect. Dis.* **2009**, *48*, 1–12. [CrossRef]
6. World Health Organization. Prioritization of Pathogens to Guide Discovery, Research and Development of New Antibiotics for Drug-Resistant Bacterial Infections, Including Tuberculosis. 2017. Available online: https://www.who.int/publications/i/item/WHO-EMP-IAU-2017.12 (accessed on 17 July 2023).
7. Wolf, S.; Barth-Jakschic, E.; Birkle, K.; Bader, B.; Marschal, M.; Liese, J.; Peter, S.; Oberhettinger, P. *Acinetobacter geminorum* sp. nov., Isolated from Human Throat Swabs. *Int. J. Syst. Evol. Microbiol.* **2021**, *71*, 005018. [CrossRef] [PubMed]
8. Cosgaya, C.; Marí-Almirall, M.; Van Assche, A.; Fernández-Orth, D.; Mosqueda, N.; Telli, M.; Huys, G.; Higgins, P.G.; Seifert, H.; Lievens, B.; et al. *Acinetobacter dijkshoorniae* sp. nov., a Member of the Acinetobacter Calcoaceticus-*Acinetobacter baumannii* Complex Mainly Recovered from Clinical Samples in Different Countries. *Int. J. Syst. Evol. Microbiol.* **2016**, *66*, 4105–4111. [CrossRef] [PubMed]
9. Kang, Y.S.; Jung, J.; Jeon, C.O.; Park, W. *Acinetobacter oleivorans* sp. nov. Is Capable of Adhering to and Growing on Diesel-Oil. *J. Microbiol.* **2011**, *49*, 29–34. [CrossRef]

10. Dunlap, C.A.; Rooney, A.P. *Acinetobacter dijkshoorniae* Is a Later Heterotypic Synonym of Acinetobacter Lactucae. *Int. J. Syst. Evol. Microbiol.* **2018**, *68*, 131–132. [CrossRef]
11. Nemec, A.; Krizova, L.; Maixnerova, M.; van der Reijden, T.J.K.; Deschaght, P.; Passet, V.; Vaneechoutte, M.; Brisse, S.; Dijkshoorn, L. Genotypic and Phenotypic Characterization of the *Acinetobacter calcoaceticus–Acinetobacter baumannii* Complex with the Proposal of *Acinetobacter pittii* sp. nov. (Formerly Acinetobacter Genomic Species 3) and *Acinetobacter nosocomialis* sp. nov. (Formerly Acinetobacter Genomic Species 13TU). *Res. Microbiol.* **2011**, *162*, 393–404. [CrossRef]
12. Glover, J.S.; Ticer, T.D.; Engevik, M.A. Profiling Antibiotic Resistance in *Acinetobacter calcoaceticus*. *Antibiotics* **2022**, *11*, 978. [CrossRef] [PubMed]
13. Diakite, A.; Dubourg, G.; Raoult, D. Updating the Repertoire of Cultured Bacteria from the Human Being. *Microb. Pathog.* **2021**, *150*, 104698. [CrossRef]
14. Salzer, H.J.F.; Rolling, T.; Schmiede, S.; Klupp, E.M.; Lange, C.; Seifert, H. Severe Community-Acquired Bloodstream Infection with *Acinetobacter ursingii* in Person Who Injects Drugs. *Emerg. Infect. Dis.* **2016**, *22*, 134. [CrossRef] [PubMed]
15. Chusri, S.; Chongsuvivatwong, V.; Rivera, J.I.; Silpapojakul, K.; Singkhamanan, K.; McNeil, E.; Doi, Y. Clinical Outcomes of Hospital-Acquired Infection with *Acinetobacter nosocomialis* and *Acinetobacter pittii*. *Antimicrob. Agents Chemother.* **2014**, *58*, 4172–4179. [CrossRef] [PubMed]
16. Turton, J.F.; Shah, J.; Ozongwu, C.; Pike, R. Incidence of Acinetobacter Species Other than *A. baumannii* among Clinical Isolates of *Acinetobacter*: Evidence for Emerging Species. *J. Clin. Microbiol.* **2010**, *48*, 1445. [CrossRef]
17. Mittal, S.; Sharma, M.; Yadav, A.; Bala, K.; Chaudhary, U. *Acinetobacter lwoffii* an Emerging Pathogen in Neonatal ICU. *Infect. Disord. Drug Targets* **2015**, *15*, 184–188. [CrossRef]
18. Fitzpatrick, M.A.; Ozer, E.; Bolon, M.K.; Hauser, A.R. Influence of ACB Complex Genospecies on Clinical Outcomes in a U.S. Hospital with High Rates of Multidrug Resistance. *J. Infect.* **2015**, *70*, 144. [CrossRef]
19. Matsui, M.; Suzuki, S.; Yamane, K.; Suzuki, M.; Konda, T.; Arakawa, Y.; Shibayama, K. Distribution of Carbapenem Resistance Determinants among Epidemic and Non-Epidemic Types of *Acinetobacter* Species in Japan. *J. Med. Microbiol.* **2014**, *63*, 870–877. [CrossRef]
20. Al Atrouni, A.; Joly-Guillou, M.L.; Hamze, M.; Kempf, M. Reservoirs of Non-*baumannii* Acinetobacter Species. *Front. Microbiol.* **2016**, *7*, 49. [CrossRef] [PubMed]
21. Vijayakumar, S.; Biswas, I.; Veeraraghavan, B. Accurate Identification of Clinically Important *Acinetobacter* spp.: An Update. *Future Sci. OA* **2019**, *5*, FSO395. [CrossRef]
22. La Scola, B.; Gundi, V.A.K.B.; Khamis, A.; Raoult, D. Sequencing of the RpoB Gene and Flanking Spacers for Molecular Identification of *Acinetobacter* Species. *J. Clin. Microbiol.* **2006**, *44*, 827–832. [CrossRef]
23. Lee, M.J.; Jang, S.J.; Li, X.M.; Park, G.; Kook, J.K.; Kim, M.J.; Chang, Y.H.; Shin, J.H.; Kim, S.H.; Kim, D.M.; et al. Comparison of RpoB Gene Sequencing, 16S RRNA Gene Sequencing, GyrB Multiplex PCR, and the VITEK2 System for Identification of *Acinetobacter* Clinical Isolates. *Diagn. Microbiol. Infect. Dis.* **2014**, *78*, 29–34. [CrossRef]
24. Turton, J.F.; Woodford, N.; Glover, J.; Yarde, S.; Kaufmann, M.E.; Pitt, T.L. Identification of *Acinetobacter baumannii* by Detection of the BlaOXA-51-like Carbapenemase Gene Intrinsic to This Species. *J. Clin. Microbiol.* **2006**, *44*, 2974. [CrossRef] [PubMed]
25. Cheng, K.; Chui, H.; Domish, L.; Hernandez, D.; Wang, G. Recent Development of Mass Spectrometry and Proteomics Applications in Identification and Typing of Bacteria. *Proteomics Clin. Appl.* **2016**, *10*, 346–357. [CrossRef]
26. Marí-Almirall, M.; Cosgaya, C.; Higgins, P.G.; Van Assche, A.; Telli, M.; Huys, G.; Lievens, B.; Seifert, H.; Dijkshoorn, L.; Roca, I.; et al. MALDI-TOF/MS Identification of Species from the *Acinetobacter baumannii* (Ab) Group Revisited: Inclusion of the Novel *A. seifertii* and *A. dijkshoorniae* Species. *Clin. Microbiol. Infect.* **2017**, *23*, e1–e210. [CrossRef]
27. Li, X.; Tang, Y.; Lu, X. Insight into Identification of *Acinetobacter* Species by Matrix-Assisted Laser Desorption/Ionization Time of Flight Mass Spectrometry (MALDI-TOF MS) in the Clinical Laboratory. *J. Am. Soc. Mass. Spectrom.* **2018**, *29*, 1546–1553. [CrossRef] [PubMed]
28. Hamidian, M.; Nigro, S.J. Emergence, Molecular Mechanisms and Global Spread of Carbapenem-Resistant *Acinetobacter baumannii*. *Microb. Genom.* **2019**, *5*, e000306. [CrossRef]
29. Li, P.; Yang, C.; Xie, J.; Liu, N.; Wang, H.; Zhang, L.; Wang, X.; Wang, Y.; Qiu, S.; Song, H. *Acinetobacter calcoaceticus* from a Fatal Case of Pneumonia Harboring BlaNDM-1 on a Widely Distributed Plasmid. *BMC Infect. Dis.* **2015**, *15*, 131. [CrossRef] [PubMed]
30. Rani, F.M.; Rahman, N.I.A.; Ismail, S.; Abdullah, F.H.; Othman, N.; Alattraqchi, A.G.; Cleary, D.W.; Clarke, S.C.; Yeo, C.C. Prevalence and Antimicrobial Susceptibilities of *Acinetobacter baumannii* and Non-*baumannii* Acinetobacters from Terengganu, Malaysia and Their Carriage of Carbapenemase Genes. *J. Med. Microbiol.* **2018**, *67*, 1538–1543. [CrossRef]
31. Lee, K.; Kim, M.N.; Choi, T.Y.; Cho, S.E.; Lee, S.; Whang, D.H.; Yong, D.; Chong, Y.; Woodford, N.; Livermore, D.M. Wide Dissemination of OXA-Type Carbapenemases in Clinical *Acinetobacter* spp. Isolates from South Korea. *Int. J. Antimicrob. Agents* **2009**, *33*, 520–524. [CrossRef]
32. Tietgen, M.; Kramer, J.S.; Brunst, S.; Djahanschiri, B.; Wohra, S.; Higgins, P.G.; Weidensdorfer, M.; Riedel-Christ, S.; Pos, K.M.; Gonzaga, A.; et al. Identification of the Novel Class D β-Lactamase OXA-679 Involved in Carbapenem Resistance in *Acinetobacter calcoaceticus*. *J. Antimicrob. Chemother.* **2019**, *74*, 1494–1502. [CrossRef]

33. Lasarte-Monterrubio, C.; Guijarro-Sánchez, P.; Bellés, A.; Vázquez-Ucha, J.C.; Arca-Suárez, J.; Fernández-Lozano, C.; Bou, G.; Beceiro, A. Carbapenem Resistance in *Acinetobacter nosocomialis* and *Acinetobacter junii* Conferred by Acquisition of BlaOXA-24/40 and Genetic Characterization of the Transmission Mechanism between *Acinetobacter* Genomic Species. *Microbiol. Spectr.* **2022**, *10*, e02734-21. [CrossRef]
34. Singkham-In, U.; Chatsuwan, T. Mechanisms of Carbapenem Resistance in *Acinetobacter pittii* and *Acinetobacter nosocomialis* Isolates from Thailand. *J. Med. Microbiol.* **2018**, *67*, 1667–1672. [CrossRef] [PubMed]
35. Mo, X.M.; Pan, Q.; Seifert, H.; Xing, X.W.; Yuan, J.; Zhou, Z.Y.; Luo, X.Y.; Liu, H.M.; Xie, Y.L.; Yang, L.Q.; et al. First Identification of Multidrug-Resistant *Acinetobacter bereziniae* Isolates Harboring BlaNDM-1 from Hospitals in South China. *Heliyon* **2023**, *9*, e12365. [CrossRef]
36. Tavares, L.C.B.; Cunha, M.P.V.; De Vasconcellos, F.M.; Bertani, A.M.D.J.; De Barcellos, T.A.F.; Bueno, M.S.; Santos, C.A.; Sant'Ana, D.A.; Ferreira, A.M.; Mondelli, A.L.; et al. Genomic and Clinical Characterization of IMP-1-Producing Multidrug-Resistant *Acinetobacter bereziniae* Isolates from Bloodstream Infections in a Brazilian Tertiary Hospital. *Microb. Drug Resist.* **2020**, *26*, 1399–1404. [CrossRef]
37. Cayô, R.; Rodrigues-Costa, F.; Matos, A.P.; Carvalhaes, C.G.; Dijkshoorn, L.; Gales, A.C. Old Clinical Isolates of *Acinetobacter seifertii* in Brazil Producing OXA-58. *Antimicrob. Agents Chemother.* **2016**, *60*, 2589. [CrossRef] [PubMed]
38. Montaña, S.; Palombarani, S.; Carulla, M.; Kunst, A.; Rodriguez, C.H.; Nastro, M.; Vay, C.; Ramirez, M.S.; Almuzara, M. First Case of Bacteraemia Due to *Acinetobacter schindleri* Harbouring BlaNDM-1 in an Immunocompromised Patient. *New Microbes New Infect.* **2018**, *21*, 28. [CrossRef]
39. Cayô, R.; Streling, A.P.; Nodari, C.S.; Matos, A.P.; De Paula Luz, A.; Dijkshoorn, L.; Pignatari, A.C.C.; Gales, A.C. Occurrence of IMP-1 in Non-*baumannii Acinetobacter* Clinical Isolates from Brazil. *J. Med. Microbiol.* **2018**, *67*, 628–630. [CrossRef]
40. Park, Y.K.; Jung, S.I.; Park, K.H.; Kim, S.H.; Ko, K.S. Characteristics of Carbapenem-Resistant *Acinetobacter* spp. Other than *Acinetobacter baumannii* in South Korea. *Int. J. Antimicrob. Agents* **2012**, *39*, 81–85. [CrossRef] [PubMed]
41. Cui, C.Y.; Chen, C.; Liu, B.T.; He, Q.; Wu, X.T.; Sun, R.Y.; Zhang, Y.; Cui, Z.H.; Guo, W.Y.; Jia, Q.L.; et al. Co-Occurrence of Plasmid-Mediated Tigecycline and Carbapenem Resistance in *Acinetobacter* spp. from Waterfowls and Their Neighboring Environment. *Antimicrob. Agents Chemother.* **2020**, *64*, 02502-19. [CrossRef]
42. Kimura, Y.; Harada, K.; Shimizu, T.; Sato, T.; Kajino, A.; Usui, M.; Tamura, Y.; Tsuyuki, Y.; Miyamoto, T.; Ohki, A.; et al. Species Distribution, Virulence Factors, and Antimicrobial Resistance of *Acinetobacter* spp. Isolates from Dogs and Cats: A Preliminary Study. *Microbiol. Immunol.* **2018**, *62*, 462–466. [CrossRef]
43. Baraka, A.; Traglia, G.M.; Montaña, S.; Tolmasky, M.E.; Ramirez, M.S. An *Acinetobacter* Non-*baumannii* Population Study: Antimicrobial Resistance Genes (ARGs). *Antibiotics* **2021**, *10*, 16. [CrossRef] [PubMed]
44. Nemec, A.; Radolfova-Krizova, L.; Maixnerova, M.; Vrestiakova, E.; Jezek, P.; Sedo, O. Taxonomy of Haemolytic and/or Proteolytic Strains of the Genus *Acinetobacter* with the Proposal of *Acinetobacter courvalinii* sp. nov. (Genomic Species 14 Sensu Bouvet & Jeanjean), *Acinetobacter dispersus* sp. nov. (Genomic Species 17), *Acinetobacter modestus* sp. nov., *Acinetobacter proteolyticus* sp. nov. and *Acinetobacter vivianii* sp. nov. *Int. J. Syst. Evol. Microbiol.* **2016**, *66*, 1673–1685. [CrossRef]
45. Dey, D.K.; Park, J.; Kang, S.C. Genotypic, Phenotypic, and Pathogenic Characterization of the Soil Isolated *Acinetobacter courvalinii*. *Microb. Pathog.* **2020**, *149*, 104287. [CrossRef]
46. Poirel, L.; Figueiredo, S.; Cattoir, V.; Carattoli, A.; Nordmann, P. *Acinetobacter* Radioresistens as a Silent Source of Carbapenem Resistance for *Acinetobacter* spp. *Antimicrob. Agents Chemother.* **2008**, *52*, 1252–1256. [CrossRef]
47. Kuzmenkov, A.Y.; Trushin, I.V.; Vinogradova, A.G.; Avramenko, A.A.; Sukhorukova, M.V.; Malhotra-Kumar, S.; Dekhnich, A.V.; Edelstein, M.V.; Kozlov, R.S. AMRmap: An Interactive Web Platform for Analysis of Antimicrobial Resistance Surveillance Data in Russia. *Front. Microbiol.* **2021**, *12*, 620002. [CrossRef]
48. Gkorezis, P.; Rineau, F.; Van Hamme, J.; Franzetti, A.; Daghio, M.; Thijs, S.; Weyens, N.; Vangronsveld, J. Draft Genome Sequence of Acinetobacter Oleivorans PF1, a Diesel-Degrading and Plant-Growth-Promoting Endophytic Strain Isolated from Poplar Trees Growing on a Diesel-Contaminated Plume. *Genome Announc.* **2015**, *3*, e01430-14. [CrossRef] [PubMed]
49. Deems, A.; Du Prey, M.; Dowd, S.E.; McLaughlin, R.W. Characterization of the Biodiesel Degrading *Acinetobacter oleivorans* Strain PT8 Isolated from the Fecal Material of a Painted Turtle (*Chrysemys picta*). *Curr. Microbiol.* **2021**, *78*, 522–527. [CrossRef] [PubMed]
50. Wang, P.; Wei, H.; Ke, T.; Fu, Y.; Zeng, Y.; Chen, C.; Chen, L. Characterization and Genome Analysis of *Acinetobacter oleivorans* S4 as an Efficient Hydrocarbon-Degrading and Plant-Growth-Promoting rhizobacterium. *Chemosphere* **2023**, *331*, 138732. [CrossRef]
51. Park, J.H.; Jang, Y.; Yoon, I.; Kim, T.S.; Park, H. Comparison of Autof Ms1000 and Bruker Biotyper MALDI-TOF MS Platforms for Routine Identification of Clinical Microorganisms. *Biomed. Res. Int.* **2021**, *2021*, 6667623. [CrossRef]
52. Kozlov, R.S.; Azizov, I.S.; Dekhnich, V.; Ivanchik, N.V.; Kuzmenkov, Y.; Martinovich; Mikotina, V.; Sukhorukova, V.; Trushin, I.V.; Edelstein, V. In Vitro Activity of Biapenem and Other Carbapenems against Russian Clinical Isolates of *Pseudomonas aeruginosa*, *Acinetobacter* spp., and *Enterobacterales*. *Klin. Mikrobiol. Antimikrobn. Himioter.* **2021**, *23*, 280–291. [CrossRef]
53. Shek, E.A.; Sukhorukova, M.V.; Edelstein, M.V.; Skleenova, E.Y.; Ivanchik, N.V.; Shajdullina, E.R.; Kuzmenkov, A.Y.; Dekhnich, A.V.; Kozlov, R.S.; Semyonova, N.V.; et al. Antimicrobial Resistance, Carbapenemase Production, and Genotypes of Nosocomial *Acinetobacter* spp. Isolates in Russia: Results of Multicenter Epidemiological Study "MARATHON 2015–2016". *Klin. Mikrobiol. Antimikrobn. Himioter.* **2019**, *21*, 171–180. [CrossRef]

54. Jayol, A.; Poirel, L.; Brink, A.; Villegas, M.V.; Yilmaz, M.; Nordmann, P. Resistance to Colistin Associated with a Single Amino Acid Change in Protein PmrB among *Klebsiella pneumoniae* Isolates of Worldwide Origin. *Antimicrob. Agents Chemother.* 2014, 58, 4762–4766. [CrossRef] [PubMed]
55. Brovedan, M.; Repizo, G.D.; Marchiaro, P.; Viale, A.M.; Limansky, A. Characterization of the Diverse Plasmid Pool Harbored by the BlaNDM-1-Containing *Acinetobacter bereziniae* HPC229 Clinical Strain. *PLoS ONE* 2019, 14, e0220584. [CrossRef]
56. Brovedan, M.; Marchiaro, P.M.; Morán-Barrio, J.; Revale, S.; Cameranesi, M.; Brambilla, L.; Viale, A.M.; Limansky, A.S. Draft Genome Sequence of *Acinetobacter bereziniae* HPC229, a Carbapenem-Resistant Clinical Strain from Argentina Harboring BlaNDM-1. *Genome Announc.* 2016, 4, 00117-16. [CrossRef]
57. Kamolvit, W.; Higgins, P.G.; Paterson, D.L.; Seifert, H. Multiplex PCR to Detect the Genes Encoding Naturally Occurring Oxacillinases in *Acinetobacter* spp. *J. Antimicrob. Chemother.* 2014, 69, 959–963. [CrossRef]
58. Marqué, S.; Poirel, L.; Héritier, C.; Brisse, S.; Blasco, M.D.; Filip, R.; Coman, G.; Naas, T.; Nordmann, P. Regional Occurrence of Plasmid-Mediated Carbapenem-Hydrolyzing Oxacillinase OXA-58 in *Acinetobacter* spp. in Europe. *J. Clin. Microbiol.* 2005, 43, 4885–4888. [CrossRef] [PubMed]
59. Coelho, J.; Woodford, N.; Afzal-Shah, M.; Livermore, D. Occurrence of OXA-58-like Carbapenemases in *Acinetobacter* spp. Collected over 10 Years in Three Continents. *Antimicrob. Agents Chemother.* 2006, 50, 756–758. [CrossRef]
60. Mendes, R.E.; Bell, J.M.; Turnidge, J.D.; Castanheira, M.; Deshpande, L.M.; Jones, R.N. Codetection of BlaOXA-23-like Gene (BlaOXA-133) and BlaOXA-58 in *Acinetobacter* Radioresistens: Report from the SENTRY Antimicrobial Surveillance Program. *Antimicrob. Agents Chemother.* 2009, 53, 843–844. [CrossRef]
61. Peleg, A.Y.; Franklin, C.; Walters, L.J.; Bell, J.M.; Spelman, D.W. OXA-58 and IMP-4 Carbapenem-Hydrolyzing Beta-Lactamases in an *Acinetobacter junii* Blood Culture Isolate from Australia. *Antimicrob. Agents Chemother.* 2006, 50, 399–400. [CrossRef]
62. Huang, L.Y.; Lu, P.L.; Chen, T.L.; Chang, F.Y.; Fung, C.P.; Siu, L.K. Molecular Characterization of Beta-Lactamase Genes and Their Genetic Structures in *Acinetobacter* Genospecies 3 Isolates in Taiwan. *Antimicrob. Agents Chemother.* 2010, 54, 2699–2703. [CrossRef]
63. Feng, Y.; Yang, P.; Wang, X.; Zong, Z. Characterization of *Acinetobacter johnsonii* Isolate XBB1 Carrying Nine Plasmids and Encoding NDM-1, OXA-58 and PER-1 by Genome Sequencing. *J. Antimicrob. Chemother.* 2016, 71, 71–75. [CrossRef] [PubMed]
64. Jiang, N.; Zhang, X.; Zhou, Y.; Zhang, Z.; Zheng, X. Whole-Genome Sequencing of an NDM-1- and OXA-58-Producing *Acinetobacter towneri* Isolate from Hospital Sewage in Sichuan Province, China. *J. Glob. Antimicrob. Resist.* 2019, 16, 4–5. [CrossRef] [PubMed]
65. Suzuki, Y.; Endo, S.; Nakano, R.; Nakano, A.; Saito, K.; Kakuta, R.; Kakuta, N.; Horiuchi, S.; Yano, H.; Kaku, M. Emergence of IMP-34- and OXA-58-Producing Carbapenem-Resistant *Acinetobacter colistiniresistens*. *Antimicrob. Agents Chemother.* 2019, 63, e02633-18. [CrossRef] [PubMed]
66. Hendrickx, A.P.A.; Schade, R.P.; Landman, F.; Bosch, T.; Schouls, L.M.; van Dijk, K. Comparative Analysis of IMP-4- and OXA-58-Containing Plasmids of Three Carbapenemase-Producing *Acinetobacter ursingii* Strains in the Netherlands. *J. Glob. Antimicrob. Resist.* 2022, 31, 207–211. [CrossRef] [PubMed]
67. Fávaro, L.D.S.; de Paula-Petroli, S.B.; Romanin, P.; Tavares, E.D.R.; Ribeiro, R.A.; Hungria, M.; de Oliveira, A.G.; Yamauchi, L.M.; Yamada-Ogatta, S.F.; Carrara-Marroni, F.E. Detection of OXA-58-Producing *Acinetobacter bereziniae* in Brazil. *J. Glob. Antimicrob. Resist.* 2019, 19, 53–55. [CrossRef]
68. Ang, G.Y.; Yu, C.Y.; Cheong, Y.M.; Yin, W.F.; Chan, K.G. Emergence of ST119 *Acinetobacter pittii* Co-Harbouring NDM-1 and OXA-58 in Malaysia. *Int. J. Antimicrob. Agents* 2016, 47, 168–169. [CrossRef]
69. Strateva, T.; Sirakov, I.; Savov, E.; Mitov, I. First Detection of an OXA-58 Carbapenemase-Producing *Acinetobacter nosocomialis* Clinical Isolate in the Balkan States. *J. Glob. Antimicrob. Resist.* 2018, 13, 123–124. [CrossRef]
70. Tognim, M.C.B.; Gales, A.C.; Penteado, A.P.; Silbert, S.; Sader, H.S. Dissemination of IMP-1 Metallo- Beta -Lactamase-Producing *Acinetobacter* Species in a Brazilian Teaching Hospital. *Infect. Control Hosp. Epidemiol.* 2006, 27, 742–747. [CrossRef]
71. Lee, K.; Kim, C.K.; Hong, S.G.; Choi, J.; Song, S.; Koh, E.; Yong, D.; Jeong, S.H.; Yum, J.H.; Docquier, J.D.; et al. Characteristics of Clinical Isolates of *Acinetobacter* Genomospecies 10 Carrying Two Different Metallo-Beta-Lactamases. *Int. J. Antimicrob. Agents* 2010, 36, 259–263. [CrossRef]
72. Hu, H.; Hu, Y.; Pan, Y.; Liang, H.; Wang, H.; Wang, X.; Hao, Q.; Yang, X.; Yang, X.; Xiao, X.; et al. Novel Plasmid and Its Variant Harboring Both a Bla(NDM-1) Gene and Type IV Secretion System in Clinical Isolates of *Acinetobacter lwoffii*. *Antimicrob. Agents Chemother.* 2012, 56, 1698–1702. [CrossRef] [PubMed]
73. Wang, Y.; Wu, C.; Zhang, Q.; Qi, J.; Liu, H.; Wang, Y.; He, T.; Ma, L.; Lai, J.; Shen, Z.; et al. Identification of New Delhi Metallo-β-Lactamase 1 in *Acinetobacter lwoffii* of Food Animal Origin. *PLoS ONE* 2012, 7, e37152. [CrossRef]
74. Yamamoto, M.; Nagao, M.; Matsumura, Y.; Hotta, G.; Matsushima, A.; Ito, Y.; Takakura, S.; Ichiyama, S. Regional Dissemination of *Acinetobacter* Species Harbouring Metallo-β-Lactamase Genes in Japan. *Clin. Microbiol. Infect.* 2013, 19, 729–736. [CrossRef]
75. Alattraqchi, A.G.; Mohd Rani, F.; Rahman, N.I.A.; Ismail, S.; Cleary, D.W.; Clarke, S.C.; Yeo, C.C. Complete Genome Sequencing of *Acinetobacter baumannii* AC1633 and *Acinetobacter nosocomialis* AC1530 Unveils a Large Multidrug-Resistant Plasmid Encoding the NDM-1 and OXA-58 Carbapenemases. *mSphere* 2021, 6, e01076-20. [CrossRef]
76. Chen, Y.; Guo, P.; Huang, H.; Huang, Y.; Wu, Z.; Liao, K. Detection of Co-Harboring OXA-58 and NDM-1 Carbapenemase Producing Genes Resided on a Same Plasmid from an *Acinetobacter pittii* Clinical Isolate in China. *Iran. J. Basic Med. Sci.* 2019, 22, 106–111. [CrossRef]

77. Cheikh, H.B.; Domingues, S.; Silveira, E.; Kadri, Y.; Rosário, N.; Mastouri, M.; Da Silva, G.J. Molecular Characterization of Carbapenemases of Clinical *Acinetobacter baumannii-calcoaceticus* Complex Isolates from a University Hospital in Tunisia. *3 Biotech.* **2018**, *8*, 297. [CrossRef]
78. Zhou, S.; Chen, X.; Meng, X.; Zhang, G.; Wang, J.; Zhou, D.; Guo, X. "Roar" of BlaNDM-1 and "Silence" of BlaOXA-58 Co-Exist in *Acinetobacter pittii*. *Sci. Rep.* **2015**, *5*, 8976. [CrossRef] [PubMed]
79. Wang, J.; Wang, H.; Cai, K.; Yu, P.; Liu, Y.; Zhao, G.; Chen, R.; Xu, R.; Yu, M. Evaluation of Three Sample Preparation Methods for the Identification of Clinical Strains by Using Two MALDI-TOF MS Systems. *J. Mass Spectrom.* **2021**, *56*, e4696. [CrossRef] [PubMed]
80. Clinical and Laboratory Standards Institute (CLSI). *Methods for the Identification of Cultured Microorganisms Using Matrix-Assisted Laser Desorption/Ionization Time-of-Flight Mass Spectrometry*, 1st ed.; CLSI supplement M58; CLSI: Wayne, PA, USA, 2017.
81. Diancourt, L.; Passet, V.; Nemec, A.; Dijkshoorn, L.; Brisse, S. The Population Structure of *Acinetobacter baumannii*: Expanding Multiresistant Clones from an Ancestral Susceptible Genetic Pool. *PLoS ONE* **2010**, *5*, e10034. [CrossRef]
82. Bartual, S.G.; Seifert, H.; Hippler, C.; Luzon, M.A.D.; Wisplinghoff, H.; Rodríguez-Valera, F. Development of a Multilocus Sequence Typing Scheme for Characterization of Clinical Isolates of *Acinetobacter baumannii*. *J. Clin. Microbiol.* **2005**, *43*, 4382. [CrossRef]
83. Gundi, V.A.K.B.; Dijkshoorn, L.; Burignat, S.; Raoult, D.; La Scola, B. Validation of Partial RpoB Gene Sequence Analysis for the Identification of Clinically Important and Emerging *Acinetobacter* Species. *Microbiology* **2009**, *155*, 2333–2341. [CrossRef]
84. Tamura, K.; Stecher, G.; Kumar, S. MEGA11: Molecular Evolutionary Genetics Analysis Version 11. *Mol. Biol. Evol.* **2021**, *38*, 3022–3027. [CrossRef] [PubMed]
85. Letunic, I.; Bork, P. Interactive Tree Of Life (ITOL) v5: An Online Tool for Phylogenetic Tree Display and Annotation. *Nucleic Acids Res.* **2021**, *49*, W293–W296. [CrossRef] [PubMed]
86. ISO 20776-1:2019; Susceptibility Testing of Infectious Agents and Evaluation of Performance of Antimicrobial Susceptibility Test Devices—Part 1: Broth Micro-Dilution Reference Method for Testing the In Vitro Activity of Antimicrobial Agents against Rapidly Growing Aerobic Bacteria Involved in Infectious Diseases. ISO: Geneva, Switzerland, 2019.
87. The European Committee on Antimicrobial Susceptibility Testing. EUCAST Reading Guide for Broth Microdilution v. 4.0. 2022. Available online: https://www.eucast.org/fileadmin/src/media/PDFs/EUCAST_files/Disk_test_documents/2022_manuals/Reading_guide_BMD_v_4.0_2022.pdf (accessed on 17 July 2023).
88. The European Committee on Antimicrobial Susceptibility Testing. Breakpoint Tables for Interpretation of MICs and Zone Diameters. Version 13.1. 2023. Available online: http://www.eucast.org (accessed on 17 July 2023).
89. Clinical and Laboratory Standards Institute (CLSI). *Performance Standards for Antimicrobial Susceptibility Testing*, 33rd ed.; CLSI supplement M100; CLSI: Wayne, PA, USA, 2023.
90. Argimón, S.; Abudahab, K.; Goater, R.J.E.; Fedosejev, A.; Bhai, J.; Glasner, C.; Feil, E.J.; Holden, M.T.G.; Yeats, C.A.; Grundmann, H.; et al. Microreact: Visualizing and Sharing Data for Genomic Epidemiology and Phylogeography. *Microb. Genom.* **2016**, *2*, e000093. [CrossRef] [PubMed]

**Disclaimer/Publisher's Note:** The statements, opinions and data contained in all publications are solely those of the individual author(s) and contributor(s) and not of MDPI and/or the editor(s). MDPI and/or the editor(s) disclaim responsibility for any injury to people or property resulting from any ideas, methods, instructions or products referred to in the content.

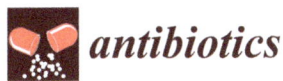

Article

# Cracking the Code: Unveiling the Diversity of Carbapenem-Resistant *Klebsiella pneumoniae* Clones in the Arabian Peninsula through Genomic Surveillance

Amani H Al Fadhli [1,*], Shaimaa F. Mouftah [2,3], Wafaa Y. Jamal [4], Vincent O. Rotimi [5] and Akela Ghazawi [2,*]

1. Laboratory Sciences, Department of Medical, Faculty of Allied Health Sciences, Health Sciences Center (HSC), Kuwait University, Jabriya 24923, Kuwait
2. Department of Medical Microbiology and Immunology, College of Medicine and Health Sciences, United Arab Emirates University, Al Ain 15551, United Arab Emirates; 201590053@uaeu.ac.ae
3. Department of Biomedical Sciences, University of Science and Technology, Zewail City of Science and Technology, Giza 12578, Egypt
4. Department of Microbiology, College of Medicine, Kuwait University, Jabriya 24923, Kuwait; wafaa.jamal@ku.edu.kw
5. Center for Infection Control and Patient Safety, College of Medicine University of Lagos, Idi-Araba 102215, Nigeria; bunmivr@yahoo.com
* Correspondence: amani@ku.edu.kw (A.H.A.F.); akelag@uaeu.ac.ae (A.G.)

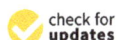

**Citation:** Al Fadhli, A.H.; Mouftah, S.F.; Jamal, W.Y.; Rotimi, V.O.; Ghazawi, A. Cracking the Code: Unveiling the Diversity of Carbapenem-Resistant *Klebsiella pneumoniae* Clones in the Arabian Peninsula through Genomic Surveillance. *Antibiotics* **2023**, *12*, 1081. https://doi.org/10.3390/antibiotics12071081

Academic Editor: Andrey Shelenkov

Received: 14 May 2023
Revised: 11 June 2023
Accepted: 14 June 2023
Published: 21 June 2023

**Copyright:** © 2023 by the authors. Licensee MDPI, Basel, Switzerland. This article is an open access article distributed under the terms and conditions of the Creative Commons Attribution (CC BY) license (https://creativecommons.org/licenses/by/4.0/).

**Abstract:** The rise of antimicrobial resistance is a global challenge that requires a coordinated effort to address. In this study, we examined the genetic similarity of carbapenem-resistant *Klebsiella pneumoniae* (CRKP) in countries belonging to the Gulf Cooperation Council (GCC) to gain a better understanding of how these bacteria are spreading and evolving in the region. We used in silico genomic tools to investigate the occurrence and prevalence of different types of carbapenemases and their relationship to specific sequence types (STs) of CRKP commonly found in the region. We analyzed 720 publicly available genomes of multi-drug resistant *K. pneumoniae* isolates collected from six GCC countries between 2011 and 2020. Our findings showed that ST-14 and ST-231 were the most common STs, and 51.7% of the isolates carried $bla_{OXA-48-like}$ genes. Additionally, we identified rare carbapenemase genes in a small number of isolates. We observed a clonal outbreak of ST-231 in Oman, and four Saudi isolates were found to have colistin resistance genes. Our study offers a comprehensive overview of the genetic diversity and resistance mechanisms of CRKP isolates in the GCC region that could aid in developing targeted interventions to combat this pressing global issue.

**Keywords:** genomic surveillance; CRKP; clone divergence; Arabian Peninsula

## 1. Introduction

Antimicrobial resistance is a growing serious threat to human health and projected to reach an all-time high by 2050, resulting in millions of deaths and a massive economic burden [1,2]. Enterobacterales, including *Klebsiella pneumoniae*, are opportunistic pathogens responsible for many hospital-acquired infections [3]. Their broad spectrum of diseases and increasing resistance to antibiotics account for almost one-third of infections caused by Gram-negative bacteria. [3,4]. Resistance to carbapenems, the last resort class of antibiotics, is a major concern, especially in *K. pneumoniae* [5]. Studies suggest that the mortality rate associated with carbapenem-resistant *K. pneumoniae* (CRKP) may exceed 75% depending on factors such as age and disease profile [1,6]. The production of enzymes by genes that mediate different mechanisms of resistance in CRKP isolates effectively degrades carbapenems, rendering the bacteria non-susceptible [7]. *Klebsiella pneumoniae* carbapenemase (KPC), located on self-conjugative plasmids, is the most problematic class A carbapenemase due to its ability to spread widely [8]. The most common KPC enzyme alleles are KPC-2 and KPC-3 that are distributed globally [7,9]. Class B carbapenemases, metallo-β-lactamases

(MBLs), are the second most significant enzymes in CRKP and can hydrolyze almost all β-lactam antibiotics, including carbapenems [10,11]. The most prevalent MBLs are IMP, VIM, NDM, GIM, and SIM which are located on genetic mobile elements that can transfer between bacteria. VIM and NDM are the most common globally, including in the Gulf [7,12]. NDM-1 is highly transferrable and can hydrolyze all β-lactams except aztreonam. It is primarily found in India [13]. VIM has more than 24 allelic variations in over 60 species [14]. Class D β-lactamases, such as the OXA-48-like enzyme, are commonly present in the Enterobacterales family and have significantly contributed to the rise of carbapenem resistance in the past decade [15]. The most significant reservoirs of these enzymes are India, the Middle East, and North African countries [16]. OXA-48 variants, including OXA-48, OXA-181, OXA-232, OXA-204, OXA-162, OXA-163, and OXA-244 have been identified [17].

CRKP is a major concern in the Gulf region, with specific clonal lineages identified, including the famous CC258 clone (ST258, ST11, ST340, ST437, and ST512) and other clones such as CG14/15, CG17/20, CG29, CG37, CG43, CG101, CG147, CG152, CG231, CG307, and CG490 [18]. However, the mechanisms of resistance and locally prevalent clones have only been explored through small-scale, local research. Studies such as [12,19–30] have contributed to our understanding of CRKP in the Gulf region. These studies have provided important information about the prevalence of specific clones and their resistance mechanisms in the region. However, larger-scale studies are needed to fully understand the impact of CRKP in the Gulf region and to develop effective prevention and treatment strategies.

Previous studies on the mechanisms of antimicrobial resistance (AMR) have focused on identifying only a few genes or mutations, while whole-genome sequencing (WGS) technology has improved the identification of various genetic bases of phenotypic variation, including point mutation, mobile genetic elements, and chromosomally encoded factors that contribute to the development of resistance, particularly to multiple antibiotics, leading to the emergence of MDR pathogens [31]. WGS data also allow identification of the evolutionary histories of homogeneous clusters using single nucleotide polymorphisms (SNPs) and the upscaling of multilocus sequence typing (MLST) perception using core genome MLST (cgMLST) analysis that provides better resolution and serves as the foundation for a universally curated nomenclature scheme accessible via various databases, enabling local and global epidemiological investigations [32,33].

To gain a better understanding of the genetic makeup of CRKP in the Gulf region, we employed cutting-edge techniques such as whole-genome sequencing and cgMLST analysis. Our investigation involved a comprehensive analysis of publicly available CRKP genomes that allowed us to identify the prevalence of various types of carbapenemases and their relationship with different sequence types (STs). By leveraging the power of in silico analysis, we were able to decipher the genetic relatedness of CRKP isolates in the Gulf Cooperation Council Countries region (GCCC) and gain insights into their evolution and spread. Our findings could pave the road to develop effective strategies to tackle the threat of CRKP and other multi-drug resistant pathogens in the GCCC and beyond.

## 2. Results

*2.1. Prevalence and Distribution of Carbapenem-Resistant K. pneumoniae Sequence Types (STs)*

As shown in Table 1, ST-14 represented 14.58% (105 out of 720) of the total isolates collected across all participant countries. The prevalence rates of ST-14 in the individual countries were UAE ($n$ = 54, 7.5%), Saudi Arabia ($n$ = 43, 6.0%), Qatar ($n$ = 4, 0.6%), Oman (3, 0.4%), and Bahrain ($n$ = 1, 0.1%). Of the 105 ST-14 isolates, 80% (84) carried at least one common carbapenemase gene. ST-231 was the second most common, accounting for 12.6% (91) of the total isolates. Amongst these 91 isolates, 74.7% (68) were found in Oman, 9.9% (9) in UAE, 8.8% (8) in Kuwait, and 6.6% (6) in Qatar (Table 1). Interestingly, ST-231 was absent in the Saudi Arabia collection. Moreover, various carbapenemase genes were detected among many isolates of this ST (73.6%; 67 out of 91) as shown in Table 1.

Table 1. Characterization of 720 *K. pneumoniae* isolates with the most abundant STs across the six Gulf countries.

| Country | Total Number (n) | Carbapenemase Genes | | | | | | | Sequence Types (ST) | | | | | | | | | |
|---|---|---|---|---|---|---|---|---|---|---|---|---|---|---|---|---|---|---|
| | | NDM | KPC | OXA | IMP | VIM | Dual | None | ST 101 | ST 11 | ST 14 | ST 147 | ST 15 | ST 2096 | ST 231 | ST 307 | ST 45 | ST 48 |
| UAE | 98 | 27 | 6 | 30 | 0 | 0 | 21 | 14 | 0 | 6 | 54 | 10 | 7 | 0 | 9 | 0 | 0 | 1 |
| Saudi | 230 | 21 | 1 | 130 | 0 | 2 | 17 | 59 | 15 | 3 | 43 | 8 | 4 | 98 | 0 | 8 | 6 | 7 |
| Qatar | 164 | 38 | 4 | 27 | 0 | 0 | 10 | 85 | 2 | 5 | 4 | 14 | 2 | 2 | 6 | 8 | 6 | 2 |
| Oman | 212 | 77 | 0 | 76 | 0 | 0 | 21 | 38 | 8 | 62 | 3 | 37 | 10 | 0 | 68 | 2 | 0 | 0 |
| Kuwait | 15 | 2 | 0 | 3 | 0 | 0 | 1 | 9 | 0 | 0 | 0 | 0 | 2 | 0 | 8 | 0 | 0 | 0 |
| Bahrain | 1 | 0 | 0 | 1 | 0 | 0 | 0 | 0 | 0 | 0 | 1 | 0 | 0 | 0 | 0 | 0 | 0 | 0 |
| Total | 720 | 165 | 11 | 266 | 0 | 2 | 70 | 206 | 25 | 76 | 105 | 69 | 25 | 100 | 91 | 18 | 12 | 10 |
| CRKp % | 71% (514/720) | 32% (165/514) | 2% (11/514) | 51.7% (266/514) | 0 | 0.38% (2/514) | 13.6% (70/514) | 28.6% (206/720) | 88% (22/25) | 94.7% (72/76) | 80% (84/105) | 84% (58/69) | 84% (21/25) | 87% (87/100) | 73.6% (67/91) | 38.8% (7/18) | 50% (6/12) | 40% (4/10) |

The subsequent frequently occurring ST was ST-2096, which accounted for 13.9% (100). Almost all these ST-2096 isolates (98%) were exclusively found in Saudi Arabia, specifically 98 out of 230 (42.6%) isolates from Saudi Arabia collection (Table 1). This ST was not detected in any other countries, except Qatar where only two (0.9%) isolates were identified. The carbapenemase genes of this lineage detected have only been found in Saudi Arabia where 87 (88.7%) of the isolates carried these resistance genes. The two isolates from Qatar did not contain any carbapenemase genes.

Out of the 720 ST identified, 76 (10.6%) belonged to the global epidemic clone ST-11. This clone was mainly identified in Oman (81%; $n = 62$), followed by UAE (7.8%; $n = 6$) and Qatar (6.5%; $n = 5$), with only three isolates detected in Saudi Arabia (3.9%; $n = 3$) (Table 1). The majority of these ST-11 isolates, 72 out of 76 (94.7%), produced carbapenemases as shown in Table 1.

Some of the STs such as ST-15, ST-101, ST-307 and ST-48 were detected in low proportions among the collections from each of the GCC states. ST-15 accounted for 25 (3.5%) of the total isolates and was found in five out of the six Gulf countries investigated (Oman, $n = 10$; Kuwait, $n = 2$; Saudi Arabia, $n = 4$; UAE, $n = 7$; Qatar, $n = 2$), with the majority, 21 out of 25 (84%), of these isolates carrying carbapenemase genes (Table 1). ST-101, on the other hand, was associated with only three out of the six countries studied (Saudi Arabia, $n = 15$; Oman, $n = 8$; Qatar, $n = 2$) (Table 1). ST-101 carbapenemase producers (88%; 22 out of 25) were found only in isolates from Saudi Arabia ($n = 14$) and Oman ($n = 8$). Similarly, ST-307 ($n = 18$) was observed in the same three countries (Saudi Arabia, $n = 8$; Qatar, $n = 8$; Oman, $n = 2$) (Table 1). ST-48 ($n = 10$) was identified in three countries (Saudi Arabia, $n = 7$; UAE, $n = 1$; Qatar, $n = 2$), while ST-45 was equally identified in only two countries (i.e., Saudi ($n = 6$) and Qatar ($n = 6$)) (Table 1).

### 2.2. Resistome Characterization of Carbapenem-Resistant K. pneumoniae Isolates

Carbapenem resistance genes were detected in 514 out of 720 (71.3%) of isolates (Table 2) and out of which 266 (51.7%) carried various alleles of $bla_{OXA}$ genes alone and 159 (31%) carried $bla_{NDM-1}$. A total of 11% (57/514) of isolates co-produced $bla_{NDM-1}$ and multiple alleles of $bla_{OXA}$. A small number of 12 (2%) co-produced $bla_{NDM-5}$ and different alleles of $bla_{OXA}$. Rare carbapenemase genes found in this study were $bla_{KPC-2}$ ($n = 10$), $bla_{NDM-5}$ ($n = 5$), $bla_{KPC-2}$ in combination with $bla_{OXA232}$ ($n = 1$), $bla_{KPC-3}$ ($n = 1$), $bla_{NDM-7}$ ($n = 1$), and $bla_{VIM-29}$ ($n = 2$), with the latter found exclusively in Saudi Arabia.

### 2.3. Mobile Colistin Resistance Elements (mcr)

Only four isolates from Saudi Arabia, belonging to ST-2096 (one isolate), ST-14 (one isolate), and ST-3513 (two isolates), were found to contain the mcr and/or mcr-8 genes that conferred colistin resistance. The ST-14 isolate also carried a $bla_{NDM-1}$ carbapenemase gene.

### 2.4. Clonal Clustering and Relatedness of the CRKP Isolates

cgMLST analysis was performed on isolates of the most abundant STs carrying at least one carbapenemase gene. The results indicated a clonal spread of certain STs within the same country or across the Arabian Peninsula. For instance, 72 out of 76 ST-11 isolates were carbapenemase producers, and five clusters and six singletons were identified. All clusters were made up of isolates from the same country. Cluster 1 consisted of 54 isolates (from Oman with less than 10 allele differences and KL14 as the dominant capsular type) (Figure 1). The majority of these isolates ($n = 21$) carried the $bla_{NDM-1}$ gene, and nine had both $bla_{NDM-1}$ and $bla_{OXA-232}$ genes and clustered with one isolate with $bla_{OXA-232}$, indicating clonal spread. Cluster 2 includes isolates from UAE with different carbapenemase genes and the same capsular type KL24. Other capsular and O antigen types were also present.

**Table 2.** Carbapenem resistance genes identified among the 514 CRKP isolates across the Arabian Peninsula.

| Carbapenem Resistance Genes | Total Isolates (n) | Percentage (%) |
|---|---|---|
| KPC-2 | 10 | 1.94 |
| KPC-2/OXA-232 | 1 | 0.19 |
| KPC-3 | 1 | 0.19 |
| NDM-1 | 159 | 30.93 |
| NDM-1/OXA-162 | 4 | 0.77 |
| NDM-1/OXA-181 | 1 | 0.19 |
| NDM-1/OXA-232 | 31 | 6.03 |
| NDM-1/OXA-48 | 21 | 4.08 |
| NDM-5 | 5 | 0.97 |
| NDM-5/OXA-181 | 3 | 0.58 |
| NDM-5/OXA-232 | 6 | 1.16 |
| NDM-5/OXA-48 | 3 | 0.58 |
| NDM-7 | 1 | 0.19 |
| OXA-162 | 5 | 0.97 |
| OXA-181 | 19 | 3.69 |
| OXA-232 | 143 | 27.82 |
| OXA-48 | 99 | 19.26 |
| VIM-29 | 2 | 0.38 |

*2.5. Clusters and Singletons Associated with ST-14 and ST-147*

cgMLST analysis of 84 ST-14 carbapenemase producers revealed six clusters and eight singletons associated with ten different types of carbapenemase genes as shown in Figure 2. Most clusters contained isolates from the same country, with Cluster 1 being the largest (31.3%) and all from Saudi Arabia. Within this cluster, 10 isolates had $bla_{NDM-1}$ and KL2; KL64 was the most common capsular type (Figure 2; Table 3). Cluster 2 contained isolates from UAE, Qatar, and Bahrain with different carbapenemase genes, while Cluster 3 had isolates from UAE and Oman. These findings suggest a clonal spread of this lineage with a high capability of acquiring different resistance genes and disseminating across different geographic locations.

cgMLST analysis of 58 ST-147 isolates found four clusters and 14 singletons, with eight different types of carbapenemase genes present. KL64 capsular type and O2a antigen were most common (Table 3). Cluster 1 and 2 had the most MST nodes, with isolates from different countries. The most frequent genes identified were $bla_{NDM-1}$ in Cluster 1 and $bla_{NDM-5}$ and/or $bla_{OXA-181}$ in Cluster 2. Singletons from different locations were closely related with less than 45 allele differences, indicating a clonal expansion of this clone

*2.6. Outbreaks Associated with ST-231 and ST-2096 CRKP*

ST-231 isolates were found to be predominantly from Oman, with only a few from Kuwait, and all carried the $bla_{OXA-232}$ gene. These isolates had the KL51 capsular type and O1 antigen (Table 3, Figure 3). ST-231 was found to be able to accommodate various carbapenem resistance genes as seen in Clusters 2 and 3, which contained isolates from different origins carrying different genes (Figure 3). Similarly, a clonal outbreak of ST-2096 CRKP was observed in Saudi Arabia in 2018, with most isolates having the KL64 capsular type and O1 antigen carrying either $bla_{OXA-48}$ or $bla_{OXA-232}$ genes. Cluster 1 contained the majority of isolates and had 67 MST nodes, with 19 carrying $bla_{OXA-48}$ and 61 carrying $bla_{OXA-232}$ (Table 3).

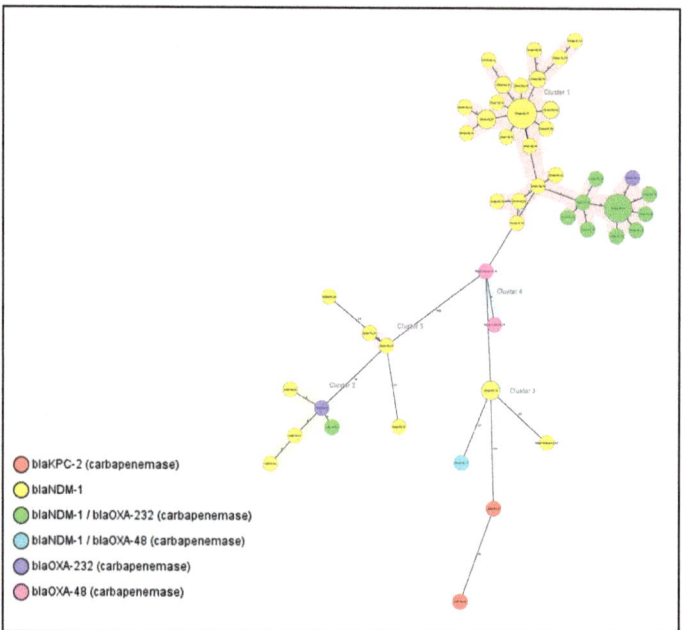

**Figure 1.** Minimum spanning tree (MST) of the 72 carbapenemase producers, ST-11 isolates. Distance based on the number of differences of the 2358 alleles in *K. pneumoniae* sensu-lato cgMLST. MST cluster distance threshold set at 15. Nodes labelled by column: Country of isolation and capsular type. Nodes colored by column: Carbapenem resistance gene.

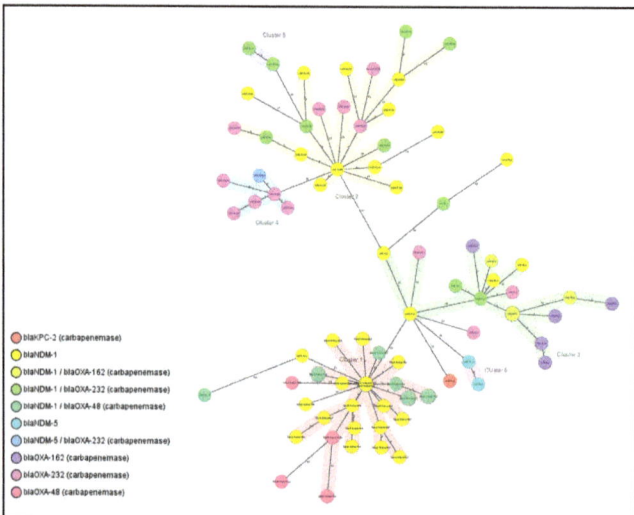

**Figure 2.** Minimum spanning tree (MST) of the 84 isolates (ST-14 carbapenemase producers). Distance based on the number of differences of the 2358 alleles in *K. pneumoniae* sensu-lato cgMLST. MST Cluster distance threshold set at 15. Nodes labelled by column: Country of isolation and capsular type. Nodes colored by column: Carbapenem resistance gene.

Table 3. Prevalence of capsular type (K locus) and O antigens among major clones of the whole isolate collections.

|  |  | ST-14 | ST-231 | ST-2096 | ST-11 | ST-147 | ST-15 | ST-101 | ST-45 |
|---|---|---|---|---|---|---|---|---|---|
| Capsular type | KL5 | 1% | -- | -- | -- | -- | -- | -- | -- |
|  | KL2 | 61% | -- | -- | -- | -- | 4% | -- | -- |
|  | KL10 | -- | -- | -- | -- | 4% | -- | -- | -- |
|  | KL14 | -- | -- | -- | 76% | -- | -- | -- | -- |
|  | KL15 | -- | -- | -- | 8% | -- | -- | -- | -- |
|  | KL16 | 1% | -- | -- | -- | -- | -- | -- | -- |
|  | KL17 | -- | -- | -- | -- | -- | -- | 88% | -- |
|  | KL19 | -- | -- | -- | -- | -- | 24% | -- | -- |
|  | KL24 | -- | -- | -- | 12% | -- | 20% | -- | 8% |
|  | KL43 | -- | -- | -- | -- | -- | -- | -- | 50% |
|  | KL47 | -- | -- | -- | 1% | -- | -- | -- | -- |
|  | KL48 | -- | -- | -- | -- | -- | 24% | -- | -- |
|  | KL50 | 1% | -- | 2% | -- | -- | -- | -- | -- |
|  | KL51 | -- | 100% | -- | -- | -- | -- | -- | -- |
|  | KL52 | -- | -- | -- | -- | -- | -- | -- | 8% |
|  | KL64 | 30% | -- | 93% | 1% | 94% | 4% | 4% |  |
|  | KL102 | -- | -- |  |  |  | 4% |  | 8% |
|  | KL107 | -- | -- | 4% | 1% | 1% | -- | 4% | 8% |
|  | KL112 | -- | -- | -- | -- | -- | 16% | -- | -- |
|  | KL127 | -- | -- | -- | -- | -- | -- | -- | 8% |
|  | KL135 | 1% | -- | -- | -- | -- | -- | -- | -- |
|  | KL166 | -- | -- | 1% | -- | -- | 4% | -- | -- |
| O antigen | O1 | 85% | 99% | 96% | -- | -- | 92% | 92% | -- |
|  | O2a | 10% | 1% | 3% | 13% | 91% | 4% | 4% | 67% |
|  | O3 | 1% | -- | -- | 41% | 4% | 4% | -- | 8% |
|  | O4 | -- | -- | -- | 8% | -- | -- | -- |  |
|  | OL101 | -- | -- | -- | 1% | -- | -- | -- | 25% |
|  | OL102 | -- | -- | 1% | 1% | 3% | -- | -- | -- |
|  | OL104 | -- | -- | -- | 36% | -- | -- | -- | -- |

### 2.7. Clustering of Isolates among ST-15, ST-101, and ST-45 Lineages

In the ST-15 and CR-Kp-ST-101 lineages, carbapenemase producer isolates were grouped into clusters and singletons. Most isolates were from the same country except for Cluster 1. ST-15's Cluster 1 included isolates from UAE and Kuwait with the $bla_{NDM-1}$ gene, while ST-101's Cluster 1 had isolates from Saudi Arabia and Oman with the $bla_{OXA-48}$ gene. Different carbapenemase gene combinations were identified within each lineage. O1 was the predominant O antigen in ST-15 isolates, while KL17 capsular type and O1 antigen were common in ST-101 isolates. ST-45 was associated with $bla_{OXA-48}$ and only two capsular types (KL43 and KL102) and one O antigen type (O2a) (Table 3).

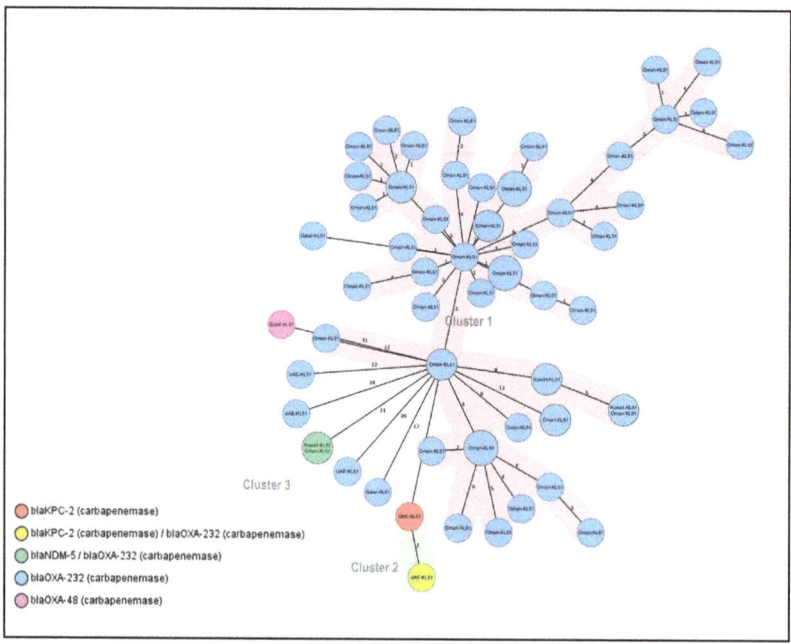

**Figure 3.** Minimum spanning tree (MST) of the 67 isolates (ST-231 carbapenemase producers). Distance based on the number of differences of the 2358 alleles in *K. pneumoniae* sensu-lato cgMLST. MST Cluster distance threshold set at 15. Nodes labelled by column: Country of isolation and capsular type. Nodes colored by column: Carbapenem resistance gene.

## 3. Discussion

This study marks a cutting-edge initiative to investigate the genomic epidemiology of CRKP in the GCC countries. The findings revealed a dangerous clan that possesses both hyper-virulent and drug-resistant traits (specific STs and capsular types). Given the widespread distribution of these clones, they pose a significant public health risk [34]. Therefore, genetic epidemiology data from this study can provide insights into the evolution and complexity of these clones. Notably, the study identified that most of the isolates belonged to the ST14 clone, which has been previously recognized as a global threat [17,35].

The OXA-48-like carbapenemases are well known for causing outbreaks that affect specific sequence types, including ST14. Recently, Mouftah and colleagues (2021) reported the prevalence of this clone along with its associated clonal transmission and potential for horizontal gene transfer among isolates from 13 hospitals in the United Arab Emirates, Bahrain, and Saudi Arabia [36]. This clone has been detected in various regions globally, including Europe, the Mediterranean, China, North America, Oceania, and South Africa [17,35]. Several studies have also identified ST14 as one of the most common sequence types of NDM-1-producing *K. pneumoniae* (NPKP) [37–39]. It seems that our findings have been further substantiated as it appears that most of our isolates carried the NDM-1 and OXA-48 carbapenemase genes. Moreover, *K. pneumoniae* ST14 from the Arabian Peninsula also exhibited specific traits, such as the KL64 capsular locus and O1 antigens [36]. Alarmingly, an apparent outbreak of this clone in UAE with dominance of Hv capsular KL2 and KL64 has been identified based on cgMLST analysis [40,41]. In a related occurrence, an outbreak that initially took place in Saudi Arabia spread to Qatar with the dominance of KL2. Given that this clone has demonstrated an ability to carry multiple types of carbapenemase genes, it is clear that this Hv clone is becoming increasingly dominant and thus requires strict monitoring measures.

It is interesting to note that in our study, despite ST231 being the most common sequence type reported in previous cases of $bla_{OXA-232}$-harboring *K. pneumoniae* [42], ST231 was in fact the second most prevalent sequence type. Additionally, we observed a higher occurrence of ST231 in Oman, which is not commonly seen in other countries in the region. Through our cgMLST analysis, we were able to identify an outbreak of this clone in Oman that had not been previously documented. Despite being located in different regions, this lineage has been strongly associated with locus type KL51 while carrying various carbapenemase genes as reported in other studies [43–45]. A recent study conducted in India also revealed a strong correlation between KL51 and ST231 in the phylogenetic tree of 307 isolates [46].

Our study revealed that a significant proportion of the *K. pneumoniae* isolates from Saudi Arabia were highly virulent (capsular serotype KL64) [40,41] and resistant, with the clonal complex 14 dominant sequence type being ST2096. These findings align with a previous analysis of *K. pneumoniae* where an analysis of *K. pneumoniae* dissemination and transmission patterns identified a two-year outbreak of ST2096 beginning in December 2016 [47]. Additionally, we discovered that the epidemic clone ST11 was present in four out of six GCC countries, posing a significant threat to human health due to its carbapenem-resistant and highly transmissibility [48]. Recently, five CRKP isolates from the Oman outbreak were confirmed to belong to ST11 clones and were closely related to Chinese isolates from the Bigsdb (Bacterial Isolate Genome Sequence Database) [49]. Studies on ST diversification have yielded conflicting results, but most countries have prioritized monitoring the occurrences of ST11, ST15, and ST14 [50]. Notably, ST11 and ST14 were the most commonly reported STs in Asia, Europe, America, Africa, and Oceania, with ST11 being a common type in many studies [51–53]. Essentially, this means that the clone has the impressive power to gather diverse resistance genes as it spreads. In addition, scrutinizing the capsular locus divulged that all ST11 *K. pneumoniae* had unique K types including KL64. These discoveries align with prior research conducted in China where a thorough examination of 364 ST-11 isolates was carried out and published by Liu et al., 2022 [54].

The most common carbapenemases found in this collection were NDM and OXA-48-like enzymes, which are commonly found in CRE from the Arabian Peninsula, according to studies conducted by Jamal et al., 2016; Sonnevend et al., 2015; and Memish et al., 2015 [12,23,26]. The Arabian Peninsula and the Indian subcontinent have close socioeconomic interactions, resulting in similar resistance patterns. ST11 and ST258 strains, which are typically found in China and the US, are prevalent in both regions with a low incidence of KPC enzymes. However, KPC was detected in this collection, specifically in the ST15 clones rather than ST11 clones, as reported by Boyd et al., 2020 [55]. To our surprise, our ST101 isolate possessed the carbapenemase gene $bla_{VIM-29}$, and this finding is significant as this clone has never been documented as producing VIM-29 before.

Our study revealed an intriguing aspect: the detection of $bla_{KPC-3}$ exclusively among the ST258 clones from Qatar isolates. While KPC was previously rare in the Arabian Peninsula, a small number of isolates associated with recent medical care abroad were found to carry the gene according to Abid et al., 2021 [56]. These findings have significant regional and global implications, given Qatar's demographics and its status as a major international travel hub. Although KPC is prevalent overseas, its emergence in the region requires attention due to its potent hydrolytic action and potential for dissemination.

Our findings indicate that only isolates from Saudi Arabia contain mobile colistin resistance elements (*mcr*). A recent study on the prevalence and molecular epidemiology of colistin-resistant Gram-negative bacilli (GNB) in Saudi Arabia revealed that while colistin still works well against GNB isolates locally, high levels of colistin resistance have been detected among major GNB such as *K. pneumoniae* [57]. Local data suggest that religious gatherings play a crucial role in triggering the acquisition of colistin resistance, and underscoring the importance of screening for colistin resistance determinants to prevent the spread of colistin-resistant GNB. Due to the absence of the most effective broad-spectrum antimicrobial agents, it is anticipated that colistin resistance will become more widespread shortly. Furthermore, mutations in the *mgrB* gene and insertion sequence transpositions were the most common mechanisms of colistin resistance among *K. pneumoniae* in the Middle East as well as in other regions [27,57].

Our analysis using cgMLST analysis showed that the most prevalent capsular type among *K. pneumoniae* was KL2, belonging to the ST14 clonal lineage. This finding is worrisome as this clonal lineage is associated with severe infections such as septicemia, pyogenic liver abscess syndrome, and pneumonia [58,59]. It has been suggested that both virulence and drug resistance are important for the pathogenesis of *K. pneumoniae* infections [60,61]. In hospital and community environments, *K. pneumoniae* clonal lineages have varying abilities to acquire resistance and virulence genes [62]. Therefore, it is crucial to have genomic surveillance in close geographic areas to understand the local epidemiology of *K. pneumoniae* infections in the Arabian Peninsula. Our cgMLST analysis also revealed distinct differences in the dominant high-risk STs of *K. pneumoniae* circulating in the GCC countries, with ST-11 being more prevalent in Oman, ST-14 in Saudi Arabia and the UAE, ST-147 in Qatar, Oman, and the UAE, and ST231 in Oman and Kuwait. Our study reveals that ST231 strains of *Klebsiella* had the highest presence of capsule genes/loci with KL51 being the most prevalent type [63]. On the other hand, the ST101 isolates of *K. pneumoniae* had KL17 capsular type and O1 antigen, which is consistent with previous reports linking pandemic ST101 with variants of KL17 and O1v1 [64]. Notably, the O1 antigen has been strongly linked to the virulence of *K. pneumoniae* in causing pyogenic liver abscesses [65].

Our study revealed a wide distribution of high-risk STs (ST-11, ST-14, ST-147, and ST-15) across each country in the region, which is consistent with previous observations [62,66]. These STs are prevalent in Asian countries, particularly India and the Philippines [67], which have a high percentage of workers in the Gulf region, suggesting that there may be multiple origins for the circulating lineages. The emergence of these high-risk clones may involve a complex phenomenon, including international transfer of successful clones and local dissemination of genetically flexible clones. Our cgMLST analysis revealed an association between some clones (ST-11, ST-14, ST-147, and ST-15) and carbapenemase genes (NDM-1), resulting in regional and local accessory gene sharing. Furthermore, the sharing of accessory genes within a local gene pool is increasing. These findings suggest that high-risk lineages are co-circulating and may have followed divergent evolutionary paths.

## 4. Materials and Methods

Demographic data. The population of the GCCC is one of the highest growing populations in the world owing primarily to immigration. The GCCC region includes six countries: (https://worldpopulationreview.com/country-rankings/gulf-countries (accessed on 20 January 2022).

Selection of bacterial isolates and data collection. Publicly available raw sequence reads of 720 MDR *K. pneumoniae* isolates were downloaded from the European Nucleotide Archives (ENA) ENA Browser (ebi.ac.uk) (accessed on 20 January 2022). All isolates were of clinical origin, collected between 2011 and 2020, and reported from the six GCCC, namely, Saudi Arabia, $n$ = 230; Oman, $n$ = 212; Qatar, $n$ = 164; UAE, $n$ = 98; Kuwait, $n$ = 15; and Bahrain, $n$ = 1; see Table 1. To ensure high-quality, raw sequencing reads were quality-trimmed and filtered using Trimmomatic (version 0.33) [68]. De novo assembly of reads was performed using SPAdes (ve3.12.0) [69]. The mean number of contigs was 175 (range: 33–2278) for a mean total genome size of 5.6 Mbp (range: 5.0–6.3 Mbp). The mean N50 contig length was 222,214 (range: 5290–729,359) and the mean G+C content was 57% (range: 56–58.2%) (Supplementary Table S1).

In silico antibiotic resistance and virulence gene analysis. The assembled contigs were then annotated, and known antibiotic resistance genes (ARGs) were detected using ResFinder (http://cge.cbs.dtu.dk/services/ResFinder/ (accessed on 15 April 2022)) [70]. The capsular type and O antigen serotype were identified using Pathogen watch (Pathogenwatch | A Global Platform for Genomic Surveillance (accessed on 15 April 2022), the

Kaptive online tool (http://kaptive.holtlab.net/ (accessed on 15 April 2022) [71], and Kleborate database (https://github.com/katholt/Kleborate (accessed on 15 April 2022) [72].

Multi-locus sequence typing (MLST). Assembled genomes were typed using both the '*Klebsiella pneumoniae*' database from PubMLST (https://pubmlst.org/abaumannii/ (accessed on 15 May 2022) and Ridom SeqSphere+ v.8.3.5 software (Ridom GmbH, Münster, Germany) [73], and sequence types (STs) were identified using both the Pasteur and Oxford schemes.

Core genome MLST (cgMLST) characterization and phylogenetic analysis. cgMLST analysis was performed using a well-defined scheme available in Ridom SeqSphere+ v.8.3.5 software (Ridom GmbH, Münster, Germany), according to the '*K. pneumoniae* sensu lato cgMLST' version 1.0 scheme (https://www.cgmlst.org/ncs/schema/2187931/ (accessed on 25 September 2022). This included 2358 genes of the *K. pneumoniae* core genome (cgMLST) and 2526 genes of the *K. pneumoniae* accessory genome (wgMLST; total of 4891 targets). Seqsphere+ tool mapped the reads against the reference genome using BWA v 0.6.2 software (parameters setting: minimum coverage of five and Phred value > 30) and defined the cgMLST gene alleles. A combination of all these alleles in each isolate formed an allelic profile that was utilized to create a minimum spanning tree (MST) using Ridom SeqSphere+ with the 'pairwise ignore missing values; % column difference' parameter. A threshold was set at $\leq 15$ allelic differences paired with a cluster alert quality threshold of at least 90% good cgMLST targets to define the clusters.

**Supplementary Materials:** The following supporting information can be downloaded at: https://www.mdpi.com/article/10.3390/antibiotics12071081/s1. Table S1: Genomic characterization, epidemiology, and carbapenemase genes description of 720 Klebsiella pneumoniae collected from six countries around the Arabian Peninsula.

**Author Contributions:** Conceptualization, A.H.A.F., S.F.M. and A.G.; methodology, S.F.M., A.H.A.F. and A.G.; software, S.F.M.; formal analysis, A.H.A.F., S.F.M. and A.G.; investigation, A.H.A.F., S.F.M. and A.G.; writing—original draft preparation, A.G., S.F.M. and A.H.A.F.; writing—review and editing, A.H.A.F., S.F.M., A.G., W.Y.J. and V.O.R.; visualization, S.F.M. and A.G.; project administration, A.H.A.F., S.F.M. and A.G. All authors have read and agreed to the published version of the manuscript.

**Funding:** This research did not receive any specific grant from funding agencies in the public, commercial, or not-for-profit sectors.

**Institutional Review Board Statement:** Not applicable.

**Informed Consent Statement:** Not applicable.

**Data Availability Statement:** Raw genome sequence data examined in this study are publicly available from the European Nucleotide Archive under the accession numbers stated in Supplementary Table S1. Using the Short Read Archive (SRA) database, metadata on collection date are also available, and the sequencing was done with Illumina platforms (Supplementary Table S1).

**Conflicts of Interest:** The authors declare no conflict of interest.

# References

1. Vivas, R.; Dolabella, S.S.; Barbosa, A.A.T.; Jain, S. Prevalence of *Klebsiella pneumoniae* carbapenemase—And New Delhi metallo-beta-lactamase-positive K. pneumoniae in Sergipe, Brazil, and combination therapy as a potential treatment option. *Rev. Soc. Bras. Med. Trop.* **2020**, *53*, e20200064. [CrossRef] [PubMed]
2. O'Neill, J. Tackling Drug Resistant Infections Globally: Final Report and Recommendations. Review on Antimicrobial Resistance. Wellcome Trust and HM Government. 2016. Available online: https://amr-review.org/sites/default/files/160525_Final%20paper_with%20cover.pdf (accessed on 14 May 2023).
3. Feil, E.J. Enterobacteriaceae: Joining the dots with pan-European epidemiology. *Lancet Infect. Dis.* **2017**, *17*, 118–119. [CrossRef] [PubMed]
4. Perez, F.; Villegas, M.V. The role of surveillance systems in confronting the global crisis of antibiotic-resistant bacteria. *Curr. Opin. Infect. Dis.* **2015**, *28*, 375–383. [CrossRef]
5. Han, R.; Shi, Q.; Wu, S.; Yin, D.; Peng, M.; Dong, D.; Zheng, Y.; Guo, Y.; Zhang, R.; Hu, F. Dissemination of Carbapenemases (KPC, NDM, OXA-48, IMP, and VIM) Among Carbapenem-Resistant Enterobacteriaceae Isolated From Adult and Children Patients in China. *Front. Cell. Infect. Microbiol.* **2020**, *10*, 314. [CrossRef] [PubMed]

6. Tischendorf, J.; de Avila, R.A.; Safdar, N. Risk of infection following colonization with carbapenem-resistant Enterobactericeae: A systematic review. *Am. J. Infect. Control* **2016**, *44*, 539–543. [CrossRef]
7. Hammoudi Halat, D.; Ayoub Moubareck, C. The Current Burden of Carbapenemases: Review of Significant Properties and Dissemination among Gram-Negative Bacteria. *Antibiotics* **2020**, *9*, 186. [CrossRef]
8. Naas, T.; Dortet, L.; Iorga, B.I. Structural and Functional Aspects of Class A Carbapenemases. *Curr. Drug Targets* **2016**, *17*, 1006–1028. [CrossRef]
9. Moghnia, O.H.; Rotimi, V.O.; Al-Sweih, N.A. Preponderance of blaKPC-Carrying Carbapenem-Resistant Enterobacterales among Fecal Isolates from Community Food Handlers in Kuwait. *Front. Microbiol.* **2021**, *12*, 737828. [CrossRef]
10. Jeon, J.H.; Lee, J.H.; Lee, J.J.; Park, K.S.; Karim, A.M.; Lee, C.R.; Jeong, B.C.; Lee, S.H. Structural basis for carbapenem-hydrolyzing mechanisms of carbapenemases conferring antibiotic resistance. *Int. J. Mol. Sci.* **2015**, *16*, 9654–9692. [CrossRef]
11. Walsh, T.R.; Toleman, M.A.; Poirel, L.; Nordmann, P. Metallo-beta-lactamases: The quiet before the storm? *Clin. Microbiol. Rev.* **2005**, *18*, 306–325. [CrossRef]
12. Jamal, W.Y.; Albert, M.J.; Rotimi, V.O. High Prevalence of New Delhi Metallo-β-Lactamase-1 (NDM-1) Producers among Carbapenem-Resistant Enterobacteriaceae in Kuwait. *PLoS ONE* **2016**, *11*, e0152638. [CrossRef]
13. Zhang, H.; Hao, Q. Crystal structure of NDM-1 reveals a common β-lactam hydrolysis mechanism. *FASEB J.* **2011**, *25*, 2574–2582. [CrossRef] [PubMed]
14. Wu, W.; Feng, Y.; Tang, G.; Qiao, F.; McNally, A.; Zong, Z. NDM Metallo-β-Lactamases and Their Bacterial Producers in Health Care Settings. *Clin. Microbiol. Rev.* **2019**, *32*, e00115-8. [CrossRef]
15. Poirel, L.; Potron, A.; Nordmann, P. OXA-48-like carbapenemases: The phantom menace. *Int. J. Antimicrob. Agents* **2012**, *67*, 1597–1606. [CrossRef]
16. Potron, A.; Rondinaud, E.; Poirel, L.; Belmonte, O.; Boyer, S.; Camiade, S.; Nordmann, P. Genetic and biochemical characterisation of OXA-232, a carbapenem-hydrolysing class D β-lactamase from Enterobacteriaceae. *Int. J. Antimicrob. Agents* **2013**, *41*, 325–329. [CrossRef] [PubMed]
17. Pitout, J.D.D.; Peirano, G.; Kock, M.M.; Strydom, K.A.; Matsumura, Y. The Global Ascendency of OXA-48-Type Carbapenemases. *Clin. Microbiol. Rev.* **2019**, *33*, e00102-19. [CrossRef] [PubMed]
18. Dong, N.; Yang, X.; Chan, E.W.; Zhang, R.; Chen, S. Klebsiella species: Taxonomy, hypervirulence and multidrug resistance. *EbioMedicine* **2022**, *79*, 103998. [CrossRef]
19. Abd El Ghany, M.; Sharaf, H.; Al-Agamy, M.H.; Shibl, A.; Hill-Cawthorne, G.A.; Hong, P.Y. Genomic characterization of NDM-1 and 5, and OXA-181 carbapenemases in uropathogenic *Escherichia coli* isolates from Riyadh, Saudi Arabia. *PLoS ONE* **2018**, *13*, e0201613. [CrossRef]
20. Al-Agamy, M.H.; Aljallal, A.; Radwan, H.H.; Shibl, A.M. Characterization of carbapenemases, ESBLs, and plasmid-mediated quinolone determinants in carbapenem-insensitive *Escherichia coli* and *Klebsiella pneumoniae* in Riyadh hospitals. *J. Infect. Public Health* **2018**, *11*, 64–68. [CrossRef]
21. Al-Baloushi, A.E.; Pál, T.; Ghazawi, A.; Sonnevend, A. Genetic support of carbapenemases in double carbapenemase producer *Klebsiella pneumoniae* isolated in the Arabian Peninsula. *Acta Microbiol. Immunol. Hung.* **2018**, *65*, 135–150. [CrossRef] [PubMed]
22. Alotaibi, F.E.; Bukhari, E.E.; Al-Mohizea, M.M.; Hafiz, T.; Essa, E.B.; AlTokhais, Y.I. Emergence of carbapenem-resistant Enterobacteriaceae isolated from patients in a university hospital in Saudi Arabia. Epidemiology, clinical profiles and outcomes. *J. Infect. Public Health* **2017**, *10*, 667–673. [CrossRef] [PubMed]
23. Memish, Z.A.; Assiri, A.; Almasri, M.; Roshdy, H.; Hathout, H.; Kaase, M.; Gatermann, S.G.; Yezli, S. Molecular characterization of carbapenemase production among gram-negative bacteria in Saudi Arabia. *Microb. Drug Resist.* **2015**, *21*, 307–314. [CrossRef] [PubMed]
24. Moubareck, C.A.; Mouftah, S.F.; Pál, T.; Ghazawi, A.; Halat, D.H.; Nabi, A.; AlSharhan, M.A.; AlDeesi, Z.O.; Peters, C.C.; Celiloglu, H.; et al. Clonal emergence of *Klebsiella pneumoniae* ST14 co-producing OXA-48-type and NDM carbapenemases with high rate of colistin resistance in Dubai, United Arab Emirates. *Int. J. Antimicrob. Agents* **2018**, *52*, 90–95. [CrossRef] [PubMed]
25. Pál, T.; Ghazawi, A.; Darwish, D.; Villa, L.; Carattoli, A.; Hashmey, R.; Aldeesi, Z.; Jamal, W.; Rotimi, V.; Al-Jardani, A.; et al. Characterization of NDM-7 Carbapenemase-Producing *Escherichia coli* Isolates in the Arabian Peninsula. *Microb. Drug Resist.* **2017**, *23*, 871–878. [CrossRef]
26. Sonnevend, Á.; Ghazawi, A.A.; Hashmey, R.; Jamal, W.; Rotimi, V.O.; Shibl, A.M.; Al-Jardani, A.; Al-Abri, S.S.; Tariq, W.U.; Weber, S.; et al. Characterization of Carbapenem-Resistant Enterobacteriaceae with High Rate of Autochthonous Transmission in the Arabian Peninsula. *PLoS ONE* **2015**, *10*, e0131372. [CrossRef]
27. Uz Zaman, T.; Albladi, M.; Siddique, M.I.; Aljohani, S.M.; Balkhy, H.H. Insertion element mediated mgrB disruption and presence of ISKpn28 in colistin-resistant *Klebsiella pneumoniae* isolates from Saudi Arabia. *Infect. Drug Resist.* **2018**, *11*, 1183–1187. [CrossRef]
28. Zowawi, H.M.; Sartor, A.L.; Balkhy, H.H.; Walsh, T.R.; Al Johani, S.M.; AlJindan, R.Y.; Alfaresi, M.; Ibrahim, E.; Al-Jardani, A.; Al-Abri, S.; et al. Molecular characterization of carbapenemase-producing *Escherichia coli* and *Klebsiella pneumoniae* in the countries of the Gulf cooperation council: Dominance of OXA-48 and NDM producers. *Antimicrob. Agents Chemother.* **2014**, *58*, 3085–3090. [CrossRef]
29. Al-Abdely, H.; AlHababi, R.; Dada, H.M.; Roushdy, H.; Alanazi, M.M.; Alessa, A.A.; Gad, N.M.; Alasmari, A.M.; Radwan, E.E.; Al-Dughmani, H.; et al. Molecular characterization of carbapenem-resistant Enterobacterales in thirteen tertiary care hospitals in Saudi Arabia. *Ann. Saudi Med.* **2021**, *41*, 63–70. [CrossRef]

30. Sonnevend, Á.; Abdulrazzaq, N.; Ghazawi, A.; Thomsen, J.; Bharathan, G.; Makszin, L.; Rizvi, T.A.; Pál, T.; UAE CRE Study Group. The first nationwide surveillance of carbapenem-resistant Enterobacterales in the United Arab Emirates-increased association of *Klebsiella pneumoniae* CC14 clone with Emirati patients. *Int. J. Infect. Dis.* **2022**, *120*, 103–112. [CrossRef]
31. Zhao, Y.; Zhang, M.; Qiu, S.; Wang, J.; Peng, J.; Zhao, P.; Zhu, R.; Wang, H.; Li, Y.; Wang, K.; et al. Antimicrobial activity and stability of the D-amino acid substituted derivatives of antimicrobial peptide polybia-MPI. *AMB Express* **2016**, *6*, 122. [CrossRef]
32. Zhang, J.; Xiong, Y.; Rogers, L.; Carter, G.P.; French, N. Genome-by-genome approach for fast bacterial genealogical relationship evaluation. *Bioinformatics* **2018**, *34*, 3025–3027. [CrossRef]
33. Jolley, K.A.; Bray, J.E.; Maiden, M.C.J. Open-access bacterial population genomics: BIGSdb software, the PubMLST.org website and their applications. *Wellcome Open Res.* **2018**, *3*, 124. [CrossRef] [PubMed]
34. Pei, N.; Li, Y.; Liu, C.; Jian, Z.; Liang, T.; Zhong, Y.; Sun, W.; He, J.; Cheng, X.; Li, H.; et al. Large-Scale Genomic Epidemiology of *Klebsiella pneumoniae* Identified Clone Divergence with Hypervirulent Plus Antimicrobial-Resistant Characteristics Causing Within-Ward Strain Transmissions. *Microbiol. Spectr.* **2022**, *10*, e0269821. [CrossRef] [PubMed]
35. Findlay, J.; Hopkins, K.L.; Loy, R.; Doumith, M.; Meunier, D.; Hill, R.; Pike, R.; Mustafa, N.; Livermore, D.M.; Woodford, N. OXA-48-like carbapenemases in the UK: An analysis of isolates and cases from 2007 to 2014. *J. Antimicrob. Chemother.* **2017**, *72*, 1340–1349. [CrossRef]
36. Mouftah, S.F.; Pál, T.; Higgins, P.G.; Ghazawi, A.; Idaghdour, Y.; Alqahtani, M.; Omrani, A.S.; Rizvi, T.A.; Sonnevend, Á. Diversity of carbapenem-resistant *Klebsiella pneumoniae* ST14 and emergence of a subgroup with KL64 capsular locus in the Arabian Peninsula. *Eur. J. Clin. Microbiol. Infect. Dis.* **2021**, *10*, 1–9. [CrossRef] [PubMed]
37. Giske, C.G.; Fröding, I.; Hasan, C.M.; Turlej-Rogacka, A.; Toleman, M.; Livermore, D.; Woodford, N.; Walsh, T.R. Diverse sequence types of *Klebsiella pneumoniae* contribute to the dissemination of blaNDM-1 in India, Sweden, and the United Kingdom. *Antimicrob. Agents Chemother.* **2012**, *56*, 2735–2738. [CrossRef]
38. Navon-Venezia, S.; Kondratyeva, K.; Carattoli, A. Klebsiella pneumoniae: A major worldwide source and shuttle for antibiotic resistance. *FEMS Microbiol. Rev.* **2017**, *4*, 252–275. [CrossRef]
39. Yoon, E.J.; Yang, J.W.; Kim, J.O.; Lee, H.; Lee, K.J.; Jeong, S.H. Carbapenemase-producing Enterobacteriaceae in South Korea: A report from the National Laboratory Surveillance System. *Future Microbiol.* **2018**, *13*, 771–783. [CrossRef]
40. Holt, K.E.; Wertheim, H.; Zadoks, R.N.; Baker, S.; Whitehouse, C.A.; Dance, D.; Jenney, A.; Connor, T.R.; Hsu, L.Y.; Severin, J.; et al. Genomic analysis of diversity, population structure, virulence, and antimicrobial resistance in *Klebsiella pneumoniae*, an urgent threat to public health. *Proc. Natl. Acad. Sci. USA* **2015**, *112*, E3574–E3581. [CrossRef]
41. Lee, I.R.; Molton, J.S.; Wyres, K.L.; Gorrie, C.; Wong, J.; Hoh, C.H.; Teo, J.; Kalimuddin, S.; Lye, D.C.; Archuleta, S.; et al. Differential host susceptibility and bacterial virulence factors driving Klebsiella liver abscess in an ethnically diverse population. *Sci. Rep.* **2016**, *6*, 29316. [CrossRef]
42. Shankar, C.; Mathur, P.; Venkatesan, M.; Pragasam, A.K.; Anandan, S.; Khurana, S.; Veeraraghavan, B. Rapidly disseminating blaOXA-232 carrying *Klebsiella pneumoniae* belonging to ST231 in India: Multiple and varied mobile genetic elements. *BMC Microbiol.* **2019**, *19*, 137. [CrossRef]
43. Arabaghian, H.; Salloum, T.; Alousi, S.; Panossian, B.; Araj, G.F.; Tokajian, S. Molecular Characterization of Carbapenem Resistant Klebsiella pneumoniae and *Klebsiella quasipneumoniae* Isolated from Lebanon. *Sci. Rep.* **2019**, *9*, 531. [CrossRef]
44. Blundell-Hunter, G.; Enright, M.C.; Negus, D.; Dorman, M.J.; Beecham, G.E.; Pickard, D.J.; Wintachai, P.; Voravuthikunchai, S.P.; Thomson, N.R.; Taylor, P.W. Characterisation of Bacteriophage-Encoded Depolymerases Selective for Key *Klebsiella pneumoniae* Capsular Exopolysaccharides. *Front. Cell. Infect. Microbiol.* **2021**, *11*, 686090. [CrossRef]
45. Koskinen, K.; Penttinen, R.; Örmälä-Odegrip, A.M.; Giske, C.G.; Ketola, T.; Jalasvuori, M. Systematic Comparison of Epidemic and Non-Epidemic Carbapenem Resistant *Klebsiella pneumoniae* Strains. *Front. Cell. Infect. Microbiol.* **2021**, *11*, 599924. [CrossRef]
46. Nagaraj, G.; Shamanna, V.; Govindan, V.; Rose, S.; Sravani, D.; Akshata, K.P.; Shincy, M.R.; Venkatesha, V.T.; Abrudan, M.; Argimón, S.; et al. High-Resolution Genomic Profiling of Carbapenem-Resistant *Klebsiella pneumoniae* Isolates: A Multicentric Retrospective Indian Study. *Clin. Infect. Dis.* **2021**, *73* (Suppl. S4), S300–S307. [CrossRef] [PubMed]
47. Hala, S.; Antony, C.P.; Alshehri, M.; Alsaedi, A.; Thaqafi, O.A.; Al-Ahmadi, G.J.; Kaaki, M.; Alazmi, M.A.; Alhaj-Hussein, T.B.; Yasen, M.; et al. An Emerging Clone (ST2096) of *Klebsiella pneumoniae* Clonal Complex 14 With Enhanced Virulence Causes an Outbreak in Saudi Arabia. *J. Infect. Public Health* **2020**, *13*, 363–364. [CrossRef]
48. Gu, D.; Dong, N.; Zheng, Z.; Gu, D.; Dong, N.; Zheng, Z.; Lin, D.; Huang, M.; Wang, L.; Chan, E.W.; et al. A fatal outbreak of ST11 carbapenem-resistant hypervirulent *Klebsiella pneumoniae* in a Chinese hospital: A molecular epidemiological study. *Lancet Infect. Dis.* **2018**, *18*, 37–46. [CrossRef] [PubMed]
49. Balushi, M.A.; Kumar, R.; Al-Rashdi, A.; Ratna, A.; Al-Jabri, A.; Al-Shekaili, N.; Rani, R.; Sumri, S.A.; Al-Ghabshi, L.; Al-Abri, S.; et al. Genomic analysis of the emerging carbapenem-resistant *Klebsiella pneumoniae* sequence type 11 harbouring Klebsiella pneumoniae carbapenemase (KPC) in Oman. *J. Infect. Public Health* **2022**, *15*, 1089–1096. [CrossRef]
50. Safavi, M.; Bostanshirin, N.; Hajikhani, B.; Yaslianifard, S.; van Belkum, A.; Goudarzi, M.; Hashemi, A.; Darban-Sarokhalil, D.; Dadashi, M. Global genotype distribution of human clinical isolates of New Delhi metallo-β-lactamase-producing Klebsiella pneumoniae; A systematic review. *J. Glob. Antimicrob.* **2020**, *23*, 420–429. [CrossRef]
51. Jiang, Y.; Wei, Z.; Wang, Y.; Hua, X.; Feng, Y.; Yu, Y. Tracking a hospital outbreak of KPC-producing ST11 *Klebsiella pneumoniae* with whole genome sequencing. *Clin. Microbiol. Infect.* **2015**, *21*, 1001–1007. [CrossRef]

52. Chen, C.M.; Guo, M.K.; Ke, S.C.; Lin, Y.P.; Li, C.R.; Vy Nguyen, H.T.; Wu, L.T. Emergence and nosocomial spread of ST11 carbapenem-resistant *Klebsiella pneumoniae* co-producing OXA-48 and KPC-2 in a regional hospital in Taiwan. *J. Med. Microbiol.* **2018**, *67*, 957–964. [CrossRef] [PubMed]
53. Yu, F.; Hu, L.; Zhong, Q.; Hang, Y.; Liu, Y.; Hu, X.; Ding, H.; Chen, Y.; Xu, X.; Fang, X.; et al. Dissemination of *Klebsiella pneumoniae* ST11 isolates with carbapenem resistance in integrated and emergency intensive care units in a Chinese tertiary hospital. *J. Med. Microbiol.* **2019**, *68*, 882–889. [CrossRef]
54. Liu, C.; Yang, P.; Zheng, J.; Yi, J.; Lu, M.; Shen, N. Convergence of two serotypes within the epidemic ST11 KPC-producing *Klebsiella pneumoniae* creates the "Perfect Storm" in a teaching hospital. *BMC Genom.* **2022**, *23*, 693. [CrossRef] [PubMed]
55. Boyd, S.E.; Livermore, D.M.; Hooper, D.C.; Hope, W.W. Metallo-β-Lactamases: Structure, Function, Epidemiology, Treatment Options, and the Development Pipeline. *Antimicrob. Agents Chemother.* **2020**, *64*, e00397-20. [CrossRef] [PubMed]
56. Abid, F.B.; Tsui, C.; Doi, Y.; Deshmukh, A.; McElheny, C.L.; Bachman, W.C.; Fowler, E.L.; Albishawi, A.; Mushtaq, K.; Ibrahim, E.B.; et al. Molecular characterization of clinical carbapenem-resistant Enterobacterales from Qatar. *Eur. J. Clin. Microbiol.* **2021**, *40*, 1779–1785. [CrossRef]
57. Aris, P.; Robatjazi, S.; Nikkhahi, F.; Amin Marashi, S.M. Molecular mechanisms and prevalence of colistin resistance of *Klebsiella pneumoniae* in the Middle East region: A review over the last 5 years. *J. Glob. Antimicrob. Resist.* **2020**, *22*, 625–630. [CrossRef]
58. Siri, G.P.; Sithebe, N.P.; Ateba, C.N. Identification of Klebsiella species isolated from Modimola dam (Mafikeng) Northwest Province South Africa. *Afr. J. Microbiol. Res.* **2011**, *5*, 3958–3963.
59. Fang, C.T.; Lai, S.Y.; Yi, W.C.; Hsueh, P.R.; Liu, K.L.; Chang, S.C. *Klebsiella pneumoniae* genotype K1, An emerging pathogen that causes septic ocular or central nervous system complications from pyogenic liver abscess. *Clin. Infect. Dis.* **2007**, *45*, 284–293. [CrossRef]
60. Vila, A.; Cassata, A.; Pagella, H.; Amadio, C.; Yeh, K.M.; Chang, F.Y.; Siu, L.K. Appearance of *Klebsiella pneumoniae* liver abscess syndrome in Argentina: Case report and review of molecular mechanisms of pathogenesis. *Open Microbiol. J.* **2011**, *5*, 107–113. [CrossRef]
61. Da Silva, G.J.; Mendonça, N. Association between antimicrobial resistance and virulence in *Escherichia coli*. *Virulence* **2012**, *3*, 18–28. [CrossRef]
62. Wyres, K.L.; Lam, M.M.C.; Holt, K.E. Population genomics of *Klebsiella pneumoniae*. *Nat. Rev. Microbiol.* **2020**, *18*, 344–359. [CrossRef]
63. Al Fadhli, A.H.; Jamal, W.Y.; Rotimi, V.O. Elucidating the virulence genes harboured by carbapenemase- and non-carbapenemase-producing carbapenem-resistant *Klebsiella pneumoniae* rectal isolates from patients admitted to intensive care units using whole-genome sequencing in Kuwait. *J. Med. Microbiol.* **2022**, *71*, 10. [CrossRef] [PubMed]
64. Roe, C.C.; Vazquez, A.J.; Esposito, E.P.; Zarrilli, R.; Sahl, J.W. Diversity, Virulence, and Antimicrobial Resistance in Isolates From the Newly Emerging *Klebsiella pneumoniae* ST101 Lineage. *Front. Microbiol.* **2019**, *10*, 542. [CrossRef]
65. Hsieh, P.F.; Lin, T.L.; Yang, F.L.; Wu, M.C.; Pan, Y.J.; Wu, S.H.; Wang, J.T. Lipopolysaccharide O1 antigen contributes to the virulence in *Klebsiella pneumoniae* causing pyogenic liver abscess. *PLoS ONE* **2012**, *7*, e33155. [CrossRef]
66. Castanheira, M.; Costello, A.J.; Deshpande, L.M.; Jones, R.N. Expansion of clonal complex 258 KPC-2-producing *Klebsiella pneumoniae* in Latin American hospitals: Report of the SENTRY Antimicrobial Surveillance Program. *Antimicrob. Agents Chemother.* **2012**, *56*, 1668–1671. [CrossRef] [PubMed]
67. Argimón, S.; David, S.; Underwood, A.; Abrudan, M.; Wheeler, N.E.; Kekre, M.; Abudahab, K.; Yeats, C.A.; Goater, R.; Taylor, B.; et al. Rapid Genomic Characterization and Global Surveillance of Klebsiella Using Pathogenwatch. *Clin. Infect. Dis.* **2021**, *73*, S325–S335. [CrossRef]
68. Bolger, A.M.; Lohse, M.; Usadel, B. Trimmomatic: A flexible trimmer for Illumina sequence data. *Bioinformatics* **2014**, *30*, 2114–2120. [CrossRef] [PubMed]
69. Bankevich, A.; Nurk, S.; Antipov, D.; Gurevich, A.A.; Dvorkin, M.; Kulikov, A.S.; Lesin, V.M.; Nikolenko, S.I.; Pham, S.; Prjibelski, A.D.; et al. SPAdes: A new genome assembly algorithm and its applications to single-cell sequencing. *J. Comput. Biol.* **2012**, *19*, 455–477. [CrossRef] [PubMed]
70. Bortolaia, V.; Kaas, R.S.; Ruppe, E.; Roberts, M.C.; Schwarz, S.; Cattoir, V.; Philippon, A.; Allesoe, R.L.; Rebelo, A.R.; Florensa, A.F.; et al. ResFinder 4.0 for predictions of phenotypes from genotypes. *J. Antimicrob. Chemother.* **2020**, *75*, 3491–3500. [CrossRef] [PubMed]
71. Wyres, K.L.; Wick, R.R.; Gorrie, C.; Jenney, A.; Follador, R.; Thomson, N.R.; Holt, K.E. Identification of *Klebsiella capsule* synthesis loci from whole genome data. *Microb. Genom.* **2016**, *2*, e000102. [CrossRef] [PubMed]
72. Lam, M.M.C.; Wick, R.R.; Watts, S.C.; Cerdeira, L.T.; Wyres, K.L.; Holt, K.E. A genomic surveillance framework and genotyping tool for *Klebsiella pneumoniae* and its related species complex. *Nat. Commun.* **2021**, *12*, 4188. [CrossRef] [PubMed]
73. Jünemann, S.; Sedlazeck, F.J.; Prior, K.; Albersmeier, A.; John, U.; Kalinowski, J.; Mellmann, A.; Goesmann, A.; von Haeseler, A.; Stoye, J.; et al. Updating benchtop sequencing performance comparison. *Nat. Biotechnol.* **2013**, *31*, 294–296. [CrossRef] [PubMed]

**Disclaimer/Publisher's Note:** The statements, opinions and data contained in all publications are solely those of the individual author(s) and contributor(s) and not of MDPI and/or the editor(s). MDPI and/or the editor(s) disclaim responsibility for any injury to people or property resulting from any ideas, methods, instructions or products referred to in the content.

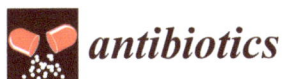

Article

# Molecular Characterization and Epidemiology of Antibiotic Resistance Genes of β-Lactamase Producing Bacterial Pathogens Causing Septicemia from Tertiary Care Hospitals

Mohammad Riaz Khan [1], Sadiq Azam [1], Sajjad Ahmad [2,3,*], Qaisar Ali [1], Zainab Liaqat [1], Noor Rehman [4], Ibrar Khan [1,*], Metab Alharbi [5] and Abdulrahman Alshammari [5]

1. Centre of Biotechnology and Microbiology, University of Peshawar, Peshawar 25120, Pakistan
2. Department of Computer Science, Virginia Tech, Blacksburg, WV 24061, USA
3. Department of Health and Biological Sciences, Abasyn University, Peshawar 25000, Pakistan
4. Department of Pathology, Khyber Teaching Hospital, Peshawar 25120, Pakistan
5. Department of Pharmacology and Toxicology, College of Pharmacy, King Saud University, P.O. Box 2455, Riyadh 11451, Saudi Arabia
* Correspondence: sajjademaan8@gmail.com (S.A.); ibrarkhan1984@uop.edu.pk (I.K.)

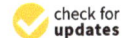

**Citation:** Khan, M.R.; Azam, S.; Ahmad, S.; Ali, Q.; Liaqat, Z.; Rehman, N.; Khan, I.; Alharbi, M.; Alshammari, A. Molecular Characterization and Epidemiology of Antibiotic Resistance Genes of β-Lactamase Producing Bacterial Pathogens Causing Septicemia from Tertiary Care Hospitals. *Antibiotics* **2023**, *12*, 617. https://doi.org/10.3390/antibiotics12030617

Academic Editor: Andrey Shelenkov

Received: 25 February 2023
Revised: 14 March 2023
Accepted: 16 March 2023
Published: 20 March 2023

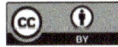

**Copyright:** © 2023 by the authors. Licensee MDPI, Basel, Switzerland. This article is an open access article distributed under the terms and conditions of the Creative Commons Attribution (CC BY) license (https:// creativecommons.org/licenses/by/ 4.0/).

**Abstract:** Septicemia is a systematic inflammatory response and can be a consequence of abdominal, urinary tract and lung infections. Keeping in view the importance of Gram-negative bacteria as one of the leading causes of septicemia, the current study was designed with the aim to determine the antibiotic susceptibility pattern, the molecular basis for antibiotic resistance and the mutations in selected genes of bacterial isolates. In this study, clinical samples (n = 3389) were collected from potentially infected male (n = 1898) and female (n = 1491) patients. A total of 443 (13.07%) patients were found to be positive for bacterial growth, of whom 181 (40.8%) were Gram-positive and 262 (59.1%) were Gram-negative. The infected patients included 238 males, who made up 12.5% of the total number tested, and 205 females, who made up 13.7%. The identification of bacterial isolates revealed that 184 patients (41.5%) were infected with *Escherichia coli* and 78 (17.6%) with *Pseudomonas aeruginosa*. The clinical isolates were identified using Gram staining biochemical tests and were confirmed using polymerase chain reaction (PCR), with specific primers for *E. coli* (USP) and *P. aeruginosa* (oprL). Most of the isolates were resistant to aztreonam (ATM), cefotaxime (CTX), ampicillin (AMP) and trimethoprim/sulfamethoxazole (SXT), and were sensitive to tigecycline (TGC), meropenem (MEM) and imipenem (IPM), as revealed by high minimum inhibitory concentration (MIC) values. Among the antibiotic-resistant bacteria, 126 (28.4%) samples were positive for ESBL, 105 (23.7%) for AmpC β-lactamases and 45 (10.1%) for MBL. The sequencing and mutational analysis of antibiotic resistance genes revealed mutations in TEM, SHV and AAC genes. We conclude that antibiotic resistance is increasing; this requires the attention of health authorities and clinicians for proper management of the disease burden.

**Keywords:** septicemia; *Escherichia coli*; *Pseudomonas aeruginosa*; antibiotic resistance; antibiotic resistance genes; mutational analysis

## 1. Introduction

Blood is a connective tissue which forms about 8% of total body weight; 5–7 L of blood is present in an average human body. The main components of blood are plasma (liquid portions 55%) and cells (45%): white blood cells, platelets and leucocytes [1,2]. Blood functions as the transportation medium for nutrients and aids in the excretion of waste materials by specialized organs. In vertebrates, blood is important for the maintenance of the body's temperature [3].

Blood is a sterile medium, but its contamination with pathogens or toxins leads to blood stream infections (BSIs), which are some of the leading causes of mortality and morbidity around the globe. BSIs are associated with fatal health conditions, which require admission to intensive care units [4]. In the United States, BSIs have been correlated with various risk factors, including exposure to microorganisms and the use of central venous catheters [5]. Causative agents for septicemia vary from region to region; it can be caused by both Gram-positive and Gram-negative bacteria, the most common of these being *E. coli, P. aeruginosa, Staphylococcus aureus, Klebsiella pneumonia* and *Salmonella typhi* [6]. Among these, the Gram-negative bacteria most associated with septicemia is *E. coli* [7–9].

The most common classes of antibiotics used to treat BSIs are penicillin, cephalosporins, aminoglycosides, glycopeptides, lincosamides, tetracyclines, fluoroquinolones and carbapenems. Due to overuse and misuse of antibiotics, bacteria have developed resistance to them, resulting in global health hazards [10,11]. Drug resistance in *E. coli* and other Gram-negative bacteria continues to rise, resulting in the emergence of multidrug-resistant strains. Treating the infections caused by these pathogens is a challenging issue [12]. An estimated 700,000 patients die globally each year due to high antibiotic resistance, and this number continues to rise [13]. A study in 2017 reported a total of 48.9 million cases of morbidity and 11 million of mortality worldwide, which constitutes a total of 20% mortality. Of the total, 85% of the cases of sepsis, including those of sepsis associated with death, were reported in low-middle income countries, and in Pakistan 60% of sepsis cases were fatal because of the infection being caused by multidrug-resistant strains and the misuse of antibiotics [14,15]. A study on neonatal sepsis in Sub-Saharan Africa revealed that *E. coli* accounted for 10% of the reported cases and was mostly resistant to aminoglycosides and β-lactams [16].

Determining the common pathogens and the antimicrobial susceptibility pattern causing septicemia is essential in order to select appropriate antibiotic therapies to decrease mortality and morbidity [17]. Keeping in view the importance of Gram-negative bacteria as one of the leading causes of septicemia, the current study was designed with the aim to determine the antibiotic susceptibility pattern, the molecular basis for antibiotic resistance and the mutations in selected genes of the bacterial isolates in Peshawar, Khyber-Pakhtunkhwa, Pakistan.

## 2. Results

Out of the total blood samples (n = 3389) from males and females of various age groups, 443 (13.07%) were found to be positive for bacterial growth. A total of 238 (12.5%) positive samples were from male patients and 205 (13.7%) were from female patients. Of the 443 bacterial isolates, 59.1% (n = 262) were identified as Gram-negative. The highest number of bacterial isolates were of *E. coli*, 184 (41.5%), followed by *P. aeruginosa*, 78 (17.6%). The highest ratio of *E. coli* (n = 184) was observed in the age group 41–60 years, at 50 (27.1%), followed by 21–40 years, at 48 (26.01%). Similarly, the highest ratio of *P. aeruginosa* (n = 78) was observed in patients older than 60 years, 16 (50%), followed by 41–60 years, 7 (21.8%), as mentioned in Table 1.

**Table 1.** Frequency and percentage (in parenthesis) distribution of various bacterial isolates from blood samples.

| Parameters | | *E. coli* (n = 184) | *P. aeruginosa* (n = 78) |
|---|---|---|---|
| | | Frequency (%) | Frequency (%) |
| Gender | Male | 65 (35.3) | 60 (76.9) |
| | Female | 119 (64.7) | 18 (23.1) |
| Age Groups | 00 to 10 | 37 (20.10) | 02 (2.56) |
| | 11 to 20 | 26 (14.13) | 04 (5.12) |
| | 21 to 40 | 48 (26.01) | 18 (23.07) |
| | 41 to 60 | 50 (27.1) | 28 (35.8) |
| | Above 60 | 23 (12.5) | 26 (33.3) |
| | Total | 184 (100) | 78 (100) |

## 2.1. Identification of Bacterial Isolates

All the isolates were identified by being cultured on MacConkey and blood agar media, followed by Gram staining (pink color colonies under microscope), API strips (as per API codes and reading scales) and on the molecular level by USP for *E. coli* and oprL for *P. aeruginosa* (Figure 1).

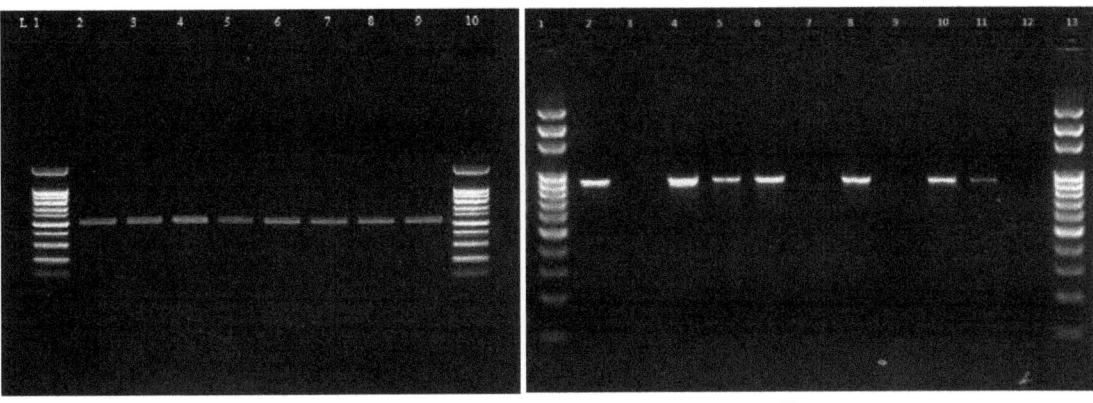

**Figure 1.** Products of PCR for the detection of USP (884 bp) gene (**A**) and oprL (504 bp) (**B**) on 1.5% EB-stained agarose gel amplified from *E. coli* and *P. aeruginosa*, where L1 and 1 are 100 bp DNA ladders.

## 2.2. Antibiotic Susceptibility Pattern of Clinical Isolates

The resulting antibiotic sensitivity patterns of identified *E. coli* and *P. aeruginosa* revealed resistance to AMP, SXT and CIP, and sensitivity to MEM, IPM and TOB (Table 2).

**Table 2.** Antibiotic susceptibility patterns of *E. coli* and *P. aeruginosa* against selected antibiotics.

| Antibiotics | *E. coli* (n = 184) | | *P. aeruginosa* (n = 78) | |
|---|---|---|---|---|
| | Sensitive (%) | Resistant (%) | Sensitive (%) | Resistant (%) |
| AMP (ampicillin) | 13 (7.06) | 171 (92.9) | 08 (10.5) | 70 (89.7) |
| FOX (cefoxitin) | 91 (49.4) | 93 (50.5) | 08 (10.2) | 70 (89.7) |
| AMC (amoxicillin) | 76 (41.3) | 108 (58.6) | 08 (10.2) | 70 (89.7) |
| SCF (cefoperazone-sulbactam) | 134 (72.8) | 50 (27.1) | 27 (34.6) | 51 (65.3) |
| TZP (piperacillin-tazobactam) | 117 (63.5) | 67 (36.4) | 62 (79.4) | 16 (20.5) |
| FEP (cefepime) | 70 (38) | 114 (62) | 35 (44.8) | 43 (55.1) |
| CTX (cefotaxime) | 70 (38) | 114 (62) | 29 (37.1) | 49 (62.8) |
| CAZ (ceftazidime) | 70 (38) | 114 (62) | 42 (53.8) | 36 (46.1) |
| ATM (aztreonam) | 78 (42.3) | 106 (57.6) | 23 (29.48) | 55 (70.5) |
| MEM (meropenem) | 157 (85.3) | 27 (14.6) | 74 (94.8) | 04 (5.12) |
| IPM (imipenem) | 157 (85.3) | 27 (14.6) | 74 (94.8) | 04 (5.12) |
| CN (gentamicin) | 104 (56.5) | 80 (43.4) | 28 (35.8) | 50 (64.1) |
| AK (Amikacin) | 137 (74.4) | 47 (25.5) | 20 (25.6) | 58 (74.3) |
| TOB (tobramycin) | 93 (50.5) | 91 (49.4) | 31 (39.7) | 47 (60.2) |
| DO (doxycycline) | 70 (38.0) | 114 (62) | 33 (42.3) | 45 (57.6) |
| CIP (ciprofloxacin) | 45 (24.4) | 139 (75.5) | 40 (51.2) | 38 (48.7) |
| SXT (trimethoprim/sulfamethoxazole) | 21 (11.4) | 163 (88.5) | 33 (42.3) | 45 (57.6) |

## 2.3. Determination of Minimum Inhibitory Concentration

The potency of the antibiotics depends on their minimum inhibitory concentration (MIC) values. The higher the MIC value, the less potent the antibiotic, and vice versa. The

ESBLs, MBLs and AmpC β-lactamases producing *E. coli* and *P. aeruginosa* isolates were highly resistant to CTX and CAZ with high MIC values as well as non-β-lactam drugs. SXT, CIP, DO, CN and AK were susceptible to MEM and to TGC with low MIC values (Tables 3 and 4).

Table 3. MICs of selected antibiotic disks against ESBLs, MBLs and AmpC β-lactamases producing *E. coli*.

| Antibiotics | ESBLs | | MBLs | | AmpC | |
|---|---|---|---|---|---|---|
| | MIC90/MIC50 (μg/mL) | MIC Range (μg/mL) | MIC90/MIC50 (μg/mL) | MIC Range (μg/mL) | MIC90/MIC50 (μg/mL) | MIC Range (μg/mL) |
| CTX | 256/128 | 4–256 | 128/256 | 4–256 | 128/256 | 4–256 |
| CAZ | 256/64 | 16–256 | 64/256 | 16–256 | 64/256 | 16–256 |
| MEM | 0.75/0.125 | 0.023–1 | 4/32 | 3–256 | 0.19/0.75 | 0.023–1 |
| IPM | 0.75/0.19 | 0.023–1 | 4/32 | 3–96 | 0.19/1.0 | 0.023–1 |
| CN | 16/4 | 0.064–140 | 16/16 | 4–16 | 4/16 | 0.064–140 |
| AK | 256/8 | 0.19–256 | 16/256 | 1–256 | 8/256 | 0.19–256 |
| DO | 192/16 | 0.125–256 | 16/192 | 1–256 | 16/128 | 0.125–256 |
| CIP | 256/24 | 0.25–256 | 32/256 | 0.094–256 | 24/256 | 0.25–256 |
| SXT | 256/24 | 0.19–256 | 32/32 | 0.064–32 | 24/256 | 0.19–256 |
| TGC | 1.5/0.25 | 0.023–2 | 0.5/1.5 | 0.023–8 | 0.50/1.5 | 0.023–2 |

Table 4. MICs of selected antibiotic disks against ESBLs, MBLs and AmpC β-lactamases producing *P. aeruginosa*.

| Antibiotics | ESBLs | | MBLs | | AmpC | |
|---|---|---|---|---|---|---|
| | MIC90/MIC50 (μg/mL) | MIC Range (μg/mL) | MIC90/MIC50 (μg/mL) | MIC Range (μg/mL) | MIC90/MIC50 (μg/mL) | MIC Range (μg/mL) |
| CTX | 16/256 | 0.16–256 | 12/256 | 0.023–256 | 12/256 | 0.023–256 |
| CAZ | 128/256 | 2–256 | 64/256 | 1.5–256 | 64/256 | 1.5–256 |
| MEM | 0.38/1 | 0.016–1 | 2/16 | 0.023–26 | 0.75/1 | 0.023–1 |
| IPM | 0.50/1 | 0.012–1 | 2/16 | 0.016–16 | 0.50/1 | 0.012–1 |
| CN | 4/16 | 0.064–140 | 8/16 | 0.064–64 | 8/16 | 0.064–64 |
| AK | 12/256 | 0.25–256 | 8/128 | 0.094–128 | 8/128 | 0.094–128 |
| DO | 32/192 | 0.125–256 | 32/192 | 0.125–192 | 32/192 | 0.125–192 |
| CIP | 24/256 | 0.19–256 | 24/192 | 0.19–256 | 24/92 | 0.19–256 |
| SXT | 24/256 | 1.0–256 | 8/64 | 1.5–64 | 8/64 | 1.5–64 |
| TGC | 0.50/2 | 0.032–2 | 0.75/2.0 | 0.047–2 | 0.75/2 | 0.047–2 |

### 2.4. Phenotypic and Genotypic Identification of β-Lactamase Producers

All the positive isolates (n = 443) were screened phenotypically and genotypically for β-lactamase production. Out of 443 positive samples, 126 (28.4%) were ESBL positive, 105 (23.7%) were AmpC β-lactamase producers and 45 (10.1%) were MBL producers (Table 5).

Table 5. Distribution of antibiotic-resistant genes in bacterial isolates.

| Organisms | ESBL (%) | AmpC β-Lactamase (%) | MBL (%) |
|---|---|---|---|
| *P. aeruginosa* | 46 (58.9) | 38 (48.7) | 15 (19.2) |
| *E. coli* | 80 (43.4) | 67 (36.4) | 30 (16.3) |
| Total | 126 (28.4) | 105 (23.7) | 45 (10.1) |

### 2.5. Characterization of ESBLs Gene(s), MBLs and AmpC β-Lactamase Resistance Genes

Of the total 80 phenotypically detected *E. coli* isolates for ESBL production, 74 (92.5%) were positive for one or more ESBL genes. The most common gene detected was CTX-M, 56 (70%), followed by TEM, 51 (63.7%) and SHV, 28 (35%). However, in *P. aeruginosa*, the most prevalent gene was TEM (73.9%), followed by SHV (63.0%) and CTX-M (34.7%). Among the 30 phenotypically identified MBL producers, *E. coli*, 11 (36.6%) showed the presence of targeted MBLs genes, with NDM1 being the most common, 9 (30%) isolates. Similarly, the NDM1 gene were observed in 3 (20%) clinically isolated *P. aeruginosa*. Among the AmpC β-lactamases in *E. coli* isolates, the highest prevalence was of AmpC gene, 57 (85%), followed by CIT gene, 11 (16.4%) and the Bla-DHA gene, 8 (11.9%). Similarly in

*P. aeruginosa*, AmpC was detected in 35 (92.1%) isolates, followed by 31 (81.5%) for CIT, 17 (44.7%) for DHA and 5 (13.1%) for the ACC gene (Table 6 and Figure 2).

**Table 6.** Distribution of ESBLs, MBL and AmpC β-lactamase resistance genes.

| Genes | *Escherichia coli* | | *Pseudomonas aeruginosa* | |
|---|---|---|---|---|
| | Negative (%) | Positive (%) | Negative (%) | Positive (%) |
| *ESBL* genes | | | | |
| Bla-CTX—M | 24 (30) | 56 (70) | 30 (65.2) | 16 (73.9) |
| Bla-TEM | 29 (36.2) | 51 (63.7) | 12 (26) | 34 (73.9) |
| Bla-SHV | 52 (65) | 28 (35) | 17 (36.9) | 29 (34.7) |
| Bla-OXA1 | 05 (6.25) | 75 (93.75) | 3 (6.52) | 43 (93.47) |
| MBL genes | | | | |
| Bla-NDM-1 | 21(70) | 09 (30) | 12 (80) | 03 (20) |
| AmpC β-Lactamases genes | | | | |
| Bla-AmpC | 10 (14.9) | 57 (85) | 03 (7.89) | 35 (92.1) |
| Bla-CIT | 56 (83.5) | 11 (16.4) | 07 (31) | 31 (81.5) |
| Bla-DHA | 59 (88) | 08 (11.9) | 21 (55.2) | 17 (44.7) |
| Bla-ACC | 67 (100) | 00 | 33 (86.3) | 05 (13.1) |

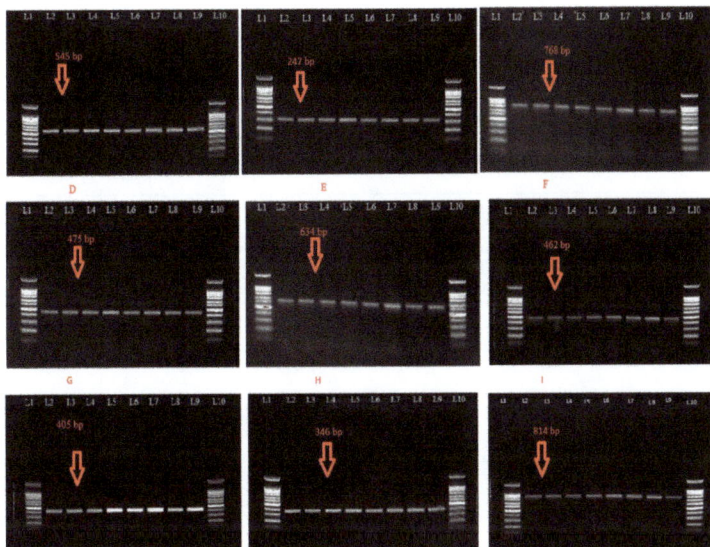

**Figure 2.** (**A**): Gel image of CTX-M gene (545 bp); L2-9: positive isolates, L1/L10: 100 bp DNA ladder, (**B**): gel image of TEM gene (247 bp); L2-9: positive isolates, L1/L10: 100 bp DNA ladder (**C**): gel image of SHV gene (768 bp); L2-L9: positive isolates, L1/L13: 100 bp DNA ladder, (**D**): gel image of NDM-1 gene (475 bp); L1/L10: 100-bpDNA ladder, L2-9: positive isolates, (**E**): gel image of AmpC gene (634 bp); L1/L10: 100-bp DNA ladder, L2-09: positive isolates (**F**): gel image of CIT gene (462 bp); L1/L10: 100-bp DNA ladder, L2-09: positive isolates, (**G**): gel image of DHA gene (405 bp); L1/L10: 100-bp DNA ladder, L2-09: positive isolates, (**H**): gel image of AAC gene (346 bp); L1/L10: 100-bp DNA ladder, L2-09: positive isolates. (**I**): gel image of OXA-1 gene (814 bp); L1/L10: 100-bp DNA ladder, L2-09: positive isolates.

### 2.6. Mutational Analysis ESBLs Gene(s), MBLs and AmpC β-Lactamase Resistance Genes

The sequencing data were analyzed using various bioinformatics tools; mutations were detected in Bla-TEM, Bla-SHV, Bla-ACC, Bla-NDM1, Bla-OXA1 and Bla-AAD genes but not in CTXM, AMP, CIT and DHA (Table 7). The effects of these mutations, as predicted by I-mutant software 3.0, are presented in Table 8.

Table 7. Mutations detected in the selected antibiotic-resistant genes.

| Antibiotic Resistance Genes | Position | Mutation |
|---|---|---|
| Bla-TEM | 31 | Deletion of G |
| Bla-SHV | 34 | Deletion of T |
|  | 101 | Insertion of G |
| Bla-ACC | 13 and 14 | Deletion of T and G |
|  | 24 | T to A |
|  | 30 and 31 | Deletion of G and T |
|  | 73 | C to A |
|  | 163 | C to A |
| Bla-NDM1 | 40–43 | Deletion of C, C, G, G |
|  | 46 | Deletion of G |
|  | 219 | C to G |
|  | 322 | C to G |
|  | 362 | G to C |
|  | 576 and 577 | Deletion of C and A |
|  | 579 | Deletion of C |
| Bla-OXA1 | 49 | Deletion of C |
|  | 51 | Deletion of A |
|  | 327 | C to T |
| Bla-AAD | 67 | Deletion of T |

Table 8. The I-Mutant software prediction result for selected antibiotic-resistant genes.

| Wild Type | New Type | I-Mutant Prediction Effect | Reliability Index (RI) | pH | Temperature |
|---|---|---|---|---|---|
| | | Bla TEM-1 gene | | | |
| A | G | Decrease | 2 | 7 | 25 |
| | | Bla SHV gene | | | |
| G | T | Decrease | 3 | 7 | 25 |
| G | V | Increase | 2 | 7 | 25 |
| | | Bla ACC | | | |
| N | V | Increase | 4 | 7 | 25 |
| N | L | Increase | 4 | 7 | 25 |
| N | A | Increase | 1 | 7 | 25 |
| C | V | Increase | 0 | 7 | 25 |
| N | I | Increase | 1 | 7 | 25 |
| T | A | Decrease | 6 | 7 | 25 |
| C | A | Decrease | 3 | 7 | 25 |
| | | Bla NDM1 | | | |
| T | V | Increase | 2 | 7 | 25 |
| G | V | Increase | 1 | 7 | 25 |
| A | V | Increase | 3 | 7 | 25 |
| T | L | Increase | 1 | 7 | 25 |
| T | V | Increase | 3 | 7 | 25 |
| A | G | Decrease | 0 | 7 | 25 |
| T | G | Increase | 0 | 7 | 25 |
| T | C | Increase | 1 | 7 | 25 |
| | | Bla AAD1 | | | |
| G | V | Increase | 2 | 7 | 25 |

## 3. Discussion

Antibiotic resistance is a major health threat and is responsible for high morbidity and mortality around the globe. Gram-negative bacteria have developed ways to combat the available antibiotics, making bacterial infections hard to treat. In the current study, the results confirmed this phenomenon, which is affecting community health and the economy. In the current study, 41.5% prevalence of *E. coli* was reported, which is similar to other findings [14]. The positivity ratios of infection of *E coli* were 64.7% in female patients and 35.3% in male patients. In our study, 27.1% of *E. coli* isolates were reported in the age group of 41–60 years; this may be due to weakened immune systems or to frequent exposure. This was followed by 26.01% in 21–40 years, which is in contrast to the reported literature [15]. The *E. coli* isolates of this study showed resistance to AMP, CTX, CAZ, CIP and LEV and sensitivity towards SCF, CO, MEM, TGC, AK, FOS and TZP, in agreement with the literature [16]. The prevalence rate of *P. aeruginosa* in the current study is 17.6%, 23.1% of this was in female patients and 76.9% in male patients, as supported by the reported study [17]. A 2016 study conducted in Pakistan found *P. aeruginosa* in 13% of septicemia patients, 55.8% males and 44.2% females. The prevalence of *P. aeruginosa* in our study at 17.6% implies that it has increased in the last few years. This directly indicates an increase in antibiotic resistance in Pakistan [18]. In the current study, ESBL genes in *E. coli* isolates were screened, in which CTX-M was detected in 70%, TEM in 63.7% and SHV in 35%. Another reported study had lower prevalence of CTX-M (57.7%), TEM (20.3%) and SHV (15.4%) [19]. Similar to that study, in the current study, 36.6% of the MBL targeted genes were detected, in which NDM1 gene prevalence was almost 30%. An Indian study reported the same results of MBL Ec with 28% prevalence of NDM-1 [20]. In this study, AmpC β-lactamase was found in 85.0%, CIT gene in 16.4% and DHA gene in 11.9% of the total clinical isolates, which supported earlier reported studies [21,22]. The mutations in the selected gene may offer a molecular explanation for the antibiotic resistance in the isolates of the current study.

## 4. Conclusions

The findings of this study have several key implications for health policymakers, clinicians and researchers. These findings highlight the need to update infection-prevention measures to be better able to manage the diseases caused by *E. coli* and *P. aeruginosa*. The increase in antibiotic resistance is an alarming situation, and necessitates a rationalization of the treatment strategy to control BSIs. The unavailability of newer drugs, and the constant increase in antibiotic resistance have led to the use of limited drugs such as colistin by physicians. This has resulted in a condition called pan-drug resistance, necessitating the discovery of new antimicrobial drugs.

## 5. Materials and Methods

The study was conducted in the Khyber Teaching Hospital Peshawar, Hayatabad Medical Complex Peshawar and the Center of Biotechnology and Microbiology, University of Peshawar, using standard microbiological procedures. A total of 3389 blood samples were collected from suspected septicemic patients in EDTA tubes aseptically, from both sexes and from various age groups, and were processed by automated blood culture systems. An overview of the whole methodology is represented in Scheme 1. Informed consent was obtained from all patients on a prescribed proforma before taking blood samples.

### 5.1. Isolation and Identification

The samples were cultured on MacConkey (Merck, Rahway, NJ, USA) and blood agar (Merck, Rahway, NJ, USA) media followed by incubation at 37 °C for 24 h [23]. The isolates were identified using Gram staining (Merck, Rahway, NJ, USA) and biochemically by API kits (Biomerieux, Marcy-Etoile France) [24,25].

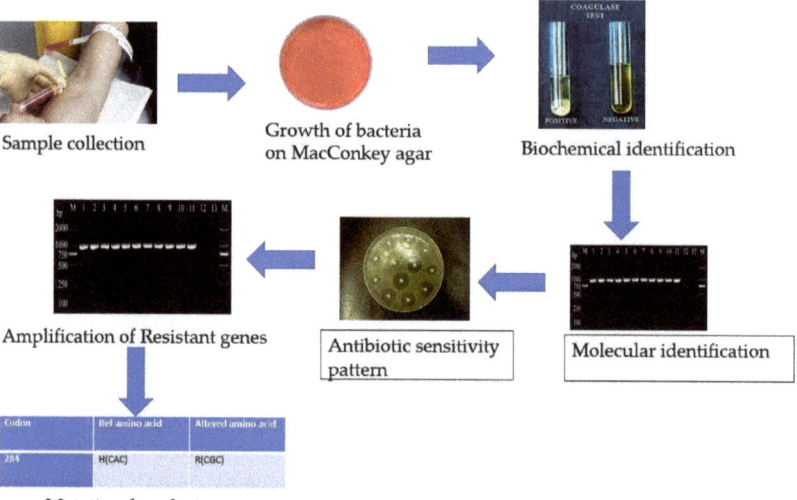

Scheme 1. Flowchart of the methodology used in the study.

*5.2. Molecular-Level Identification*

For molecular-level identification of the bacterial isolates (USP for *E. coli* and oprL for *P. aeruginosa*) and detection of antibiotic-resistant genes (Table 9), DNA of the bacterial isolates was extracted using Thermo Scientific GeneJET Genomic DNA purification kits as per the manufacturer's protocol. The extracted DNA was confirmed by gel electrophoresis (1% agarose gel in 1X triacetate EDTA buffer) and visualized by a gel documentation system.

Table 9. Sequences of primers along with optimized conditions used in the current study.

| Gene | Primer Sequence | Gene Size (bp) | Optimized Condition Annealing (°C/s): | Cycle |
|---|---|---|---|---|
| Marker genes of *E. coli* and *P. aeruginosa* | | | | |
| USP | F: ATCACCGTGGTGACCGCATGTCGC<br>R: CACCACGATGCCATGTTCATCTGC | 884 | 54/30 | 35 |
| oprL | F: ATGGAAATGCTGAAATTCGGC<br>R: CTTCTTCAGCTCGACGCGCG | 504 | 55/30 | 35 |
| *ESBL* genes | | | | |
| Bla-TEM | F: TTAACTGGCGAACTACTTAC<br>R: GTCTATTTCGTTCATCCATA | 247 | 54/30 | 35 |
| Bla-SHV | F: TCGCCTGTGTATTATCTCCC<br>R: CGCAGATAAATCACCACAATG | 768 | 52/30 | 35 |
| Bla-CTX-M | F: ATGTGCAGCACCAGTAAAGT<br>R: ACCGCGATATCGTTGGTGG | 545 | 54/30 | 35 |
| Bla-OXA-1 | F: ACACAATACATATCAACTTCGC<br>R: AGTGTGTTTAGAATGGTGATC | 814 | 57/30 | 35 |
| *MBLs* genes | | | | |
| Bla-NDM1 | F: GGGCAGTCGCTTCCAACGGT<br>R: GTAGTGCTCAGTGTCGGCAT | 475 | 54/30 | 35 |
| *AmpC β-lactamase genes* | | | | |
| Bla-AmpC | F: CCCCGCCTTATAGAGCAACAA<br>R: TCAATGGTCGACTTCACACC | 634 | 54/30 | 35 |
| Bla-ACC | F: AACAGCCTCAGCAGCCGGTTA<br>R: TTCGCCGCAATCATCCCTAGC | 346 | 54/30 | 35 |
| Bla-CIT | F: TGGCCAGAACTGACAGGCAAA<br>R: TTTCTCCTGAACGTGGCTGGC | 462 | 54/30 | 35 |
| Bla-DHA | F: AACTTTCACAGGTGTGCTGGGT<br>R: CCGTACGCATACTGGCTTTGC | 405 | 54/30 | 35 |

*5.3. Antimicrobial Susceptibility Testing*

The Kirby–Bauer disk diffusion method [21] was used to determine the antibiotic sensitivity pattern of the identified bacterial isolates against selected antibiotic disks (Table 10) as per Clinical Laboratory and Standard Institute (CLSI) guidelines. The pure cultures of the bacterial isolates (0.5 McFarland standard) were inoculated on sterile Muller–Hinton agar (MHA) media, and the antibiotic disks were applied, followed by 24 h of incubation at 37 °C. The zones of inhibition were measured and were evaluated as resistant (R), intermediate (I) and sensitive (S), as per CLSI guidelines [19].

**Table 10.** Antibiotic disks along with the concentration used in the study.

| S. No | Name of Antibiotic | Concentration (µg/mL) | Inhibition Value (mm) | |
|---|---|---|---|---|
| | | | Sensitive | Resistant |
| 1 | AMC | 20/10 | ≥18 | ≤13 |
| 2 | AMP | 10 | ≥17 | ≤13 |
| 3 | SCF | 75/30 | ≥21 | ≤15 |
| 4 | TZP | 100/10 | ≥21 | ≤17 |
| 5 | FEP | 30 | ≥25 | ≤18 |
| 6 | CTX | 30 | ≥26 | ≤22 |
| 7 | FOX | 30 | ≥18 | ≤24 |
| 8 | CAZ | 30 | ≥21 | ≤27 |
| 9 | ATM | 30 | ≥21 | ≤27 |
| 10 | MEM | 10 | ≥23 | ≤29 |
| 11 | IPM | 10 | ≥23 | ≤29 |
| 12 | GEN | 10 | ≥15 | ≤23 |
| 13 | TOB | 10 | ≥15 | ≤23 |
| 14 | AMK | 30 | ≥17 | ≤14 |
| 15 | DO | 30 | ≥14 | ≤10 |
| 16 | CIP | 5 | ≥26 | ≤21 |
| 17 | SXT | 1.25/23.75 | ≥16 | ≤10 |

*5.4. Minimum Inhibitory Concentration*

The minimum inhibitory concentrations (MICs) of the selected antibiotics were determined using MIC strips (Table 11). The strips were placed along with inoculation of the pure isolates on sterilized MHA media, followed by overnight incubation at 37 °C [24].

**Table 11.** E-strips used in the current study for determination of MIC.

| E-Strips | Symbols | Resistant | Sensitive |
|---|---|---|---|
| E-CT (Cefotaxime) | CTX | ≥4 | ≤1 |
| E-TZ (Ceftazidime) | CAZ | ≥16 | ≤4 |
| E-MP (Meropenem) | MEM | ≥4 | ≤1 |
| E-IP (Imipenem) | IPM | ≥4 | ≤1 |
| E-GM (Gentamicin) | CN | ≥16 | ≤4 |
| E-AK (Amikacin) | AK | ≤4 | ≤16 |
| E-DC (Doxycycline) | DO | ≥16 | ≤4 |
| E-CL (Ciprofloxacin) | CIP | ≥1 | ≤0.25 |
| E-TS (Co-Trimoxazole) | SXT | ≥4 | ≤2.38 |
| E-TGC (Tigecycline) | TGC | | ≤2 |

*5.5. Detection of Antibiotic-Resistant Genes by Polymerase Chain Reaction*

The selected antibiotic resistance genes, as per antibiotic resistance pattern, were amplified by polymerase chain reaction (PCR) using specific primers (Table 9). The PCR contained 12.5 µL of Taq Master Mix (Thermo Fisher Scientific™, Waltham, MA, USA), 11.5 µL nuclease-free water, 0.5 µL of forward and reverse primers (oligo nucleotide Microgen, Seoul, Korea) each and 2 µL of DNA sample. Under optimized conditions

(Table 9), the selected genes were amplified, run on gel electrophoresis and visualized using a gel documentation system.

*5.6. DNA Sequencing and Mutational Analysis*

The amplified PCR products of antibiotic-resistant genes were purified using a purification kit (Thermo Scientific™ GeneJET PCR Purification Kit, Waltham, MA, USA) and sequenced at Rehman Medical Institute (RMI), Peshawar, Pakistan. The FASTA sequences of the selected genes were retrieved from the GenBank–National Center for Biotechnology Information (NCBI) database after sequencing. Basic Local Alignment Search Tool (BLAST) and BioEdit 7.2 software were used to compare the FASTA sequences of the selected genes to confirm their presence in bacterial isolates and their mutational analysis [24]. The data were further analyzed for non-synonymous mutations, and I-Mutant software was used to predict the pathogenic effects of the identified mutations [25].

*5.7. Statistical Analysis*

A chi-square analysis was conducted using SPSS version 20 to find the association between the expected value of *E. coli* and the observed $p \leq 0.05$. The number of samples (n) was set at 150 and the degree of freedom was taken at n-1. For comparative analysis, one-way analysis of variance (ANOVA) was performed among the continuous values of antibiotics with *E. coli*, and $p \leq 0.05$ values were considered statistically significant.

**Author Contributions:** I.K. designed the study, supervised it and helped in the manuscript preparation. M.R.K. carried out the lab work and data curation and contributed to manuscript preparation. S.A. (Sadiq Azam) helped in the project design and review of the manuscript. Z.L. helped in the experimental design of the work. Q.A. helped in the review of the manuscript to finalize it. N.R. helped in the conceptualization of the work and in the review of the manuscript to finalize it. S.A. (Sajjad Ahmad) helped in the formal analysis of the work. M.A. and A.A. helped in the review and editing and in funding acquisition. All authors have read and agreed to the published version of the manuscript.

**Funding:** The authors express their gratitude to the Researchers Supporting Project (number RSP2023R462), King Saud University, Riyadh, Saudi Arabia.

**Institutional Review Board Statement:** The study was approved by the Institution Research and Ethical Review Board (IREB) of Khyber Medical College, Peshawar (document no. 122/ADR/KMC).

**Informed Consent Statement:** Informed consent was obtained from all the patients on a prescribed proforma before taking blood samples.

**Data Availability Statement:** All the data analyzed or generated in the study are provided in the manuscript to the best understanding of the authors.

**Conflicts of Interest:** The authors declare no conflict of interest.

# References

1. Liew, C.C.; Ma, J.; Tang, H.C.; Zheng, R.; Dempsey, A.A. The peripheral blood transcriptome dynamically reflects system wide biology: A potential diagnostic tool. *J. Lab. Clin. Med.* **2006**, *147*, 126–132. [CrossRef] [PubMed]
2. Abdel-Dayem, M.; Al Zou'bi, R.; Hani, R.B.; Amr, Z.S. Microbiological and parasitological investigation among food handlers in hotels in the dead sea area, Jordan. *J. Microbiol. Immunol. Infect.* **2014**, *47*, 377–380. [CrossRef] [PubMed]
3. Mack, J.P.; Miles, J.; Stolla, M. Cold-stored platelets: Review of studies in humans. *Transfus. Med. Rev.* **2020**, *34*, 221–226. [CrossRef] [PubMed]
4. Diekema, D.J.; Beekmann, S.E.; Chapin, K.C.; Morel, K.A.; Munson, E.; Doern, G.V. Epidemiology and outcome of nosocomial and community-onset bloodstream infection. *J. Clin. Microbiol.* **2003**, *41*, 3655–3660. [CrossRef]
5. Jarvis, W.R. The evolving world of healthcare-associated bloodstream infection surveillance and prevention: Is your system as good as you think. *Infect. Control Hosp. Epidemiol.* **2002**, *23*, 236–238. [CrossRef]
6. Choileain, N.N.; Redmond, H.P. Cell response to surgery. *Arch. Surg.* **2006**, *141*, 1132–1140. [CrossRef]
7. Wong, P.H.P.; Krosigk, M.V.; Roscoe, D.L.; Lau, T.T.; Yousefi, M.; Bowie, W.R. Antimicrobial coresistance patterns of gram-negative bacilli isolated from bloodstream infections: A longitudinal epidemiological study from 2002–2011. *BMC Infect. Dis.* **2014**, *14*, 393. [CrossRef]

8. Nwadioha, S.I.; Kashibu, E.; Alao, O.O.; Aliyu, I. Bacterial isolates in blood cultures of children with suspected septicaemia in kano: A two-year study. *Niger. Postgrad. Med. J.* **2011**, *18*, 130–133.
9. Vergnano, S.; Sharland, M.; Kazembe, P.; Mwansambo, C.; Heath, P.T. Neonatal sepsis: An international perspective. *Arch. Dis. Child. Fetal Neonatal Ed.* **2005**, *90*, 220–224. [CrossRef]
10. Majeed, A.; Moser, K. Age-and sex-specific antibiotic prescribing patterns in general practice in england and wales in 1996. *Br. J. Gen. Pract.* **1999**, *49*, 735–736.
11. Holmberg, S.D.; Solomon, S.L.; Blake, P.A. Health and economic impacts of antimicrobial resistance. *Rev. Infect. Dis.* **1987**, *9*, 1065–1078. [CrossRef]
12. Rabirad, N.; Mohammadpoor, M.; Lari, A.R.; Shojaie, A.; Bayat, R.; Alebouyeh, M. Antimicrobial susceptibility patterns of the gram-negative bacteria isolated from septicemia in Children's Medical Center. *J. Prev. Med. Hyg.* **2014**, *55*, 23–26.
13. Dawood, S. American society of clinical oncology 2014: Updates in breast and gastrointestinal cancers. *Indian J. Med. Paediatr. Oncol.* **2014**, *35*, 176–180. [CrossRef]
14. Rudd, K.E.; Johnson, S.C.; Agesa, K.M.; Shackelford, K.A.; Tsoi, D.; Kievlan, D.R.; Naghavi, M. Global, regional, and national sepsis incidence and mortality, 1990–2017: Analysis for the Global Burden of Disease Study. *Lancet* **2020**, *395*, 200–211. [CrossRef]
15. Chaudhry, I.; Chaudhry, N.A.; Muhammad, M.; Raheela, H.; Muhammad, T. Etiological pattern of septicemia at three hospitals in lahore. *J. Coll. Physicians Surg. Pak.* **2000**, *10*, 375–379.
16. Okomo, U.; Akpalu, E.N.; Le Doare, K.; Roca, A.; Cousens, S.; Jarde, A.; Lawn, J.E.A. Etiology of invasive bacterial infection and antimicrobial resistance in neonates in Sub-Saharan Africa: A systematic review and meta-analysis in line with the STROBE-NI reporting guidelines. *Lancet Infect. Dis.* **2019**, *19*, 1219–1234. [CrossRef]
17. Mythri, B.A.; Asha, B.; Patil, A.; Divya, P.M.; Sharon, V.A. Bacteriological profile and antibiogram of neonatal septicemia in a tertiary care hospital. *Indian J. Microbiol. Res.* **2016**, *3*, 136–140. [CrossRef]
18. Mansouri, S.; Chitsaz, M.; Haji, H.R.; Mirzaei, M.; Gheyni, M.H. Determination of resistance pattern of plasmid-mediated Ampc. *Daneshvar Med.* **2009**, *16*, 61–70.
19. Reller, L.B.; Weinstein, M.; Jorgensen, J.H.; Ferraro, M.J. Antimicrobial Susceptibility testing: A review of General Principles and Contemporary Practices. *Clin. Infect. Dis.* **2009**, *49*, 1749–1755.
20. Russotto, V.; Cortegiani, A.; Graziano, G.; Saporito, L.; Raineri, S.M.; Mammina, C.; Giarratano, A. Bloodstream infections in intensive care unit patients: Distribution and antibiotic resistance of bacteria. *Infect. Drug Resist.* **2015**, *8*, 287.
21. Bauer, R.J.; Zhang, L.; Foxman, B.; Siitonen, A.; Jantunen, M.E.; Saxen, H.; Marrs, C.F. Molecular epidemiology of 3 putative virulence genes for escherichia coli urinary tract infection–usp, iha, and Iron (E. Coli). *J. Infect. Dis.* **2002**, *185*, 1521–1524. [CrossRef] [PubMed]
22. Sana, E.M. Antibacterial properties of traditional Sudanese medicinal materials against selected enteric bacterial strains. *Afr. J. Microbiol. Res.* **2020**, *14*, 555–563. [CrossRef]
23. Aryal, S.C.; Upreti, M.K.; Sah, A.K.; Ansari, M.; Nepal, K.; Dhungel, B.; Adhikari, N.; Lekhak, B.; Rijal, K.R. Plasmid-Mediated AmpC β-Lactamase CITM and DHAM Genes among Gram-Negative Clinical Isolates. *Infect. Drug Resist.* **2020**, *13*, 4249–4261. [CrossRef] [PubMed]
24. Gupta, S.; Kashyap, B. Bacteriological profile and antibiogram of blood culture isolates from a tertiary care hospital of North India. *Trop. J. Med. Res.* **2016**, *19*, 94.
25. Velazquez, E.M.; Nguyen, H.; Heasley, K.T.; Saechao, C.H.; Gil, L.M.; Rogers, A.W.; Bäumler, A.J. Endogenous enterobacteriaceae underlie variation in susceptibility to salmonella infection. *Nat. Microbiol.* **2019**, *4*, 1057–1064. [CrossRef]

**Disclaimer/Publisher's Note:** The statements, opinions and data contained in all publications are solely those of the individual author(s) and contributor(s) and not of MDPI and/or the editor(s). MDPI and/or the editor(s) disclaim responsibility for any injury to people or property resulting from any ideas, methods, instructions or products referred to in the content.

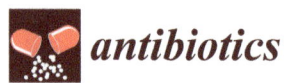 

Article

# The Diversity, Resistance Profiles and Plasmid Content of *Klebsiella* spp. Recovered from Dairy Farms Located around Three Cities in Pakistan

Samia Habib [1], Marjorie J. Gibbon [1], Natacha Couto [1,2], Khadija Kakar [3], Safia Habib [4], Abdul Samad [5], Asim Munir [6], Fariha Fatima [6], Mashkoor Mohsin [6,*] and Edward J. Feil [1,*]

1. The Milner Centre for Evolution, Department of Life Sciences, University of Bath, Bath BA2 7AY, UK
2. Centre for Genomic Pathogen Surveillance, Big Data Institute, University of Oxford, Oxford OX3 7LF, UK
3. Department of Biotechnology, Faculty of Life Sciences & Informatics, Balochistan University of Information Technology, Engineering and Management Sciences, Quetta 08763, Pakistan
4. Sardar Bahadur Khan Womens' University, Quetta 08763, Pakistan
5. Center for Advanced Studies in Vaccinology & Biotechnology (CASVAB), University of Balochistan, Quetta 08763, Pakistan
6. Institute of Microbiology, University of Agriculture, Faisalabad 38000, Pakistan
* Correspondence: mashkoormohsin@uaf.edu.pk (M.M.); e.feil@bath.ac.uk (E.J.F.)

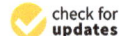

Citation: Habib, S.; Gibbon, M.J.; Couto, N.; Kakar, K.; Habib, S.; Samad, A.; Munir, A.; Fatima, F.; Mohsin, M.; Feil, E.J. The Diversity, Resistance Profiles and Plasmid Content of *Klebsiella* spp. Recovered from Dairy Farms Located around Three Cities in Pakistan. *Antibiotics* 2023, 12, 539. https://doi.org/10.3390/antibiotics12030539

Academic Editor: Andrey Shelenkov

Received: 1 February 2023
Revised: 20 February 2023
Accepted: 6 March 2023
Published: 8 March 2023

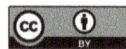

Copyright: © 2023 by the authors. Licensee MDPI, Basel, Switzerland. This article is an open access article distributed under the terms and conditions of the Creative Commons Attribution (CC BY) license (https://creativecommons.org/licenses/by/4.0/).

**Abstract:** The rise of antimicrobial resistance (AMR) in bacterial pathogens such as *Klebsiella pneumoniae* (Kp) is a pressing public health and economic concern. The 'One-Health' framework recognizes that effective management of AMR requires surveillance in agricultural as well as clinical settings, particularly in low-resource regions such as Pakistan. Here, we use whole-genome sequencing to characterise 49 isolates of *Klebisella* spp. (including 43 Kp) and 2 presumptive *Providencia rettgeri* isolates recovered from dairy farms located near 3 cities in Pakistan—Quetta ($n = 29$), Faisalabad ($n = 19$), and Sargodha ($n = 3$). The 43 Kp isolates corresponded to 38 sequence types (STs), and 35 of these STs were only observed once. This high diversity indicates frequent admixture and limited clonal spread on local scales. Of the 49 *Klebsiella* spp. isolates, 41 (84%) did not contain any clinically relevant antimicrobial resistance genes (ARGs), and we did not detect any ARGs predicted to encode resistance to carbapenems or colistin. However, four Kp lineages contained multiple ARGs: ST11 ($n = 2$), ST1391-1LV ($n = 1$), ST995 ($n = 1$) and ST985 ($n = 1$). STs 11, 1391-1LV and 995 shared a core set of five ARGs, including $bla_{CTX-M-15}$, harboured on different AMR plasmids. ST985 carried a different set of 16 resistance genes, including $bla_{CTX-M-55}$. The two presumptive *P. rettgeri* isolates also contained multiple ARGs. Finally, the four most common plasmids which did not harbour ARGs in our dataset were non-randomly distributed between regions, suggesting that local expansion of the plasmids occurs independently of the host bacterial lineage. Evidence regarding how dairy farms contribute to the emergence and spread of AMR in Pakistan is valuable for public authorities and organizations responsible for health, agriculture and the environment, as well as for industrial development.

**Keywords:** *Klebsiella pneumoniae*; One-Health; AMR; plasmids; Pakistan; agriculture

## 1. Introduction

The rise in antimicrobial resistance (AMR) is of pressing concern for public health and food security, and the role of non-clinical settings in the emergence of AMR ('One-Health') has been under increasing scrutiny [1,2]. This perspective is most pertinent in low-resource settings where there is a relatively high level of contact between humans and animals, and where antibiotic usage in agriculture is poorly regulated [3]. A recent report from the UN Environment Program [4] summarized the current evidence concerning the impact of antimicrobial resistance on human health and, specifically, the role of environmental drivers in the development and transmission of AMR between humans and animals. These drivers include antimicrobial usage, microbial diversity and anthropologic factors, in particular, the extent of sanitation infrastructure [5]. The UN report [4] also identifies three economic sectors (pharmaceuticals and other chemicals, agriculture and food, and healthcare) where effective monitoring, disclosure and transparency are critical for targeted interventions and for realigning incentives for AMR management.

Pakistan is an important case in point; more than 70% of the population of Balochistan, in the west of the country, are directly or indirectly involved in raising animals, and large-scale livestock farming is common, contributing to over 60% of agricultural output and over 11% of GDP nationally [6,7]. Moreover, farmers in Pakistan routinely use antibiotics as dietary supplements for livestock [8–10], which can accelerate the emergence and spread of multidrug-resistant (MDR) bacteria in agricultural settings. In addition to commercial losses, this has public health implications as the MDR strains may infect humans, for example, through contaminated food products, and potentially go on to cause outbreaks in healthcare settings. Insufficient monitoring of antibiotic usage and poor molecular surveillance of antimicrobial resistance in Pakistan has led to a paucity of data on the scale of AMR in a 'One Health' context and a weak evidence-base for targeted intervention measures [8].

*Klebsiella pneumoniae* (Kp) commonly colonises the guts of humans and animals as an asymptomatic commensal [11,12]. However, Kp is also an opportunistic pathogen that can cause serious infections in humans and commercially important infection in cows and other livestock. For example, Kp is a common cause of bovine mastitis, which results in significant commercial losses due to the deterioration of the taste, colour and odour of milk. Kp has also been isolated from other animal hosts, including companion animals, poultry, invertebrates and wild birds [13,14].

A key challenge in the fight against AMR is the management of resistance against third generation cephalosporins and carbapenems, conferred by genes encoding extended-spectrum β-lactamases (ESBL) or carbapenemases, respectively. Carbapenem-resistant Kp (CRKP) isolates harbouring $bla_{NDM-1}$ and $bla_{OXA-48}$ genes from clinical, environmental and animal sources have previously been detected in Pakistan [15]. However, whole-genome sequencing (WGS) has not previously been applied to characterise Kp isolates from dairy cattle in Pakistan, and there is almost no evidence regarding the diversity, spread and plasmid content of the Kp population in this context.

In this study, we aimed to generate data on the prevalence and distribution of clinically relevant antimicrobial resistance genes (ARGs) within isolates of *Klebsiella* spp. isolated from healthy dairy cattle representing distinct geographical regions in Pakistan. We generated WGS data for 49 *Klebsiella* genomes (43 Kp) and 2 isolates of *Providencia rettgeri* from dairy cattle. The samples were taken from 10 farms located around 3 cities in Pakistan: Faisalabad, Sargodha and Quetta.

## 2. Methods

### 2.1. Sampling

A total of 150 cattle rectal samples were collected in sterile charcoal swabs from 10 dairy farms with an average herd size of $n > 100$ in Faisalabad, Sargodha and Quetta in Pakistan over a one-month period from January–February 2022. Samples were collected randomly from healthy, lactating dairy cattle. The samples were shipped under refrigerated conditions to the AMR Research lab, Institute of Microbiology, University of Agriculture Faisalabad for culturing and initial processing.

### 2.2. Isolation of Klebsiella spp. and Whole-Genome Sequencing

Samples were enriched in BHI broth supplemented with amoxicillin at concentration of 10 μg/mL for overnight at 37 °C. The enriched samples were streaked on Simmons citrate agar supplemented with amoxicillin and myo-inositol at concentration of 10μg/mL and 10%, respectively (Sigma; SCAI; [16]). Amoxycillin was used to select for *Klebsiella* spp. following Thorpe et al. [14]; we did not select for other resistance phenotypes. The plates were incubated at 37 °C for 48 h. After incubation, presumptive *Klebsiella* colonies were identified on the basis of having a bright yellow colour. One colony per sample was further selected and confirmed via cultivation on UTI ChromoSelect agar (sigmaaldrich.com) at 37 °C for 24 h. After incubation, blue to purple-coloured colonies indicated the growth of *Klebsiella*. A small number of colonies were randomly chosen and further confirmed using the Vitek-2 identification system (https://www.biomerieux-usa.com/ accessed on 1 February 2022). Pure *Klebsiella* colonies were transferred to the UK with a charcoal swab for further analysis. Only a single colony from each sample was selected for sequencing.

Sequencing was carried out on the Illumina platform by MicrobesNG (Birmingham, UK), and run through their standard analysis pipeline (including genome assembly using SPAdes 3.14.4. For full protocols, including DNA extraction, see MicrobesNG Whole Genome Sequencing Service Methods. The quality of the assemblies was verified using different parameters: GC content, number of contigs, total length of assembly and N50.

*2.3. Genome Characterization*

Genome assemblies that passed QC were analysed using Kleborate v0.4.0-beta [17] to assign species and multilocus sequence type, and screened for virulence and resistance genes. Abricate v0.9.8 (https://github.com/tseemann/abricate accessed on 1 February 2022) was used for further screening for resistance genes in the ResFinder database [18] (downloaded 17 August 2022) and virulence factors in the vfdb database (downloaded 18 August 2022). We scored the presence or absence of AMR and virulence genes using a threshold of >80% nucleotide identity and coverage. Short reads were mapped to the genome of Kp isolate PAK-014, which we previously isolated from hospital wastewater in Quetta (unpublished) using Snippy v4.3.6 (https://github.com/tseemann/snippy accessed on 1 February 2022). Snippy results were used as input for FastTree v2.1.11 [19,20] to generate an approximate maximum-likelihood phylogenetic tree. The phylogenetic tree and associated metadata were visualised using Microreact v23.0.0 [21]. Kleborate output was visualised using Kleborate-viz [17].

To determine the plasmid content of the isolates, we used MOB-suite [22] to classify contigs as plasmid-borne or chromosomal. This program uses Mash distances to assign contigs to plasmids according to a closed reference database. We used the default parameters that are already optimised for *Enterobacteriaceae* plasmids. This approach identifies the accession number of the plasmid with the shortest Mash distance to a given set of contigs but, depending on the database, we recognize that substantial size or structural variation may still be present between the query contigs and the returned plasmid.

## 3. Results

*3.1. Species Assignment*

Genomes of 55 presumptive Kp from dairy cows were sequenced as described in Methods. Of these, 4 isolates were excluded because of low-quality assembly and 51 assemblies were taken forward for further analysis (summarised in Table 1 and Table S1). More detail, including the full Kleborate output, the tree and geographical information (including a map) is available via the Microreact project at https://tinyurl.com/37xn4m62, accessed on 6 January 2023. The 51 sequenced isolates were obtained from 7 separate dairy farms in Quetta ($n = 29$), in the west of Pakistan, close to the border with Afghanistan, from 2 dairy farms in Faisalabad in the northeast ($n = 19$), and from one in Sargodha ($n = 3$), which lies around 100 Km to the northwest of Faisalabad. In total, 43 of the genome assemblies were assigned by Kleborate as Kp: 24/29 from Quetta, 16/19 from Faisalabad and 3/3 from Sargodha.

Of the eight isolates that were not identified as Kp, four were *K. similipneumoniae* (three from Quetta, one from Faisalabad) and two were *K. variicola* (both from the same dairy farm in Faisalabad). We also sequenced two isolates, both from the same farm in Quetta, that were assigned as *P. rettgeri* and *Citrobacter amalonaticus*. Whilst the Kleborate species assignment for the *P. rettgeri* isolate is 'strong', and the assembly is of high quality (N50 = 792,114, contig count = 66), for the *C. amalonticus* isolate the species assignment is 'Weak', and the quality of the assembly is lower (N50 = 63,914, contig count = 469). Moreover, the total assembly size for this latter isolate is 9.29 Mb, suggesting that mixed colonies were sequenced. Providencia is in the *Proteus-Morganella* group, whereas *Citrobacter* is more closely related to *Escherichia* and *Shigella*; however, these two isolates are closely related on the tree (Figure S1). We therefore consider it likely that both are, in fact, *P. rettgeri* (Table 1).

**Table 1.** Number of isolates corresponding to each species isolated from 10 different dairy farms in the cities of Quetta, Faisalabad and Sargodha in Pakistan.

| City | Quetta | | | | | | | Sargodha | Faisalabad | |
|---|---|---|---|---|---|---|---|---|---|---|
| Dairy Farm | B | A | T | Al-K | Ak | Bi | Sa | U | SH | L |
| Total samples | 29 | | | | | | | 3 | 19 | |
| Sample size location | 1 | 1 | 6 | 4 | 4 | 7 | 6 | 3 | 16 | 3 |
| K. pneumoniae | 1 | 1 | 5 | 3 | 4 | 6 | 4 | 3 | 13 | 3 |
| K. similipneumoniae | - | - | 1 | 1 | - | 1 | - | - | 1 | - |
| K. variicola | - | - | - | - | - | - | - | - | 2 | - |
| Providencia rettgeri | - | - | - | - | - | - | 2 | - | - | - |

*3.2. Diversity by MLST and Capsule Typing*

Kleborate assigned the 43 Kp strains to 38 distinct STs, all but 3 of which were represented by a single isolate. A phylogenetic tree showing the Kp STs is provided in Figure 1, and a tree for all 51 isolates is provided in Figure S1. The tree is also available to download and explore via the Microreact project at https://tinyurl.com/37xn4m62 (accessed on 1 February 2022). The most common ST among the Kp isolates is ST37, represented by four clonal isolates. A single locus variant of ST37 (ST37-1LV) clusters closely with this clone, and a double locus variant (ST37-2LV) clusters more distantly.

To compare the Kp lineages between different farms and cities, we mapped the origin of the isolates (city and farm) onto the tree on Figure 1. The five isolates corresponding to the ST37 cluster (including the ST37-1LV isolate) were each recovered from different farms, four of which were in Quetta and one from around Faisalabad. Thus, the repeated recovery of this lineage cannot be explained simply by local clonal expansion; instead, this clone has spread between farms and cities. Similarly, the two ST11 isolates were sampled from both Quetta and Sargodha.

Just as very similar isolates are noted from different farms and cities, so a single farm can harbour a high level of diversity. The most striking example of this is the SH farm in Faisalabad, from which 16 Kp isolates were sequenced. Apart from the two isolates of ST1315, every other isolate recovered from this farm corresponded to a distinct ST representing the breadth of the tree (indicated by the green bars in Figure 1). Thus, the diversity of the isolates from this single farm mirrors the diversity present in the whole dataset.

We also considered the diversity of the Kp isolates in terms of capsule type. The *wzi* gene encodes an outer membrane protein involved in cell surface attachment, and its high level of conservation means that it has been used for rapid capsule typing (K typing) [23]. The 43 Kp isolates were represented by 27 different *wzi* allele types, and the distribution of these types was broadly consistent with that observed with MLST (Supplementary Table S1). The most common *wzi* allele was *wzi*14 (5/43, 12%), which corresponded to the cluster of four isolates of ST37 and the ST37-1LV isolate. However, there are also some discrepancies between ST and *wzi* allele. For example, the two ST11 isolates corresponded to *wzi*150, but this allele was also found in the unrelated lineage ST4075. Such a pattern could either reflect homoplasy (the independent emergence of the same *wzi* lineage in different STs) or, more likely, the horizontal transfer of the *wzi* locus.

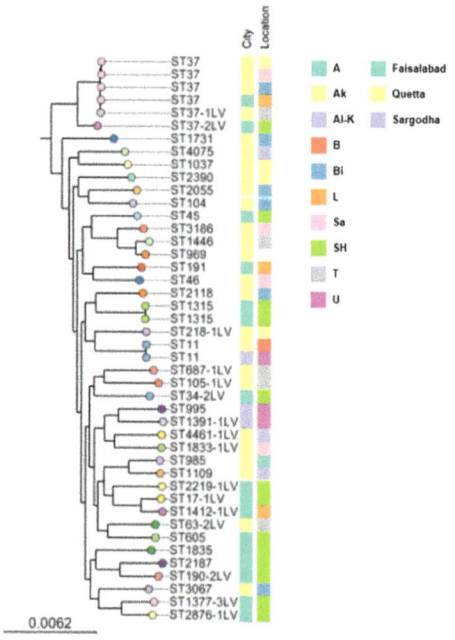

**Figure 1.** Sequence type distribution of *K. pneumoniae* among different dairy cattle farms. The location refers to the specific dairy farm. The data is available to explore via the Microreact project at https://microreact.org/project/iqM31fUDH173HKRxjpEVMi-whole-data-tree. For the exact format used in this figure, see https://microreact.org/project/7cjj9qFE8LbppJsRGXtk8f-st-distributionkp.

Similar patterns were noted with the serotype assignment, with the five isolates of the ST37 cluster being assigned as KL14. Serotypes K1 and K2, associated with hypervirulent strains, were not found, and there were five novel KL types (Supplementary Tables S1 and S2). The most common O-type in the Kp isolates was O2, which was found in the two ST11 isolates and nine other isolates of diverse Kp lineages.

### 3.3. The Presence and Distribution of Antimicrobial Resistance Genes (ARGs)

We used Kleborate and Resfinder to detect ARGs and MOB-suite to assign these ARGs to specific plasmids (see below, and Methods). Overall, the level of resistance was low; we did not detect any carbapenemase genes or genes predicted to confer resistance to colistin. Moreover, we did not detect any ARGs corresponding to the clinically relevant antibiotic classes (AGly, Flq, Sul, Tmt, Bla,, Tet, Rif, Phe, MLS) in 35/43 (81%) of the Kp isolates or in the six isolates of other *Klebsiella* species, (Supplementary Figure S2).

Two Kp isolates (ST37-1LV and ST2118) have acquired single *bla* genes ($bla_{ACT-16}$ and $bla_{CphA2}$, respectively) and the ST37-1LV isolate also contains the *fosA2* gene (predicted to confer fosfomycin resistance). However, more notably, five Kp isolates, representing four lineages, and the two presumptive *P. rettgeri* isolates contain multiple ARGs (Figures 2 and S2). Firstly, the pair of Kp ST11 isolates harbour seven ARGs conferring resistance to aminoglycosides (*aph(3")-Ib*, *aph(6)-Id*), quinolone (*qnrB1*), sulphonamides (*sul2*), trimethoprim (*dfrA14*) and β-Lactamas ($bla_{TEM-1B}$, $bla_{CTX-M-15}$). As mentioned above, the two ST11 isolates were recovered from different cities and the observation that they have identical resistance profiles suggests that they correspond to a ST11 subvariant that may be widely disseminated in Pakistan.

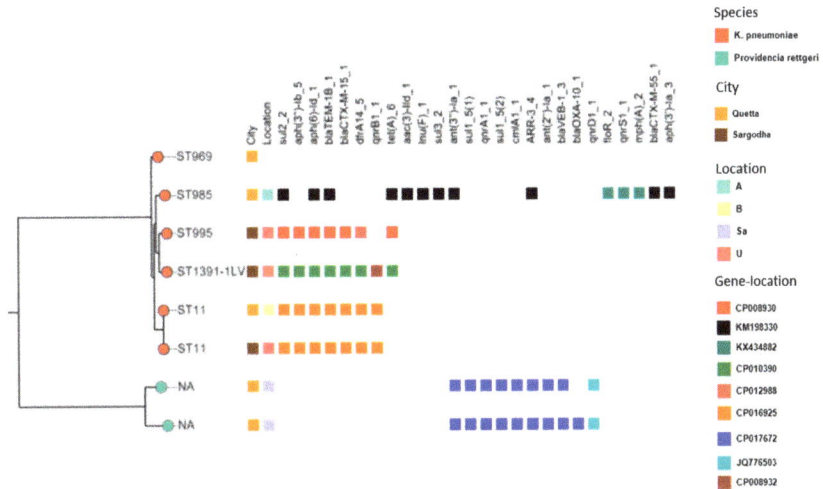

**Figure 2.** Approximate maximum-likelihood phylogenetic tree of the isolates carrying plasmids with linked resistance genes isolated from different dairy farms. The accession number of plasmids identified by MOB-suite (gene-location) and resistance genes identified using Abricate with the ResFinder database are shown. Only plasmids associated with linked resistance genes are included. See also: https://microreact.org/project/qNGWgBKZBEdnzFD6tHLuy5-linked-genes.

The second pair of Kp isolates that share identical ARG profiles are those corresponding to ST995 and ST1391-1LV. These loosely cluster on the tree and were recovered from the same farm in Sargodha. Both harbour the ARG profile of 9 genes resistant to aminoglycosides (*aph(3")-Ib*, *aph(6)-Id*), quinolones (*qnrB1*), sulphonamides (*sul2*), trimethoprim (*dfrA14*), β-Lactams (*bla*$_{SHV-106}$, *bla*$_{TEM-1B}$, *bla*$_{CTX-M-15}$) and tetracyclines (*tet(A)*). The ST985 isolate from Quetta was found to harbour 16 ARGs to aminoglycosides (*aac(3)-IId*, *ant(3")-Ia*, *aph(3')-Ia*, *aph(6)-Id*), quinolones (*qnrS1*), sulphonamide (*sul3*, *sul2*), trimethoprim (*dfrA14*), β-lactams (*bla*$_{TEM-1B}$, *bla*$_{SHV-187}$, *bla*$_{CTX-M-55}$), tetracycline (*tet(A)*), phenicols (*floR*), rifampicin (*ARR-3*) and macrolides (*lnu(F)*, *mph(A)*). Finally, the two presumptive *P. rettgeri* isolates harboured identical ARG profiles with resistance to aminoglycosides (*ant(3")-Ia*, *ant(2")-Ia*), sulphonamide (*sul1*), quinolones (*qnrA1*), chloramphenicol (*cmlA1*), rifampicin (*ARR-3_4*) and β-lactams (*bla*$_{VEB-1}$, *bla*$_{OXA-10}$). These two isolates were recovered from the same farm in Quetta.

### 3.4. The Predicted Plasmid Carriage of ARGs

The observation that different Kp lineages share identical ARG profiles suggests that these resistance traits have been acquired via one or more mobile genetic elements, namely, plasmids. To explore the presence of plasmids in our data, we followed Gibbon et al. [24] and used MOB-suite to assign contigs either as chromosomal, or matching a plasmid within the *Enterobactericae* database (see Section 2). Analysing all 51 genomes, MOB-suite returned a total of 121 plasmids; these corresponded to 71 different accession numbers (because some plasmids were found in more than one isolate) and 19 replicon types. The most common replicon type was IncFIB(K). The distribution of the plasmids and replicon types is shown in Supplementary Figures S3 and S4, respectively, although it is not possible to assign replicon types to specific plasmids. According to MOB-suite, of the 51 isolates, only 5 did not contain any plasmids. A total of 16 isolates contained 1 plasmid, 13 isolates contained 2 plasmids, 7 isolates contained 3 plasmids, 2 isolates contained 4 plasmids, 5 isolates contained 5 plasmids, 3 isolates contained 6 plasmids, and 1 isolate contained 7 plasmids.

Using MOB-suite, we assigned all contigs containing one or more ARG either to a plasmid or to the chromosome. Of the 71 different plasmids, 10 were predicted to contain at least 1 ARG; 8 of these were present in 1 of the 4 lineages containing multiple ARGs—ST11, ST985, ST995 and ST1391-1LV—with the other 2 carried by the presumptive *P. rettgeri* isolates (Figure 2). Seven of the AMR plasmids were predicted to contain multiple ARGs. For three of these plasmids, the set of ARGs were highly similar, with each sharing a core set: *sul2*, *aph(3")-Ib_5*, *aph(6)-Id_1*, *bla*$_{TEM-1B}$ and *bla*$_{CTX-M-15}$. This indicates that these genes are linked on an element that has transferred between plasmids. These three plasmids are present in the multidrug-resistant Kp lineages ST11, ST1391-1LV and ST995, whilst the plasmid in ST985 contains a different set of ARGs.

The two isolates of ST11 harbour a plasmid that matches CP106925 (pCTXM15_DHQP-1400954-like). In addition to the core set of ARGs listed above, this plasmid is also predicted to carry the ARGs *dfrA14* and *qnrB1*. This plasmid, with the same linked ARGs, has previously been found to be associated with diverse Kp lineages (ST1012, ST2167, ST48-1LV and ST495) recovered from clinical samples and wastewater in Quetta, illustrating that it is transmitting freely across the local environment (our unpublished data). Plasmid CP010390 (p6234-like) and plasmid CP008930 (pPMK1-A-like) are carried by the related multidrug-resistant isolates ST1391-1LV and ST995, respectively. These plasmids also contain the same core set of ARGs in addition to *tet*(A). The ST1391-1LV isolate additionally contains *qnrB1*. These two isolates were recovered from the same farm in Sargodha.

The third multidrug-resistant Kp lineage is ST985, which is predicted to harbour a plasmid related to KM198330 (pDGSE139-like). This plasmid harbours at least 11 ARGs, including the ESBL gene *bla*$_{CTX-M-55}$ (but not *bla*$_{CTX-M-15}$), ARR-3 and *lnu*(F). Finally, the two presumptive *P. rettgeri* isolates were predicted to carry plasmid CP017672 (pRB151-NDM-like), which harbours *ant(3")-Ia*, *sul1*, *qnrA1*, *sul1*, *cmlA1*, ARR-3, *ant(2")-Ia*, *blaVEB-1* and *bla*$_{OXA-10}$ (Figure 2).

### 3.5. The Geographical Distribution of Common Plasmids

When considered altogether, the isolates containing multiple ARGs and associated plasmids are present in multiple farms in Quetta, Sargodha and Faisalabad. However, because AMR plasmids are only found in one or two isolates, it is not possible to infer plasmid-specific patterns of spread, both with respect to geographic region or host lineage. We addressed this by considering the distribution of the most common plasmids in our data. Although none of these common plasmids contained ARGs, their prevalence makes it possible to gauge to what extent specific plasmids are circulating between diverse *Klebsiella* lineages at the level of farm or city, or else are randomly distributed (Figure 3). The most common plasmids in the dataset were CP009275 (pKV1-like) ($n = 14$), CP011627 (pCAV1374-14-like) ($n = 7$), CP013713 (J1 plasmid 2-like) ($n = 6$) and CP011633 (pCAV1374-150-like) ($n = 5$). The most common plasmid, CP009275 (pKV1-like), is most similar to one first recorded in a nitrogen fixing strain of *K. variicola* (strain DX120E) isolated from sugar cane in China [25]. This plasmid was not present in either of the two *K. variicola* isolates in our data but was present in all four *K. quasipneumoniae* subsp *pseudopneumoniae* isolates (three from Quetta, and one from Faisalabad) and in ten Kp isolates from four different farms, all in Quetta. Whilst this plasmid has spread between different *Klebsiella* species and diverse Kp lineages on different farms, it shows a non-random distribution with respect to region, as 13/14 isolates carrying this plasmid are from Quetta.

The second, third and fourth most common plasmids in the data also show associations with cities or single farms. CP011627 is present in six diverse Kp STs and the pair of ST1315 isolates. Six of the seven isolates harbouring this plasmid were recovered from the SH farm in Faisalabad, with the exception being from a farm in Quetta. Plasmid CP013713 exhibits a very similar distribution to CP011627; it is present in six Kp isolates (including the pair of ST1315 isolates and three other isolates which also contain CP011627). Five of the six isolates harbouring CP011627 were recovered from the SH farm in Faisalbad, with the exception being from a farm in Quetta. Finally, plasmid CP011633 is present in five

Kp isolates, two of which corresponded to ST37; the other three were from diverse lineages. In this case, all five isolates were recovered from three farms in Quetta. The distribution of these plasmids is summarised in Figure 3.

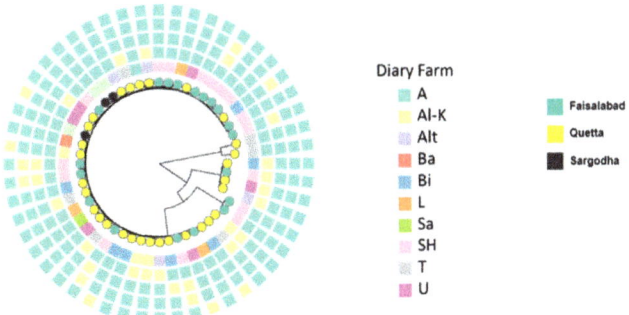

**Figure 3.** Distribution of the four most common plasmids in the *Klebsiella* isolates. The nodes indicate the region of origin (green = Faisalabad, yellow = Quetta, black = Sargodha). The inner ring indicates the specific dairy farm (legend). The next four rings indicate the presence of specific plasmids (yellow = present, green = absent). Moving outwards from the second ring, the plasmids are: CP009275, CP011627, CP013713, CP011633. The distribution of all 71 plasmids in the dataset is provided in Supplementary Figures S3 and S4.

*3.6. Virulence*

Finally, Kleborate also identifies key virulence genes in the genomes. The only virulence gene identified was *ybt*, which encodes the siderophore yersiniabactin. Five Kp isolates harboured chromosomal copies of this gene, including ST11 (both isolates) and the ST985 isolates. These lineages harboured *ybt*14 and 16, respectively. It is of concern that these lineages harbour both virulence and resistance traits. The other two isolates to harbour *ybt* are those corresponding to ST45 and ST2876. No ARGs were identified in these isolates, which were recovered from the SH farm in Faisalabad.

In sum, the WGS data revealed high levels of diversity, evidence of local plasmid spread, and the presence of Kp lineages containing multiple ARGs.

## 4. Discussion

Kp is a priority ESKAPE pathogen, and the prevalence of Kp strains exhibiting resistance to carbapenems and other β-lactam antibiotics has increased steadily on a global scale in recent years [26]. Moreover, the ecological breadth of this species makes it a pertinent model to assess the role of nonclinical settings in the emergence and spread of AMR (the so-called 'One-Health' approach). This framework may be highly informative in Pakistan, where a high level of agricultural activity is combined with poor antibiotic stewardship, and Kp strains resistant to carbapenems and third-generation cephalosporins are known to be circulating in veterinary and farm settings [15,27]. However, WGS has not been deployed on large population samples of Kp from agricultural settings in Pakistan, which makes it impossible to generate a more complete picture of the diversity, the presence of plasmids and other MGEs and the increased phylogenetic resolution for inferring patterns of spread [14]. Here, we begin to address this by presenting an analysis of genome data for 49 *Klebsiella* isolates (43 Kp) and 2 isolates of *P. rettgeri* from 10 dairy farms in the regions of Faisalabad, Sargodha and Quetta. The comparison of three distinct regions is important to understand whether Kp clones are expanding locally on single farms or regions, or whether there are geographical differences regarding the presence of distinct strains.

The data reveal a remarkably high level of diversity within the Kp population; 38 STs were recovered, but only three of these were represented by more than one isolate. This contrasts to comparable studies on European farms, which show much lower levels of Kp diversity due to clonal expansion on single farms [14,28,29]. This fundamental difference suggests that Kp in dairy farms in Pakistan may be more often acquired from diverse environmental sources and/or transmitted more freely between different farms or regions. It is particularly striking that the 16 Kp isolates recovered from the SH farm in Faisalabad correspond to 15 different STs. Whilst this indicates that the tracking of specific clones may not be a valid approach in agricultural settings in Pakistan, our data suggest that specific plasmids are circulating locally. An example is the plasmid CP106925 (pCTXM15_DHQP1400954-like), which carries multiple ARGs and is present in the ST11 isolates. This plasmid has also been noted to be associated with other STs recovered from clinical and environmental settings in Quetta (our unpublished data), which suggests it is circulating in multiple lineages in this region. Given such examples, it is possible that as additional data sets are generated and long-read sequencing becomes more routine, epidemiological surveillance may be more appropriately focused on specific AMR plasmids, rather than the underlying strains.

The majority (84%) of the isolates do not contain major ARGs and, importantly, we did not identify any carbapenemases or predicted colistin resistance. It is important to note that we did not select for resistance to carbapenems or any other antibiotics other than amoxicillin. This was in order to capture the diversity of the underlying Kp population and to gauge the prevalence of AMR. The low prevalence of AMR in our data should, therefore, not be interpreted as indicating that resistance is of negligible importance in these settings. Indeed, we recovered 4 Kp lineages (ST11, ST1391-1LV, ST995 and ST985) that contain between 7 and 16 ARGs, including ESBL-encoding genes. The ST11 and ST985 isolates also contain the important virulence factor *ybt*, which encodes yersiniabactin, although we did not detect the presence of any other key virulence gene, such as *iuc* or *rmp*A.

ST11 is a globally disseminated clone associated with carbapenemases and other resistance genes as well as virulence factors, particularly in Asia [30]. The presence of two isolates of ST11 that possess both multiple resistance and virulence genes is noteworthy given that this lineage has previously been reported from nonclinical settings in Pakistan [27]. We note that the two ST11 isolates in our data correspond to an unknown K-type, with the closest match being KL107. KL107 is common in the closely related healthcare-associated AMR clone ST258 [31], but it is very rare in ST11 [32], indicating that a novel subtype of this global lineage may be circulating in Pakistan. Kp ST37 is the most common clone in our data. Although we did not find this clone to be associated with multiple antibiotic resistance, it is known to be common in clinical and environmental settings globally, and is often associated with ARGs [33].

Although we targeted *Klebsiella* species in this study, we also sequenced two isolates which we consider are likely *P. rettgeri*. Both isolates are predicted to contain a plasmid originally isolated from *P. rettgeri*. *P. rettgeri* is related to insect pathogens, but is an opportunistic pathogen of humans known to cause urinary tract infections, particularly in immunocompromised patients, and is commonly resistant to multiple antibiotics [34]. The sequencing of these two isolates was serendipitous, as they share the same plasmid containing multiple ARGs, including $bla_{OXA-10}$, $bla_{CTX-M-55}$, *lnu*(F)—which encodes resistance to lincosamides (widely used in veterinary medicine)—and ARR-3, encoding resistance to rifampicin. In addition to being a potential public threat to humans, this species could be acting as an important reservoir of ARGs and plasmids and warrants further surveillance.

In conclusion, our study reveals a very high level of diversity among Kp strains circulating within dairy farms in Pakistan and provides evidence that this setting is a potentially significant reservoir of plasmid-borne ARGs. We acknowledge several limitations with our study. Most importantly, we were limited to short-read data and thus not able to generate closed assemblies. This has important consequences for characterising the plasmid content of the isolates. Although MOB-suite was able to identify the best matched plasmids to our contigs, without closed plasmid assemblies it is not possible to validate these inferences, directly compare the plasmids with those previously published or confirm the presence of the ARGs.

Despite these limitations, our analysis highlights the utility of whole-genome sequencing for surveying the prevalence and distribution of ARGs in dairy farms in Pakistan. The study provides valuable benchmark data, paving the way for more large-scale WGS One-Health studies in Pakistan, and raises the question as to whether surveillance is best carried out at the level of strain, ARG or AMR plasmid. The exception of ST11 aside, the high degree of Kp strain diversity uncovered in this study points to the possibility that emerging AMR carriage in dairy farms is not primarily the result of simple clonal spread, and that further focus, specifically on AMR plasmid surveillance in Pakistan, will prove informative.

**Supplementary Materials:** The following supporting information can be downloaded at: https://www.mdpi.com/article/10.3390/antibiotics12030539/s1. Table S1. Serotypes and sequence types of sequenced *Klebsiella* spp. Isolates; Table S2. Kleborate mean resistance and virulence scores of Pakistan's animal data compared to a global dataset; Figure S1. Species diversity and distribution in cattle from ten different dairy farms in Quetta, Faisalabad, and Sargodha city, Pakistan; Figure S2. AMR distribution among species; Figure S3. Approximate maximum likelihood phylogenetic tree (midpoint rooted) of the 51 isolates analysed; Figure S4. Distribution of replicons among species.

**Author Contributions:** S.H. (Samia Habib) drove the analysis of the data and preparing the paper. M.J.G. and N.C. contributed to the data analysis and preparation of the paper. K.K., S.H. (Safia Habib), A.S., A.M. and F.F. helped with sampling, microbiology and strain transportation. M.M. and E.J.F. were responsible for study design, analysis and paper preparation. All authors have read and agreed to the published version of the manuscript.

**Funding:** SamH is sponsored by a Schlumberger Foundation Faculty for the Future Fellowship. Additional funding was provided by grant MR/S004769/1 (OH-DART) from the Antimicrobial Resistance Cross Council Initiative supported by the seven United Kingdom research councils and the National Institute for Health Research. The APC was funded by the University of Bath.

**Institutional Review Board Statement:** Not Applicable.

**Informed Consent Statement:** Not Applicable.

**Data Availability Statement:** The genome data have been deposited under BioProject ID PRJNA935981.

**Acknowledgments:** Computational resources were provided by CLIMB-BIGDATA (https://www.climb.ac.uk/, accessed on 6 January 2023).

**Conflicts of Interest:** The authors declare no conflict of interest.

# References

1. Robinson, T.P.; Bu, D.P.; Carrique-Mas, J.; Fèvre, E.M.; Gilbert, M.; Grace, D.; Hay, S.I.; Jiwakanon, J.; Kakkar, M.; Kariuki, S.; et al. Antibiotic resistance is the quintessential One Health issue. *Trans. R. Soc. Trop. Med. Hyg.* **2016**, *110*, 377–380. [CrossRef] [PubMed]
2. Walsh, T.R. A one-health approach to antimicrobial resistance. *Nat. Microbiol.* **2018**, *3*, 854–855. [CrossRef] [PubMed]
3. Ikhimiukor, O.O.; Odih, E.E.; Donado-Godoy, P.; Okeke, I.N. A bottom-up view of antimicrobial resistance transmission in developing countries. *Nat. Microbiol.* **2022**, *7*, 757–765. [CrossRef] [PubMed]
4. UNEP-UN Environment Programme. Report. Bracing for Superbugs: Strengthening Environmental Action in the One Health Response to Antimicrobial Resistance. 2023. Available online: https://www.unep.org/resources/superbugs/environmental-action (accessed on 6 January 2023).
5. Collignon, P.; Beggs, J.J.; Walsh, T.R.; Gandra, S.; Laxminarayan, R. Anthropological and socioeconomic factors contributing to global antimicrobial resistance: A univariate and multivariable analysis. *Lancet Planet. Health. Elsevier* **2018**, *2*, e398–e405. [CrossRef] [PubMed]
6. Fazl, E.; Haider, S. Balochistan's Potential Livestock Sector–Need of Innovative Investment Plan. Pakistan & Gulf Economist. Available online: https://www.pakistangulfeconomist.com/2018/09/03/balochistans-potential-livestock-sector-need-of-innovative-investment-plan/ (accessed on 6 January 2023).
7. Wasim, A. No Change in Population of Camels, Horses and Mules. Dawn. Available online: https://www.dawn.com/news/1562879 (accessed on 6 January 2023).
8. Ur Rahman, S.; Mohsin, M. The under reported issue of antibiotic-resistance in food-producing animals in Pakistan. *Pak. Vet. J.* **2019**, *1*, 1–16.
9. Qamar, A.; Ismail, T.; Akhtar, S. Prevalence and antibiotic resistance of *Salmonella* spp. in South Punjab-Pakistan. *PLoS ONE* **2020**, *15*, e0232382. [CrossRef]

10. Umair, M.; Tahir, M.F.; Ullah, R.W.; Ali, J.; Siddique, N.; Rasheed, A.; Akram, M.; Zaheer, M.U.; Mohsin, M. Quantification and Trends of Antimicrobial Use in Commercial Broiler Chicken Production in Pakistan. *Antibiotics* **2021**, *10*, 598. [CrossRef]
11. Wyres, K.L.; Holt, K.E. Klebsiella pneumoniae as a key trafficker of drug resistance genes from environmental to clinically important bacteria. *Curr. Opin. Microbiol.* **2018**, *45*, 131–139. [CrossRef]
12. Wyres, K.L.; Lam, M.M.C.; Holt, K.E. Population genomics of *Klebsiella pneumoniae*. *Nat. Rev. Microbiol.* **2020**, *18*, 344–359. [CrossRef]
13. Ahlstrom, C.A.; Woksepp, H.; Sandegren, L.; Mohsin, M.; Hasan, B.; Muzyka, D.; Hernandez, J.; Aguirre, F.; Tok, A.; Söderman, J.; et al. Genomically diverse carbapenem resistant Enterobacteriaceae from wild birds provide insight into global patterns of spatiotemporal dissemination. *Sci. Total. Environ.* **2022**, *824*, 153632. [CrossRef]
14. Thorpe, H.A.; Booton, R.; Kallonen, T.; Gibbon, M.J.; Couto, N.; Passet, V.; López-Fernández, S.; Rodrigues, C.; Matthews, L.; Mitchell, S.; et al. A large-scale genomic snapshot of Klebsiella spp. isolates in Northern Italy reveals limited transmission between clinical and non-clinical settings. *Nat. Microbiol.* **2022**, *7*, 2054–2067. [CrossRef]
15. Chaudhry, T.H.; Aslam, B.; Arshad, M.I.; Alvi, R.F.; Muzammil, S.; Yasmeen, N.; Aslam, M.A.; Khurshid, M.; Rasool, M.H.; Baloch, Z. Emergence of bla NDM-1 Harboring Klebsiella pneumoniae ST29 and ST11 in Veterinary Settings and Waste of Pakistan. *Infect. Drug. Resist.* **2020**, *13*, 3033–3043. [CrossRef]
16. Van Kregten, E.; Westerdaal, N.A.; Willers, J.M. New, simple medium for selective recovery of *Klebsiella pneumoniae* and *Klebsiella oxytoca* from human feces. *J. Clin. Microbiol.* **1984**, *20*, 936–941. [CrossRef]
17. Lam, M.M.; Wick, R.R.; Watts, S.C.; Cerdeira, L.T.; Wyres, K.L.; Holt, K.E. A genomic surveillance framework and genotyping tool for *Klebsiella pneumoniae* and its related species complex. *Nat. Commun.* **2021**, *12*, 4188. [CrossRef]
18. Florensa, A.F.; Kaas, R.S.; Clausen, P.T.L.; Aytan-Aktug, D.; Aarestrup, F.M. ResFinder—an open online resource for identification of antimicrobial resistance genes in next-generation sequencing data and prediction of phenotypes from genotypes. *Microbial. Genom.* **2022**, *8*, 000748. [CrossRef]
19. Price, M.N.; Dehal, P.S.; Arkin, A.P. FastTree: Computing large minimum evolution trees with profiles instead of a distance matrix. *Mol. Biol. Evol.* **2009**, *26*, 1641–1650. [CrossRef]
20. Price, M.N.; Dehal, P.S.; Arkin, A.P. FastTree 2—Approximately maximum-likelihood trees for large alignments. *PLoS ONE* **2010**, *5*, e9490. [CrossRef]
21. Argimón, S.; Abudahab, K.; Goater, R.J.E.; Fedosejev, A.; Bhai, J.; Glasner, C. Microreact: Visualizing and sharing data for genomic epidemiology and phylogeography. *Microb. Genom.* **2016**, *2*, e000093. [CrossRef]
22. Robertson, J.; Bessonov, K.; Schonfeld, J.; Nash, J.H.E. Universal whole-sequence-based plasmid typing and its utility to prediction of host range and epidemiological surveillance. *Microb. Genom.* **2020**, *6*, 10. [CrossRef]
23. Brisse, S.; Passet, V.; Haugaard, A.B.; Babosan, A.; Kassis-Chikhani, N.; Struve, C.; Decré, D. Gene sequencing, a rapid method for determination of capsular type for *Klebsiella strains*. *J. Clin. Microbiol.* **2013**, *51*, 4073–4078. [CrossRef]
24. Gibbon, M.J.; Couto, N.; David, S.; Barden, R.; Standerwick, R.; Jagadeesan, K.; Birkwood, H.; Dulyayangkul, P.; Avison, M.B.; Kannan, A.; et al. A high prevalence of blaOXA-48 in Klebsiella (Raoultella) ornithinolytica and related species in hospital wastewater in South West England. *Microb. Genom.* **2021**, *7*, mgen000509. [CrossRef] [PubMed]
25. Lin, L.; Wei, C.; Chen, M.; Wang, H.; Li, Y.; Li, Y.; Yang, L.; An, Q. Complete genome sequence of endophytic nitrogen-fixing *Klebsiella variicola* strain DX120E. *Stand Genom. Sci.* **2015**, *10*, 22. [CrossRef] [PubMed]
26. Tacconelli, E.; Carrara, E.; Savoldi, A.; Harbarth, S.; Mendelson, M.; Monnet, D.L.; Pulcini, C.; Kahlmeter, G.; Kluytmans, J.; Carmeli, Y.; et al. Discovery, research, and development of new antibiotics: The WHO priority list of antibiotic-resistant bacteria and tuberculosis. *Lancet. Infect. Dis.* **2018**, *18*, 318–327. [CrossRef] [PubMed]
27. Aslam, B.; Chaudhry, T.H.; Arshad, M.I.; Muzammil, S.; Siddique, A.B.; Yasmeen, N.; Khurshid, M.; Amir, A.; Salman, M.; Rasool, M.H.; et al. Distribution and genetic diversity of multi-drug-resistant Klebsiella pneumoniae at the human-animal-environment interface in Pakistan. *Front. Microbiol.* **2022**, *13*, 898248. [CrossRef] [PubMed]
28. Ludden, C.; Moradigaravand, D.; Jamrozy, D.; Gouliouris, T.; Blane, B.; Naydenova, P.; Hernandez-Garcia, J.; Wood, P.; Hadjirin, N.; Radakovic, M.; et al. A One Health Study of the Genetic Relatedness of *Klebsiella pneumoniae* and Their Mobile Elements in the East of England. *Clin. Infect. Dis.* **2020**, *70*, 219–226. [CrossRef]
29. Schubert, H.; Morley, K.; Puddy, E.F.; Arbon, R.; Findlay, J.; Mounsey, O.; Gould, V.C.; Vass, L.; Evans, M.; Rees, G.M.; et al. Reduced Antibacterial Drug Resistance and blaCTX-M β-Lactamase Gene Carriage in Cattle-Associated *Escherichia coli* at Low Temperatures, at Sites Dominated by Older Animals, and on Pastureland: Implications for Surveillance. *Appl. Environ. Microbiol.* **2021**, *87*, 6. [CrossRef]
30. Liao, W.; Liu, Y.; Zhang, W. Virulence evolution, molecular mechanisms of resistance and prevalence of ST11 carbapenem-resistant *Klebsiella pneumoniae* in China: A review over the last 10 years. *J. Glob. Antimicrob. Resist.* **2020**, *23*, 174–180. [CrossRef]
31. Yu, F.; Lv, J.; Niu, S.; Du, H.; Tang, Y.W.; Pitout, J.D.; Bonomo, R.A.; Kreiswirth, B.N.; Chen, L. Multiplex PCR Analysis for Rapid Detection of *Klebsiella pneumoniae* Carbapenem-Resistant (Sequence Type 258 [ST258] and ST11) and Hypervirulent (ST23, ST65, ST86, and ST375) Strains. *J. Clin. Microbiol.* **2018**, *56*, 9. [CrossRef]
32. Zhao, J.; Liu, C.; Liu, Y.; Zhang, Y.; Xiong, Z.; Fan, Y.; Zou, X.; Lu, B.; Cao, B. Genomic characteristics of clinically important ST11 *Klebsiella pneumoniae* strains worldwide. *J. Glob. Antimicrob. Resist.* **2020**, *22*, 519–526. [CrossRef]

33. Rocha, J.; Henriques, I.; Gomila, M.; Manaia, C.M. Common and distinctive genomic features of *Klebsiella pneumoniae* thriving in the natural environment or in clinical settings. *Sci. Rep.* **2022**, *12*, 10441. [CrossRef]
34. Abdallah, M.; Balshi, A. First literature review of carbapenem-resistant Providencia. *New Microbes New Infect.* **2018**, *25*, 16–23. [CrossRef]

**Disclaimer/Publisher's Note:** The statements, opinions and data contained in all publications are solely those of the individual author(s) and contributor(s) and not of MDPI and/or the editor(s). MDPI and/or the editor(s) disclaim responsibility for any injury to people or property resulting from any ideas, methods, instructions or products referred to in the content.

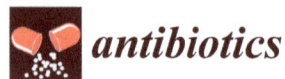 

Article

# Genomic Analysis of a Hybrid Enteroaggregative Hemorrhagic *Escherichia coli* O181:H4 Strain Causing Colitis with Hemolytic-Uremic Syndrome

Angelina A. Kislichkina [1,*], Nikolay N. Kartsev [2], Yury P. Skryabin [2], Angelika A. Sizova [1], Maria E. Kanashenko [2], Marat G. Teymurazov [2], Ekaterina S. Kuzina [3], Alexander G. Bogun [1], Nadezhda K. Fursova [2], Edward A. Svetoch [2] and Ivan A. Dyatlov [1,2,3]

[1] Department of Culture Collection, State Research Center for Applied Microbiology and Biotechnology, Territory "Kvartal A", 142279 Obolensk, Russia
[2] Department of Molecular Microbiology, State Research Center for Applied Microbiology and Biotechnology, Territory "Kvartal A", 142279 Obolensk, Russia
[3] Department of Training and Improvement of Specialists, State Research Center for Applied Microbiology and Biotechnology, Territory "Kvartal A", 142279 Obolensk, Russia
* Correspondence: angelinakislichkina@yandex.ru

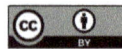

Citation: Kislichkina, A.A.; Kartsev, N.N.; Skryabin, Y.P.; Sizova, A.A.; Kanashenko, M.E.; Teymurazov, M.G.; Kuzina, E.S.; Bogun, A.G.; Fursova, N.K.; Svetoch, E.A.; et al. Genomic Analysis of a Hybrid Enteroaggregative Hemorrhagic *Escherichia coli* O181:H4 Strain Causing Colitis with Hemolytic-Uremic Syndrome. *Antibiotics* 2022, 11, 1416. https://doi.org/10.3390/antibiotics11101416

Academic Editor: Jonathan Frye

Received: 21 September 2022
Accepted: 13 October 2022
Published: 14 October 2022

**Publisher's Note:** MDPI stays neutral with regard to jurisdictional claims in published maps and institutional affiliations.

**Copyright:** © 2022 by the authors. Licensee MDPI, Basel, Switzerland. This article is an open access article distributed under the terms and conditions of the Creative Commons Attribution (CC BY) license (https://creativecommons.org/licenses/by/4.0/).

**Abstract:** Hybrid diarrheagenic *E. coli* strains combining genetic markers belonging to different pathotypes have emerged worldwide and have been reported as a public health concern. The most well-known hybrid strain of enteroaggregative hemorrhagic *E. coli* is *E. coli* O104:H4 strain, which was an agent of a serious outbreak of acute gastroenteritis and hemolytic uremic syndrome (HUS) in Germany in 2011. A case of intestinal infection with HUS in St. Petersburg (Russian Federation) occurred in July 2018. *E. coli* strain SCPM-O-B-9427 was obtained from the rectal swab of the patient with HUS. It was determined as O181:H4-, *stx2*-, and *aggR*-positive and belonged to the phylogenetic group B2. The complete genome assembly of the strain SCPM-O-B-9427 contained one chromosome and five plasmids, including the plasmid coding an aggregative adherence fimbriae I. MLST analysis showed that the strain SCPM-O-B-9427 belonged to ST678, and like *E. coli* O104:H4 strains, 2011C-3493 caused the German outbreak in 2011, and 2009EL-2050 was isolated in the Republic of Georgia in 2009. Comparison of three strains showed almost the same structure of their chromosomes: the plasmids pAA and the *stx2a* phages are very similar, but they have distinct sets of the plasmids and some unique regions in the chromosomes.

**Keywords:** *Escherichia coli*; hybrid pathotype; EHEC; EAHEC; O181

## 1. Introduction

*Escherichia coli* is a bacterium that is widely distributed as a free-living in the environment and as an important member of the large intestine microbiota in humans and warm-blooded animals [1,2]. Although most *E. coli* are harmless commensals, some strains of this species are pathogenic and can induce diseases in humans and animals [3]. Human-pathogenic *E. coli* strains exhibit a wide spectrum of clinical manifestations, which are dependent on the virulence factors [4]. The *E. coli* genome is characterized by genetic mosaicism, high variability, and the ability to exchange genetic information [5]. In most cases, this exchange is carried out by the horizontal transfer of the bacterial mobile genetic elements such as plasmids, transposons, pathogenicity islands, and bacteriophages [6,7]. Pathogenic *E. coli*, according to their localization in the macro-organism and generated pathological processes, are divided into diarrheagenic (DEC) and extraintestinal (ExPEC) pathogens [8,9]. Seven pathotypes have been described for the DEC group, including enteropathogenic *E. coli* (EPEC), enterohaemorrhagic *E. coli* (EHEC), enterotoxigenic *E. coli* (ETEC), enteroinvasive *E. coli* (EIEC), enteroaggregative *E. coli* (EAEC), diffusely adherent

E. coli (DAEC), and adherent-Invasive E. coli (AIEC), based on their virulence mechanisms, associated clinical symptoms, and consequences [10]. E. coli of different pathotypes contains the specific combinations of virulence genetic determinants located in the chromosome and plasmids [10,11].

Improvements in techniques allowing the better understanding of the genomic and virulence mechanisms among diarrheagenic E. coli led to detecting atypical hybrid E. coli strains combining genetic markers of different pathotypes [12–14]. Hybrid DEC strains carrying various combinations of virulence factors have emerged worldwide and have been reported as a public health concern [15]. The most well-known example is the E. coli O104:H4 strain, which caused a serious outbreak of acute gastroenteritis and hemolytic uremic syndrome (HUS) in Germany in 2011 [16]. This strain produced a Shiga toxin 2 (Stx2), a signature feature of the EHEC pathotype, and additionally carried a plasmid containing the genes coding to the aggregative adherence fimbriae (AAF)-mediating aggregative adherence in EAEC [17]. This bacterium was considered as a hybrid novel genetic lineage: enteroaggregative hemorrhagic E. coli (EAHEC) [18]. Even earlier, several cases of HUS and bloody diarrhea occurred in the Republic of Georgia in 2009, which were caused by stx2-positive E. coli strains of O104:H4 [19]. Comparative genome analysis showed that the Georgian strains were the nearest neighbors to the agents of the outbreak in 2011; only several structural and nucleotide differences were detected in the stx2 phage genomes, the mer/tet antibiotic resistance island, and in the prophage and plasmid profiles of the strains [20]. A case of intestinal infection with HUS happened in St. Petersburg (Russian Federation) in July 2018. The pathogenic E. coli strain was obtained from the rectal swab of a patient with HUS. The strain was identified as E. coli O181:H4-, stx2- and aggR-positive. This genetic profiling indicated that the studied E. coli belonged to EAEC and EHEC at the same time. It was positive for the chuA gene and for the fragment of TspE4.C2, which made it possible to assign them to the B2 phylogenetic group. In general, E. coli strains of the B2 phylogenetic group carry more virulence factors compared with the strains belonging to other phylogenetic groups (A, B1, D), which are associated with a more pronounced ability to colonize intestinal mucosa [21].

E. coli serogroup O181 is a relatively new; it was included in the serotyping scheme for E. coli in 2004 [22]. Sporadically, E. coli O181 were isolated from the patients with diarrhea, from meats and meat products, as well as from livestock wastewater and environmental objects [23–26]. The aim of this work is to characterize the genetic properties of the new hybrid enteroaggregative and Shiga-toxin-producing E. coli strain of O181:H4, which was isolated from the patient with HUS in Saint Petersburg, Russian Federation, in 2018.

## 2. Results

### 2.1. Bacterial Strain, Pathotype Identification, and Susceptibility to Antimicrobials

The E. coli clinical strain SCPM-O-B-9427 was isolated from a rectal swab of the patient with HUS in Saint Petersburg, Russian Federation, in 2018, and deposited in the State Collection of Pathogenic Microorganisms and Cell Cultures "SCPM-Obolensk". Pathotype identification revealed that this strain belonged to both EHEC and EAEC (EAHEC), according to commercial assay AmpliSens® Escherichioses-FRT and because it carried both stx and aggR genes, according to The European Union Reference Laboratory method. Multiplex PCR for phylogroup identification was positive for the chuA gene and for the fragment of TspE4.C2, which allows to assign the strain SCPM-O-B-9427 to the B2 phylogenetic group.

The strain SCPM-O-B-9427 was susceptible to amoxicillin/clavulanic acid, cefotaxime, ceftazidime, cefoperazone/sulbactam, cefepime, aztreonam, imipenem, meropenem, amikacin, gentamicin, netilmicin, fosfomycin, nitrofurantoin, and trimethoprim/sulfamethoxazole and resistant to ampicillin and ciprofloxacin (Table 1).

**Table 1.** Antimicrobial susceptibility of EAHEC strain SCPM-O-B-9427.

| Antimicrobials | MIC, mg/L | Interpretation |
|---|---|---|
| Ampicillin | 16 | R [1] |
| Amoxicillin/clavulanic acid | 4 | S [2] |
| Cefotaxime | ≤1 | S |
| Ceftazidime | ≤1 | S |
| Cefoperazone/sulbactam | ≤8 | S |
| Cefepime | ≤1 | S |
| Aztreonam | ≤1 | S |
| Imipenem | ≤1 | S |
| Meropenem | ≤0.25 | S |
| Amikacin | ≤2 | S |
| Gentamicin | ≤1 | S |
| Netilmicin | 2 | S |
| Ciprofloxacin | 1 | R |
| Fosfomycin | ≤16 | S |
| Nitrofurantoin | ≤16 | S |
| Trimethoprim/sulfamethoxazole | ≤20 | S |

[1] Resistant; [2] susceptible.

## 2.2. Genomic Characteristics of EAHEC Strain SCPM-O-B-9427

The complete genome assembly of the strain SCPM-O-B-9427 contained one chromosome and five plasmids, one of which is homologous with virulence plasmid pAA–pSCPM-O-B-9427-2, encoding an aggregative adherence fimbria I (AAF/I). The major genomic characteristics are summarized in Table 2 and are shown in comparison to two hybrid EAHEC strains of O104:H4: 2011C-3493, which caused large German outbreak in 2011, and 2009EL-2050, which caused the group outbreak in 2009 in Georgia. The chromosome sizes of the strains are comparable and slightly different, with identical GC content. The total numbers of genes, including RNA genes, are about the same amount, but the chromosome of the strain SCPM-O-B-9427 contained more pseudogenes.

**Table 2.** Major genome characteristics of the EAHEC strains SCPM-O-B-9427, 2011C-3493, and 2009EL-2050.

| Feature/Strain | SCPM-O-B-9427 | 2011C-3493 | 2009EL-2050 |
|---|---|---|---|
| GenBank chromosome | CP086259 | CP003289 | CP003297 |
| Region | Russian Federation | Germany | Georgia |
| Isolation year | 2018 | 2011 | 2009 |
| Serotype | O181:H4 | O104:H4 | O104:H4 |
| ST | ST678 | ST678 | ST678 |
| *stx* subtype | 2a | 2a | 2a |
| *aggDCBA* cluster | + | + | + |
| Chromosome size, bp | 5,268,110 | 5,273,097 | 5,253,138 |
| GC content of chromosome, % | 50.7 | 50.7 | 50.7 |
| Genes (total) | 5408 | 5314 | 5325 |
| CDS (total) | 5283 | 5191 | 5197 |
| Genes (RNA) | 125 | 123 | 128 |
| rRNAs | 8, 7, 7 (5S, 16S, 23S) | 8, 7, 7 (5S, 16S, 23S) | 8, 7, 7 (5S, 16S, 23S) |
| tRNAs | 95 | 92 | 97 |
| Pseudogenes (total) | 297 | 227 | 237 |
| Plasmids | - | - | p09EL50 (109,274 bp) |
|  | pB-9427-1 (83,340 bp) | pESBL-EA11 (88,544 bp) | - |
|  | pB-9427-2 (75,544 bp) | pAA-EA11 (74,213 bp) | pAA-09EL50 (74,213 bp) |
|  | pB-9427-3 (51,013 bp) | - | - |
|  | pB-9427-4 (7939 bp) | - | - |
|  | pB-9427-5 (6728 bp) | - | - |
|  | - | pG-EA11 (1549 bp) | pG-09EL50 (1549 bp) |

Note: ST, sequence type; CDS, coding sequence.

## 2.3. Genotypic Profiling of the EAHEC Strain SCPM-O-B-9427

Genoserotyping of the strain SCPM-O-B-9427 was performed by extracting the sequences of the *wzx* gene (identity 100%, AB812078) and *wzy* gene (identity 99.92%, AB812078), which confirmed the affiliation of *E. coli* SCPM-O-B-9427 with the serogroup O181. The *fliC* gene was assigned to the type H4 (identity 100%, AJ605764). The *stxA* and *stxB* genes coding Shiga toxin Stx2a subunits A and B (identity 100%, LC645441), cluster genes *aggDCBA* coding the aggregative adhesion fimbriae (AAF), and the transcriptional activator *aggR* (identity 100%, CP003291) were detected in the genome.

In silico multi-locus sequence typing (MLST) based on seven loci of house-keeping genes by the Achtman's MLST scheme database (*adk_6*, *fumC_6*, *gyrB_5*, *icd_136*, *mdh_9*, *purA_7*, *recA_7*) showed the strain SCPM-O-B-9427 belonging to ST678 [27]. The same sequence type was identified for the strain *E. coli* 2011C-3493 O104:H4 that caused the large German outbreak in 2011 and for the strain *E. coli* 2009EL-2050 O104:H4 that was isolated in the Republic of Georgia, in 2009.

Several chromosomal-located virulence genes were identified in the strain SCPM-O-B-9427 as well as in the genomes of two above-named EAHEC strains of O104:H4. The strain SCPM-O-B-9427 was positive for *aaiC* gene (coding type VI secretion protein), *capU* (hexosyltransferase homolog), *fyuA* (siderophore receptor), *gad* (glutamate decarboxylase), *iha* (adherence protein), *irp2* (high-molecular-weight protein 2 non-ribosomal peptide synthetase), *iucC* (aerobactin synthetase), *iutA* (ferric aerobactin receptor), *lpfA* (long polar fimbriae), *pic* (serine protease autotransporters of Enterobacteriaceae, SPATE), *sigA* (serine protease), and *terC* (tellurium ion resistance protein). However, the differences between three EAHEC strains were found: compared to the strains of O104:H4, the strain SCPM-O-B-9427 is negative for the *neuC* gene coding the polysialic acid capsule biosynthesis protein; and the strain 2011C-3493 is negative for the *bor* gene coding the serum resistance lipoprotein, while the strains SCPM-O-B-9427 and 2009EL-2050 are positive. In addition to the *aggDCBA* cluster and *aggR* regulator gene, other EAEC genetic determinants were detected in all three EAHEC strains: *sepA* gene (Shigella extracellular protein A), *aap* gene (dispersin), and *aat* operon (factor of adhesion). Other *E. coli* virulence genes such as *fimH*, *sfa*, *papA*, *hylA*, *cnfl*, *aer*, and *afaC* were not detected.

## 2.4. Chromosomal SNPs in the EAHEC Strains SCPM-O-B-9427, 2011C-3493, and 2009EL-2050

Chromosomes of the strains SCPM-O-B-9427, 2011C-3493, and 2009EL-2050 were compared using Snippy software for detailed genomic analysis. A comparison between the strains SCPM-O-B-9427 and 2011C-3493 revealed 1326 SNPs (959 synonymous, 242 non-synonymous, and 125 intergenic) and 26 insertions and deletions; 19 of them were intergenic. On the contrary, the difference between SCPM-O-B-9427 and 2009EL-2050 chromosomes was significantly less: 1053 SNPs were identified (793 synonymous, 180 non-synonymous, and 80 intergenic) as well as 20 insertions and deletions, and 14 of them were intergenic. Revealed SNPs were not evenly distributed along the chromosome but clustered in a few regions; the biggest one was the region coding lipopolysaccharide synthesis. The distribution of SNPs, insertions, deletions, and the chromosome complex of the strain SCPM-O-B-9427 compared to the strains 2011C-3493 and 2009EL-2050 is shown in Figure 1.

## 2.5. Chromosomal Structural Comparison of the Strains SCPM-O-B-9427, 2011C-3493, and 2009EL-2050

We studied the chromosomal architectures of the hybrid EAHEC strains SCPM-O-B-9427, 2009EL-2050, and 2011C-3493, which are very similar in overall structure, without rearrangements detected using Artemis (Figure 2). However, significant differences between genomes were revealed consisting of one extended inverted region in the genome of the strain SCPM-O-B-9427 and unique regions for each of three EAHEC strains. The features of non-homologous unique regions of the strains SCPM-O-B-9427, 2009EL-2050, and 2011C-3493 are listed in Table 3. The region R1 of the strain SCPM-O-B-9427 is not homologous to the same regions of the strains 2011C-3493 and 2009EL-2050. Since the strains belong to different serogroups, the region R2 carries genes are involved in lipopolysaccharide synthesis (O104 and O181 antigen gene clusters).

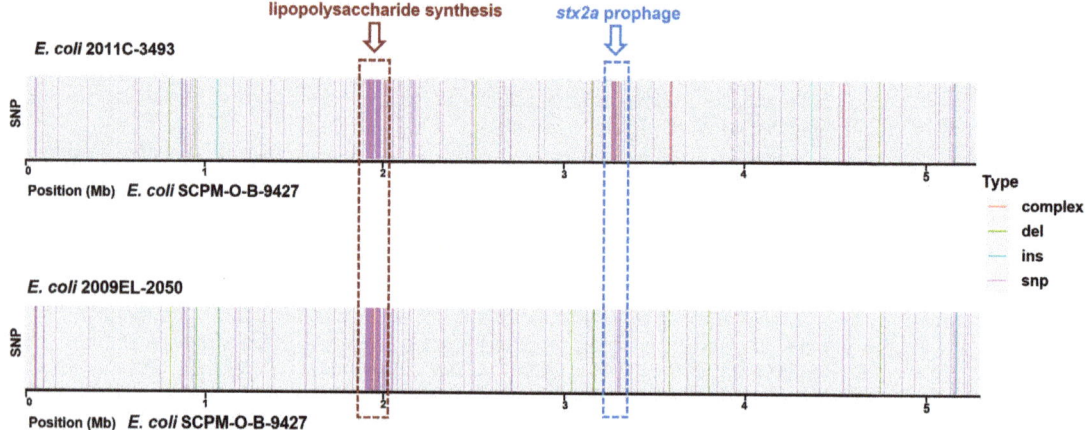

**Figure 1.** Distribution of the sequence variations at a genomic position. Chromosome mapping of EAHEC strains 2011C-3493 and 2009EL-2050 was performed against of the strain SCPM-O-B-9427 chromosome.

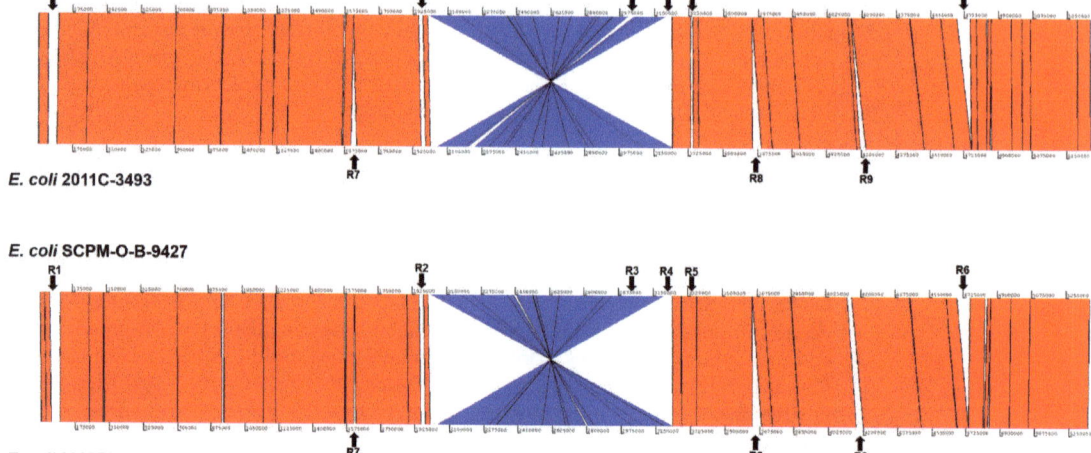

**Figure 2.** The Artemis comparison of the strain SCPM-O-B-9427 chromosome with chromosomes of the strains 2009EL-2050 and 2011C-3493. Red vertical lines correspond to the regions that are highly homologous and are oriented in the same order, and blue vertical lines depict a region whose orientation is reversed between strains. Arrows on the top and bottom indicate white lines showing that unique regions are non-homologous or are absent in another strain.

Table 3. Feature of unique regions of EAHEC strains SCPM-O-B-9427, 2009EL-2050, and 2011C-3493 detected using Artemis.

| Region | Sequence, Kbp/GC Content. % | | | Note |
| --- | --- | --- | --- | --- |
| | SCPM-O-B-9427 | 2009EL-2050 | 2011C-3493 | |
| R1 | 52.0/47.5 | 45.0/56.5 | 44.5/56.8 | Part of R1 are incomplete prophages and in the strain SCPM-O-B-9427 are related to *Enterobacteria phage* BP-4795 (NC_004813) and in other strains to *Enterobacteria phage* P1 (NC_005856). |
| R2 | 11.7/31.4 | 9.6/30.7 | 9.6/30.7 | The region contains the genes involved in lipopolysaccharide synthesis of O104 (the strains 2011C-3493 and 2009EL-2050) and O181 (the strain SCPM-O-B-9427) antigen gene clusters. |
| R3 | 33.9/52.6 | 33.9/52.6 | 32.6/53.0 | The region of the strain 2011C-3493 is related to *Bacteriophage* sp. isolate ctdA53 (BK038108) and the regions of the strains SCPM-O-B-9427 and 2009EL-2050 to *Escherichia phage* Lambda_ev017 (NC_049948). |
| R4 | 21.6/51.4 | 20.1/52.3 | 20.1/52.3 | The region contains the chromosomal genes, IS elements, and genes coding the hypothetical proteins. |
| R5 | 61.6/50.2 | 60.6/50.2 | 60.9/50.2 | The region is the *stx2a* prophage. |
| R6 | 65.6/49.2 | - | - | The region contains the chromosome genes, part of them coding the type II secretion system. |
| R7 | - | 11.0/43.3 | 27.8/45.7 | The region contains the genes related to *Enterobacteria phage* Sf6 (NC_005344). |
| R8 | - | 44.6/50.5 | 44.6/50.5 | The region contains the genes related to intact *Enterobacteria phage* lambda (NC_001416). |
| R9 | - | 14.8/53.1 | 30.2/49.0 | The region coding the chromosome genes that are partly missed in the strain 2009EL-2050. |

The strains 2011C-3493 and 2009EL-2050 are very similar genetically, and the regions of diversity with the strain SCPM-O-B-9427 are partly matched. Three unique regions (R7, 27.8 kbp; R8, 44.6 kbp; and R9, 30.2 kbp) of the strain 2011C-3493 are absent in the strain SCPM-O-B-9427; two of them were related to prophages; these prophages are truncated in the genome of the strain 2009EL-2050. Interestingly, the strains SCPM-O-B-9427 and 2009EL-2050 have a prophage (R3), which is missed in the strain 2011C-3493. The region R6 of the strain SCPM-O-B-9427 is unique and carrying the genes coding the type II secretion system; the region R4 of this strain is not homologous to the same regions of the strains 2011C-3493 and 2009EL-2050. The *stx2a* prophage (R5) is almost identical in the strains SCPM-O-B-9427 and 2009EL-2050, and there is a large number of SNPs in some genes in the strain 2011C-3493 (Table 3).

*2.6. Comparison of the stx2a Prophages Located in the Genomes of the Strains SCPM-O-B-9427, 2011C-3493, and 2009EL-2050*

We performed a comparison of the *stx2a*-carrying prophages of the strains SCPM-O-B-9427, 2011C-3493, and 2009EL-2050 using BRIG (Figure 3). The comparative analysis showed that the *stx2a* phage of the strain SCPM-O-B-9427 is highly homologous to the phage of the strain 2009EL-2050 and distinguished from that of the strain 2011C-3493. The strains SCPM-O-B-9427 and 2009EL-2050 carried a *bor* gene, which may be involved in serum complement resistance, but the strain 2011C-3493 does not have this gene. The second difference between the strain 2011C-3493 and other two strains is in sequence of putative tail fiber protein, which is 133 amino acids shorter. The third site of difference is a deletion, which perturbed homologous antirepressor proteins genes (*antA* and *antB*); the anti-termination protein gene is absent in the strain 2009EL-2050.

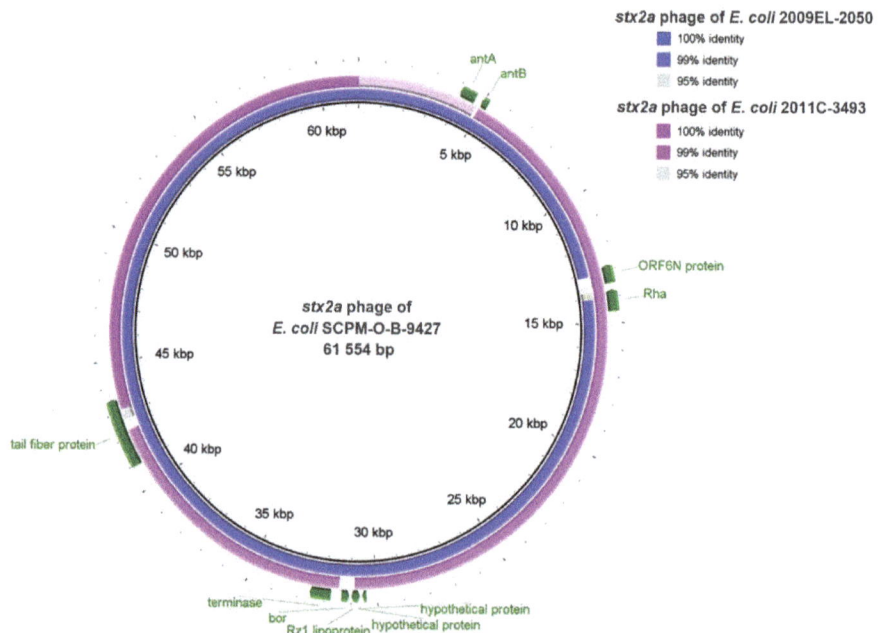

**Figure 3.** BRIG diagram of *stx2a* phages comparison. From center to outside: SCPM-O-B-9427 (black ring), 2009EL-2050 (blue ring), and 2011C-3493 (purple ring). The genes of the strain SCPM-O-B-9427 (colored green) show the regions of differences with the strains 2009EL-2050 and 2011C-3493.

Nucleotide sequence alignment of the *stx2a*-carrying phages of three EAHEC strains was carried out by Snippy. A comparison between prophages of SCPM-O-B-9427 and 2011C-3493 strains showed 198 SNPs (132 synonymous, 43 non-synonymous, and 23 intergenic) and 6 insertions and deletions, where 3 of them are intergenic. The changes of nucleotides did not affect the *stx* genes, which were the most SNPs detected in the genes coding hypothetical proteins and putative endolysin. The number of SNPs between the *stx2a* phages of the strains SCPM-O-B-9427 and 2009EL-2050 is only five. One of them is intergenic, one is a non-synonymous change in each of two genes (hypothetical protein, putative tail fiber protein), and one is a synonymous change in each of two genes (repressor protein CI, Shiga toxin 2 subunit A).

*2.7. The Plasmids of the Strain SCPM-O-B-9427*

Five plasmids were identified in the strain SCPM-O-B-9427. Plasmid sequences were compared using BLASTn to the NCBI nucleotide database to identify their closest matches, which are given in Table 4. The plasmid pB-9427-2 (CP086261) is homologous to pAA plasmid, which harbored several EAEC-specific virulence loci, including *aggDCBA* cluster, *aggR* gene, *aatPABCD* operon, *sepA* gene, and *aap* gene. Importance of pAA in disease severity has been demonstrated: it was involved in the host–pathogen interaction [28] (Berger et al., 2016). We compared the plasmid pB-9427-2 with homologous plasmids pAA-EA11 and pAA-09EL50 of the strains 2011C-3493 and 2009EL-2050. The plasmids do not have rearrangements; the size of pB-9427-2 was 1331 bp bigger due to an additional insertion caused by IS4-like element IS421 family transposase (Figure 4).

Table 4. Plasmids of the strain SCPM-O-B-9427.

| Plasmid | Accession Number | GC Contain (%) | Homolog | Query Cover (%) | Percentage of Identity (%) | Note |
|---|---|---|---|---|---|---|
| pB-9427-1 | CP086260 | 53.3 | *Escherichia coli* FDAARGOS_1300 plasmid unnamed3 (CP069999)—82,270 bp | 98 | 99.53 | F plasmid |
| pB-9427-2 | CP086261 | 47.2 | *Escherichia coli* O104:H4 FDAARGOS_348 plasmid unnamed2 (CP022087)—75,559 bp | 100 | 99.91 | pAA plasmid |
| pB-9427-3 | CP086262 | 49.6 | *Escherichia coli* SJ7 plasmid pSJ7-2 (CP051658)—53,543 bp | 94 | 99.23 | Contains genes encoding the type IV conjugative transfer system |
| pB-9427-4 | CP086263 | 41.6 | *Escherichia coli* RHBSTW-00895 plasmid pRHBSTW-00895_4 (CP056266)—7939 bp | 100 | 99.67 | Contains genes related to mobilization proteins |
| pB-9427-5 | CP086264 | 51.3 | *Shigella sonnei* 500867 plasmid pSSE2 (KP979588)—6728 bp | 100 | 100 | Contains plasmid-borne E-type colicin |

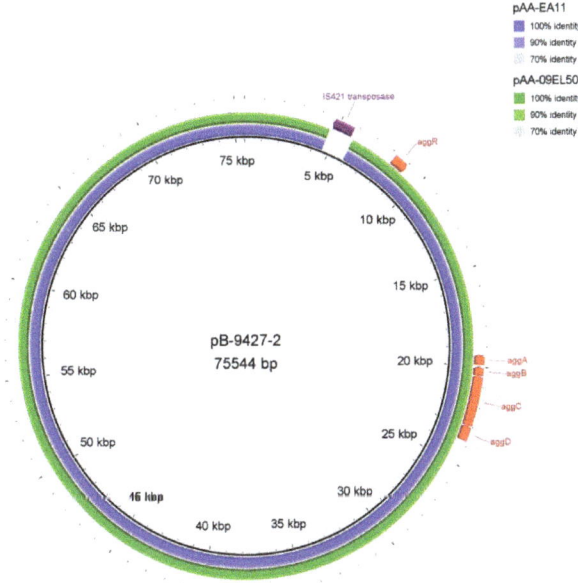

**Figure 4.** BRIG diagram of pAA plasmids comparison. From the center to outside: pB-9427-2 (black ring), pAA-09EL50 (blue ring), and pAA-EA11 (green ring). The cluster genes *aggDCBA* coding aggregative adhesion fimbriae (AAF) and transcriptional activator aggR are indicated (colored red). An additional insertion caused by IS4-like element IS421 family transposase in pB-9427-2 is shown (colored violet).

The nucleotide sequence comparison of pB-9427-2 with 2011C-3493_pAA-EA11 by Snippy showed 39 SNPs (19 synonymous, 11 non-synonymous, and 9 intergenic) and 5 insertions; and with 2009EL-2050_pAA-09EL50, it showed 35 SNPs (21 synonymous, 10 non-synonymous, and 4 intergenic) and 7 deletions (four intergenic) and 1 insertion in *finO* (conjugal transfer fertility inhibition protein). The changes of nucleotides did not affect the virulence genes, and the most SNPs were detected in *umuC* (DNA polymerase V subunit), *finO*, *traX* (conjugal transfer pilus acetylation protein), *traI* (conjugal transfer nickase/helicase), and in transposase (IS110 family protein).

Another four replicons of the strain SCPM-O-B-9427 were not homologous to the plasmids of the strains 2011C-3493 and 2009EL-2050 (pESBL-EA11, pG, and p09EL50) (Table 2). The plasmids of the strain SCPM-O-B-9427 did not carry any antibiotic resistance genes, and there were not identified any significant virulence factors on the plasmid pB-9427-5 except *celb* gene (endonuclease colicin E2).

### 2.8. Phylogenetic Analysis for E. coli O181 and O104:H4

To clarify the relationship of the hybrid EAHEC strain SCPM-O-B-9427 and several *E. coli* strains of O104:H4 and O181 found in the database NCBI, a phylogenetic tree based on the core chromosomal SNPs using Wombac was built. The tree was represented on 96,244 SNPs of 25 strains (Figure 5). The *E. coli* strains were grouped due to their sero- and MLST sequence type. The hybrid strain SCPM-O-B-9427 was very closely related to the group of O181:H4 and O104:H4 strains while not to the strains of O181 non-H4 serogroups.

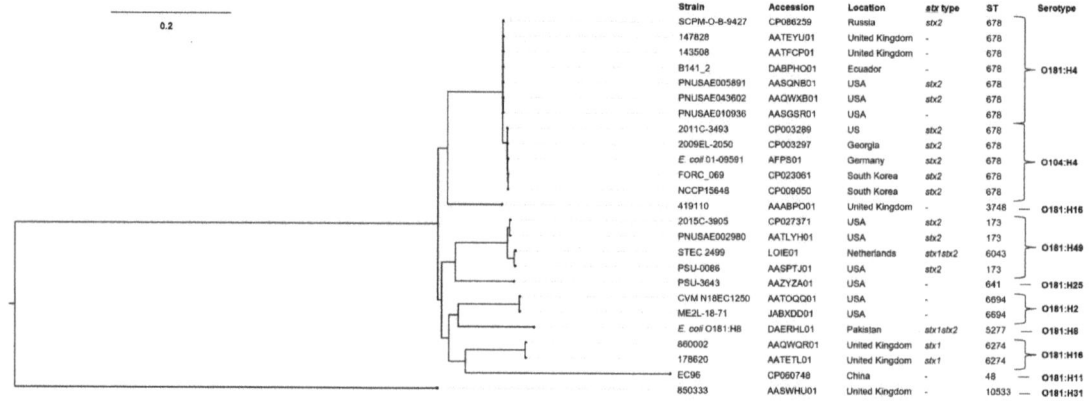

**Figure 5.** Neighbor-joining phylogenetic tree based on core SNPs, showing the phylogenetic relationship between chromosomes of EAHEC strain SCPM-O-B-9427 and *E. coli* O104:H4 and *E. coli* O181 strains. The scale bar shows the expected number of substitutions per site. Bar, 0.2 substitutions per nucleotide position.

For a better understanding of the relationship within the group of the strains belonging to ST678, a second phylogenetic tree based on 2115 core SNPs of 12 strains was built. *E. coli* strains formed three clusters: the first one included the strains of O181:H4 serotype; the second included the strains of O104:H4 serotype (caused outbreaks in Germany, 2011 and Georgia, 2009) and the third the other O104:H4 strains (Figure 6). The strains from the second and the third clades are hybrid, carrying both the *stx2* gene and *aggDCBA* cluster. The difference between the second and the third clades was the carriage of fimbriae AAF/I or fimbriae AAF/III gene cluster, respectively.

On the phylogenetic tree, the strains of O181:H4 are spaced from the center of the clade and do not form a well-defined subclade. The performed comparison of the SCPM-O-B-9427 chromosome with other *E. coli* O181:H4 genomes showed that the core SNP numbers varied from 133 to 159. Major strains carried genes coding fimbriae AAF/I; only three of them including the strain SCPM-O-B-9427 additionally carried the *stx2* genes and were attributed as EAHEC.

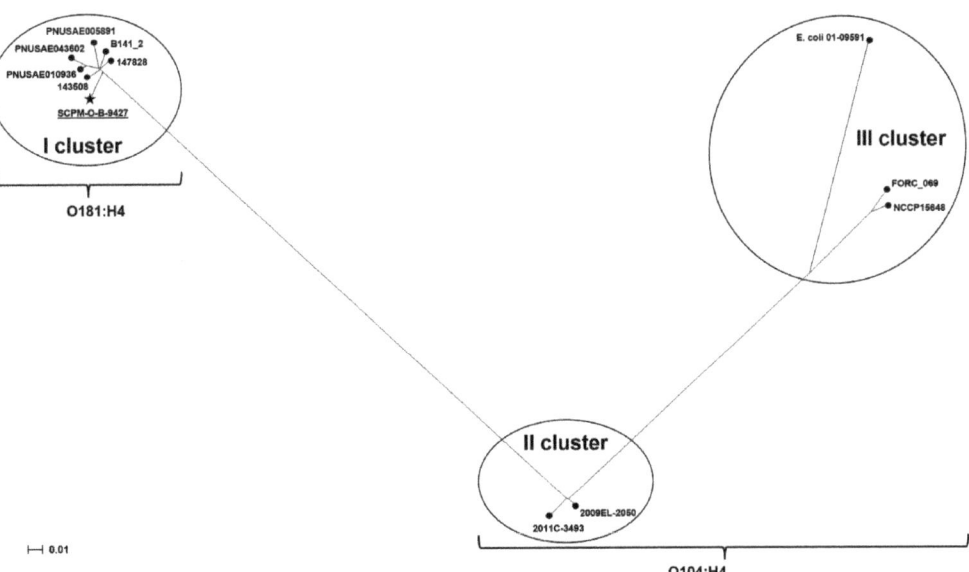

**Figure 6.** Neighbor-joining phylogenetic tree based on core SNPs, showing the phylogenetic relationship between chromosomes of EAHEC strain SCPM-O-B-9427 and *E. coli* O104:H4 and *E. coli* O181:H4 strains. The scale bar shows the expected number of substitutions per site. Bar, 0.01 substitutions per nucleotide position.

We compared the sequences of *stxA* and *stxB* genes of O181:H4 strains (Figure 6), which were attributed to the 2a type. Significant differences were revealed between named genes of the strain SCPM-O-B-9427 and other two strains of this clade, PNUSAE005891 and PNUSAE043602. The strains PNUSAE005891 and PNUSAE043602 have identical sequence of *stx2* genes. Although StxA amino acid sequences are the same for the three strains, i.e., PNUSAE005891, PNUSAE043602, and SCPM-O-B-9427, seven synonymous SNPs were identified in the *stxA* gene of the strain SCPM-O-B-9427. Moreover, two synonymous SNPs and one SNP that led to a change from alanine to valine were detected in the *stxB* gene of the strain SCPM-O-B-9427 compared to the same gene of the strains PNUSAE005891 and PNUSAE043602.

We also compared the *stx2a*-carrying phage sequence of the strain SCPM-O-B-9427 with the same phage sequences of the strains PNUSAE005891 and PNUSAE043602. In NCBI Genome, the results of whole-genome sequencing of these strains are the assemblies of contigs. In the strain PNUSAE005891, the *stxA* and *stxB* genes were located in the contig 51 (AASQNB010000051, 21,013 bp) and in the strain PNUSAE043602 in the contig 30 (AAQWXB010000030, 73,345 bp). Sequence alignment of the *stx2a* phage of the strain SCPM-O-B-9427 and the contig 30 of the strain PNUSAE043602 showed only 11% query cover (the region of *stx* genes) and 96.24% identity of this region. It was pointed out that the *stx2a*-carrying phages have a different genetic structure. BLAST search revealed the closest to the prophage of the strain PNUSAE043602 sequence of the *stx2a*-carrying phage Stx2_12E129_yecE DNA (LC567842, 46,100 bp) with 82% query cover and 94.64% identity. Comparison of the contig 30 of the strain PNUSAE043602 and assembly PNUSAE005891 revealed that the *stx2a*-carrying phage of the second strain fell to pieces, but apparently, they are the similar.

## 3. Discussion

The conception about several well-classified pathotypes of DEC *E. coli* based on the presence of specific virulence factors directly related to disease development existed before the German outbreak in 2011. This conviction collapsed due to the fact that this severe outbreak was caused by a hybrid strain bearing the virulence factors of enteroaggregative *E. coli* and Shiga-toxin-producing *E. coli* simultaneously [16,17]. After that, many studies have shown that *E. coli* strains combining genetic markers belonging to different pathotypes are more frequent than previously thought [12–15]. Hybrid DEC are associated with more serious diseases and may frequently progress to HUS, which could be explained by producing a set of proteins involved in intestinal colonization, leading to persistent diarrhea and facilitating Stx absorption [29].

We present the description of a new hybrid EAHEC O181:H4 strain obtained from the rectal swab of a HUS patient in St. Petersburg (Russian Federation) in July 2018. The strain was investigated by whole-genome sequence analysis in this study.

The genoserotyping in silico confirmed that the strain SCPM-O-B-9427 was attributed to O181:H4 serogroup and to the sequence type ST678. The same ST was identified for the strains caused the large German outbreak in 2011 and the bloody diarrhea outbreak in the Republic of Georgia in 2009, but these strains belonged to O104 serogroup [20]. Affiliation to the same ST and similar sets of virulence genes suggested a close genetic relationship between these strains belonging to different serogroups. We found six assemblies of *E. coli* O181:H4 draft genomes in the NCBI database without detailed information about isolation sources and hosts. All of them belonged to ST678 and carried the *aggR* gene, and only two possessed *stxA* and *stxB* genes. Considering these data, it was not surprising that the phylogenetic relationship of *E. coli* O181:H4 strains based on core SNPs were very closely related to *E. coli* O104:H4.

Comparison of the strain *E. coli* SCPM-O-B-9427 with *E. coli* strains 2011C-3493 and 2009EL-2050 showed almost the same structure of their chromosomes and high similarity of two pAA-carrying plasmids the major virulence factors and *stx2a*-bearing prophages. There were identified few SNPs in the homologous parts of the chromosomes. However, at the same time, they were variable from each other and have unique differences. Hence, these strains carried distinct sets of the plasmids and unique regions in the chromosomes. Thus, the compared strains are close relatives; probably, they have the same ancestor, but different genetic events occurred during their evolution.

Unfortunately, study of the EAHEC strain SCPM-O-B-9427 genetic characteristics does not allow answering the question about the origin and evolution of this pathogen. We can suppose the hypothesis about the genesis of the EAHEC strain O104:H4 that caused severe foodborne infection in Germany in 2011 [16]. The proposed development model of this strain derivation consists of the acquisition of a *stx2a*-converting prophage into an EAEC strain by transduction. The Stx-converting phages were considered as highly mobile genetic elements capable of infecting a susceptible bacterium and leading to positive Stx-conversion. However, apart from the transduction of the *stx2a* phage in an EAEC cell, it should be introduced into the chromosome in appropriate location, be properly functioned, and be stably inherited. In some cases, the infection of DEC strains by Stx-converting phages has been carried out in experiments. The emergence of hybrid EAHEC strains is not an often-occurring event, which can be explained by different susceptibility of EAEC strains to the Stx-converting phages. Probably, the EAEC of O104:H4 and O181:H4 were competent recipients of Stx-converting phages; moreover, they are very genetically close to each other. It was revealed in our study that the *stx2a* prophages of the strains SCPM-O-B-9427 and 2009EL-2050 are almost identical, while they were somewhat different from the *stx2a* prophage of the strain 2011C-3493; nevertheless, all three *stx2a* prophages are very similar. Interestingly, the *E. coli* strains PNUSAE005891 and PNUSAE043602 of the O181:H4 serotype carried different *stx2a* prophages compared to that of the strain SCPM-O-B-9427. This fact may indicate an increased sensitivity of *E. coli* of different origins to the Stx-phage infection. The forming of new hybrid DEC strains has high threat potential to humans due to the combination of the damages induced by Stx on susceptible cells and the aggregative, adherence-mediating fimbriae allowed to colonize the gastrointestinal tract, which can lead to disease worsening and the development of HUS.

*E. coli* are characterized by a high degree of genetic heterogeneity, high genome plasticity, and the ability to exchange genetic information and thereby increase virulence, to acquire drug resistance, and eventually improve the adaptation to different environments, keeping *E. coli* as a successful bacterium in various ecological niches.

Although the strain SCPM-O-B-9427 and the "Georgian strain" caused not-so-large foodborne outbreaks compared to that of the "Germany strain", some patients developed HUS. The emergence of O181:H4 EAHEC strain, phylogenetically related to the Shiga-toxin-producing *E. coli* of O104:H4, show that new genetic variants continuously formed in this bacterial species. Therefore, genetic research is essential for detecting and controlling the spread of new variants of pathogenic bacteria.

## 4. Materials and Methods

### 4.1. Bacterial Strains Used in This Study

*Escherichia coli* strain SCPM-O-B-9427 was obtained from the patient's rectal swab received from The Center of Hygiene and Epidemiology in Saint Petersburg and deposited into The State Collection of Pathogenic Microbes of The State Research Center for Applied Microbiology and Biotechnology, Obolensk. It was not needed to obtain permission from the Ethics Committee to conduct the study. The name of the strain does not contain personal data about the patient.

### 4.2. Strain Isolation, Growing, Identification, and Susceptibility Testing

A clinical case of intestinal infection was registered in Saint Petersburg, Russian Federation, in July 2018. Bacterial isolates were collected according to the Methodical Recommendations MR 4.2.2963-11 "Methods for laboratory diagnostic of the infections caused by Shiga-toxin-producing *E. coli* (STEC-cultures) and detection of STEC pathogens in food". *E. coli* isolates were grown on the nutrient media "Enrichment media for Enterobacteriaceae number 3" (SRCAMB, Obolensk, Russia) and "MacConkey agar" (HiMedia, Mumbai, Maharashtra, India) at 37 °C for 18 h. Bacterial species identification was completed using API-20 biochemical test system (Biomereux, Marcy-l'Étoile, Auvergne-Rhône-Alpes, France) and Vitek 2 Compact instrument (Biomereux, Marcy-l'Étoile, Auvergne-Rhône-Alpes, France) using VITEK 2 GN ID card (Biomereux, Marcy-l'Étoile, Auvergne-Rhône-Alpes, France). Bacterial isolates were stored in 10% glycerol at minus 70 °C.

Antimicrobial susceptibility testing was performed on Vitek2 Compact system (BioMérieux, Marcy-l'Étoile, Auvergne-Rhône-Alpes, France) using AST-N101 card (BioMérieux, Marcy-l'Étoile, Auvergne-Rhône-Alpes, France). The interpretation was made using requirements of the "The European Committee on Antimicrobial Susceptibility Testing (EUCAST), version 12.0, 2022 (http://www.eucast.org) (access on 5 September 2022). *Escherichia coli* ATCC 25922 strain was used as quality control.

### 4.3. DNA Isolation and Pathotype and Phylogroup Identification

DNA extraction was performed using a nucleic acid extraction kit AmpliSens® RIBO-prep (InterLabService, Moscow, Russia). Pathotype detection was performed using commercial assay AmpliSens® Escherichioses- FRT (InterLabService, Moscow, Russia). Detection of *stx* and *aggR* genes were completed according to The European Union Reference Laboratory method (EU Reference Laboratory VTEC, Rome, Italy, https://www.iss.it/about-eu-rl-vte) (access on 9 September 2021). Multiplex PCR for phylogroup identification was performed according to Clermont et al., 2013 [30].

### 4.4. Whole Genome Sequencing, Assembly and Annotation

DNA isolation was performed by CTAB method [31]. WGS was carried out using Nextera DNA Library Preparation Kit (Illumina, San Diego, CA, USA) and MiSeq Reagent Kits v3 (Illumina, San Diego, CA, USA) for platform Illumina MiSeq (Illumina, San Diego, CA, USA). Long reads were obtained using Rapid Barcoding Kit RBK004 and flowcell R9.4.1 on MinION platform (Oxford Nanopore, Oxford Science Park, GB). WGS was performed by running MinKNOW software v. 21.06.13 (Oxford Nanopore, Oxford Science Park, GB); basecalling was performed with Guppy v. 5.0.16 (Oxford Nanopore, Oxford Science Park, GB) with defaults parameters [32]. Short and long raw reads were used to obtain the hybrid assembly of the strain using Unicycler v. 0.4.7 software (The University of Melbourne, Victoria, Australia) with default settings that included primary filtering and quality control [33]. Annotation was carried out by NCBI Prokaryotic Genome Annotation Pipeline (PGAP) v. 5.3 (National Center for Biotechnology Information, Bethesda, MD, USA) [34].

*4.5. Whole Genome Analysis*

Serotyping and definition of virulence and resistance genes of complete genome was performed in silico using online resources SerotypeFinder 2.0 [35], VirulenceFinder 2.0 [36], ResFinder 2.0 [37] of the Center for Genomic Epidemiology (Technical University of Denmark, Kgs. Lyngby, Denmark). *In silico* multi-locus sequence typing (MLST) by the Achtman's MLST scheme database was performed with online resource MLST 2.0 of the Center for Genomic Epidemiology (Technical University of Denmark, Kgs. Lyngby, Denmark) [27]. The prophage regions in the chromosome were identified by online resource PHASTER (University of Alberta, Edmonton, AB, Canada) [38]. Web resource BLAST was used for homologous plasmids searching (National Center for Biotechnology Information, Bethesda, MD, USA) [39]. Online resource Genomics %G~C Content Calculator [40] was used to calculate GC content. Whole-genome alignments were performed using Mauve v. 2015-02-26 [41], Artemis Comparison Tool (Oxford University, Oxford, GB) [42], and BRIG v. 0.95 (https://brig.sourceforge.net/, access on 5 September 2022) [43]. Phylogenetic trees were obtained with core SNPs identified by WOMBAC (https://github.com/tseemann/wombac, access on 5 September 2022) [44] and were visualized with SplitsTree4 (https://github.com/husonlab/splitstree4, access on 5 September 2022) [45] and FigTree v. 1.4.4 (http://tree.bio.ed.ac.uk/software/figtree/, access on 5 September 2022) [46] using NJ method. Snippy software (https://github.com/tseemann/snippy, access on 5 September 2022) [47] was used to obtain variant calling into assembled chromosomes and plasmids with default parameters. The *stx2a* prophage sequences were extracted from the genomes using PHASTER (University of Alberta, Edmonton, AB, Canada) with manual detection of *att* sites by BLAST. The R package [48] with ggplot2 library (https://www.r-project.org/, access on 5 September 2022) [49] was used to calculate and visualize the distribution of SNPs, insertions, deletions, and complex in *E. coli* chromosome.

Whole-genome sequence of *E. coli* strain SCPM-O-B-9427 was submitted into GenBank database (National Center for Biotechnology Information, Bethesda, MD, USA): chromosome (CP086259) and five plasmids: pB-9427-1 (CP086260), pB-9427-2 (CP086261), pB-9427-3 (CP086262), pB-9427-4 (CP086263), and pB-9427-5 (CP086264).

Complete genomes of EAHEC strains *Escherichia coli* O104:H4 str. 2011C-3493: chromosome (CP003289), plasmid pAA-EA11 (CP003291), plasmid pESBL-EA11 (CP003290), plasmid pG-EA11 (CP003292), and *Escherichia coli* O104:H4 str. 2009EL-2050: chromosome (CP003297), plasmid pAA-09EL50 (CP003299), plasmid p09EL50 (CP003298), plasmid pG-09EL50 (CP003300) were used for comparative genomic analysis.

## 5. Conclusions

This study revealed the genetic properties of the new hybrid enteroaggregative/Shiga-toxin-producing (EAHEC) strain *E. coli* of O181:H4 (SCPM-O-B-9427) obtained from the patient with HUS in St. Petersburg (Russian Federation) in July 2018. The complete genome assembly of the strain SCPM-O-B-9427 contains one chromosome (5,268,110 bp) and five plasmids (pB-9427-1 83,340 bp; pB-9427-2 75,544 bp; pB-9427-3 51,013 bp; pB-9427-4 7939 bp; pB-9427-5 6728 bp). On the phylogenetic tree, the strain SCPM-O-B-9427 forms a close group with the strains *E. coli* O181:H4 and *E. coli* O104:H4. The comparison of the strain SCPM-O-B-9427 with *E. coli* O104:H4 strains 2011C-3493 (which caused the large German outbreak in 2011) and 2009EL-2050 (which was isolated in the Republic of Georgia in 2009) showed that all of them have the almost identical sets of virulence genes. The chromosomal architectures of the hybrid strains SCPM-O-B-9427, 2009EL-2050, and 2011C-3493 were very similar in overall structure despite one extended inverted region in the strain SCPM-O-B-9427. However, each of these strains was distinct, with extended unique regions in the genome. The comparative analysis of *stx2a* prophages, an important virulence determinant, showed that prophage of the strain SCPM-O-B-9427 is highly homologous to the prophage of the strain 2009EL-2050 and distinguished from the prophage of the strain 2011C-3493. The analysis of the plasmid pAA homologous revealed that the plasmids have no rearrangements; the size of the plasmid pB-9427-2 was 1331 bp bigger due to an additional insertion caused by IS4-like element IS421 family transposase.

Notably, the strains SCPM-O-B-9427 and 2009EL-2050 did not cause enormous outbreaks compared to the strain 2011C-3493. Therefore, hybrid strains producing Stx2 and the aggregative adherence-mediating fimbriae simultaneously could have a potential threat to humans. Combination of these virulence factors increase the pathogenic potential due to the damaging effects on the intestinal epithelium and colonization of the gastrointestinal tract. Therefore, it is necessary to undertake investigations of new genetic variants of pathogenic *E. coli* to detect their spreading among people and in environments.

**Author Contributions:** Conceptualization, A.A.K. and N.N.K.; methodology, M.E.K., M.G.T., and E.S.K.; software, Y.P.S. and A.A.S.; validation, N.K.F. and E.A.S.; formal analysis, A.A.K. and Y.P.S.; investigation, A.A.K., N.N.K., Y.P.S., and A.A.S.; resources, A.G.B.; data curation, N.N.K., M.E.K., and N.K.F.; writing—original draft preparation, A.A.K. and N.N.K.; writing—review and editing, N.K.F.; visualization, A.A.K., Y.P.S., and A.A.S.; supervision, N.K.F. and E.A.S.; project administration, N.N.K. and E.A.S.; funding acquisition, I.A.D. All authors have read and agreed to the published version of the manuscript.

**Funding:** This study was financially supported by a grant of the Ministry of Science and Higher Education of the Russian Federation (Agreement No. 075-15-2019-1671 of 31 October 2019) and The Sectoral Program of Rospotrebnadzor (2021–2025).

**Institutional Review Board Statement:** The study did not require ethical approval because it did not involve humans or animals.

**Informed Consent Statement:** Not applicable.

**Data Availability Statement:** Whole-genome sequence of *E. coli* strain SCPM-O-B-9427 was submitted into GenBank database: chromosome (CP086259) and five plasmids: pB-9427-1 (CP086260), pB-9427-2 (CP086261), pB-9427-3 (CP086262), pB-9427-4 (CP086263), and pB-9427-5 (CP086264).

**Acknowledgments:** We thank The Center of Hygiene and Epidemiology in Saint Petersburg, Russia, for providing *E. coli* clinical isolates for this study.

**Conflicts of Interest:** The authors declare that there are no conflict of interest.

# References

1. Eckburg, P.B.; Bik, E.M.; Bernstein, C.N.; Purdom, E.; Dethlefsen, L.; Sargent, M.; Gill, S.R.; Nelson, K.E.; Relman, D.A. Diversity of the human intestinal microbial flora. *Science* **2005**, *308*, 1635–1638. [CrossRef] [PubMed]
2. Stromberg, Z.R.; Johnson, J.R.; Fairbrother, J.M.; Kilbourne, J.; Van Goor, A.; Curtiss, R.; Mellata, M. Evaluation of *Escherichia coli* isolates from healthy chickens to determine their potential risk to poultry and human health. *PLoS ONE* **2017**, *12*, e0180599. [CrossRef] [PubMed]
3. Köhler, C.D.; Dobrindt, U. What defines extraintestinal pathogenic *Escherichia coli*? *Int. J. Med. Microbiol.* **2011**, *301*, 642–647. [CrossRef] [PubMed]
4. Clements, A.; Young, J.C.; Constantinou, N.; Frankel, G. Infection strategies of enteric pathogenic *Escherichia coli*. *Gut Microbes* **2012**, *3*, 71–87. [CrossRef] [PubMed]
5. Nyong, E.C.; Zaia, S.R.; Allué-Guardia, A.; Rodriguez, A.L.; Irion-Byrd, Z.; Koenig, S.; Feng, P.; Bono, J.L.; Eppinger, M. Pathogenomes of Atypical Non-shigatoxigenic *Escherichia coli* NSF/SF O157:H7/NM: Comprehensive Phylogenomic Analysis Using Closed Genomes. *Front. Microbiol.* **2020**, *11*, 619. [CrossRef]
6. Chaudhuri, R.R.; Henderson, I.R. The evolution of the *Escherichia coli* phylogeny. *Infect. Genet. Evol.* **2012**, *12*, 214–226. [CrossRef]

7. Dixit, P.D.; Pang, T.Y.; Studier, F.W.; Maslov, S. Recombinant transfer in the basic genome of *Escherichia coli*. *Proc. Natl. Acad. Sci. USA* **2015**, *112*, 9070–9075. [CrossRef]
8. Desvaux, M.; Dalmasso, G.; Beyrouthy, R.; Barnich, N.; Delmas, J.; Bonnet, R. Pathogenicity Factors of Genomic Islands in Intestinal and Extraintestinal *Escherichia coli*. *Front. Microbiol.* **2020**, *11*, 2065. [CrossRef]
9. Manges, A.R.; Geum, H.M.; Guo, A.; Edens, T.J.; Fibke, C.D.; Pitout, J. Global Extraintestinal Pathogenic *Escherichia coli* (ExPEC) Lineages. *Clin. Microbiol. Rev.* **2019**, *32*, e00135-18. [CrossRef]
10. Pakbin, B.; Brück, W.M.; Rossen, J. Virulence Factors of Enteric Pathogenic *Escherichia coli*: A Review. *Int. J. Mol. Sci.* **2021**, *22*, 9922. [CrossRef]
11. Jesser, K.J.; Levy, K. Updates on defining and detecting diarrheagenic *Escherichia coli* pathotypes. *Curr. Opin. Infect. Dis.* **2020**, *33*, 372–380. [CrossRef]
12. Bolukaoto, J.Y.; Singh, A.; Alfinete, N.; Barnard, T.G. Occurrence of Hybrid Diarrhoeagenic *Escherichia coli* Associated with Multidrug Resistance in Environmental Water, Johannesburg, South Africa. *Microorganisms* **2021**, *9*, 2163. [CrossRef]
13. Díaz-Jiménez, D.; García-Meniño, I.; Herrera, A.; García, V.; López-Beceiro, A.M.; Alonso, M.P.; Blanco, J.; Mora, A. Genomic Characterization of *Escherichia coli* Isolates Belonging to a New Hybrid aEPEC/ExPEC Pathotype O153:H10-A-ST10 eae-beta1 Occurred in Meat, Poultry, Wildlife and Human Diarrheagenic Samples. *Antibiotics* **2020**, *9*, 192. [CrossRef]
14. Valiatti, T.B.; Santos, F.F.; Santos, A.; Nascimento, J.; Silva, R.M.; Carvalho, E.; Sinigaglia, R.; Gomes, T. Genetic and Virulence Characteristics of a Hybrid Atypical Enteropathogenic and Uropathogenic *Escherichia coli* (aEPEC/UPEC) Strain. *Front. Cell. Infect. Microbiol.* **2020**, *10*, 492. [CrossRef]
15. Santos, A.; Santos, F.F.; Silva, R.M.; Gomes, T. Diversity of Hybrid- and Hetero-Pathogenic *Escherichia coli* and Their Potential Implication in More Severe Diseases. *Front. Cell. Infect. Microbiol.* **2020**, *10*, 339. [CrossRef]
16. Rasko, D.A.; Webster, D.R.; Sahl, J.W.; Bashir, A.; Boisen, N.; Scheutz, F.; Paxinos, E.E.; Sebra, R.; Chin, C.S.; Iliopoulos, D.; et al. Origins of the *E. coli* strain causing an outbreak of hemolytic-uremic syndrome in Germany. *N. Engl. J. Med.* **2011**, *365*, 709–717. [CrossRef]
17. Tietze, E.; Dabrowski, P.W.; Prager, R.; Radonic, A.; Fruth, A.; Aura, P.; Nitsche, A.; Mielke, M.; Flieger, A. Comparative genomic analysis of two novel sporadic Shiga toxin-producing *Escherichia coli* O104:H4 strains isolated 2011 in Germany. *PLoS ONE* **2015**, *10*, e0122074. [CrossRef]
18. Wald, M.; Rieck, T.; Nachtnebel, M.; Greute'laers, B.; an der Heiden, M.; Altmann, D.; Hellenbrand, W.; Faber, M.; Frank, C.; Schweickert, B.; et al. Enhanced surveillance during a large outbreak of bloody diarrhoea and haemolytic uraemic syndrome caused by Shiga toxin/verotoxin-producing *Escherichia coli* in Germany, May to June 2011. *Euro Surveill.* **2011**, *16*, 19893.
19. Chokoshvili, O.; Lomashvili, K.; Malakmadze, N.; Geleishvil, M.; Brant, J.; Imnadze, P.; Chitadze, N.; Tevzadze, L.; Chanturia, G.; Tevdoradze, T.; et al. Investigation of an outbreak of bloody diarrhea complicated with hemolytic uremic syndrome. *J. Epidemiol. Glob. Health* **2014**, *4*, 249–259. [CrossRef]
20. Ahmed, S.A.; Awosika, J.; Baldwin, C.; Bishop-Lilly, K.A.; Biswas, B.; Broomall, S.; Chain, P.S.; Chertkov, O.; Chokoshvili, O.; Coyne, S.; et al. Threat Characterization Consortium. Genomic comparison of *Escherichia coli* O104:H4 isolates from 2009 and 2011 reveals plasmid, and prophage heterogeneity, including shiga toxin encoding phage stx2. *PLoS ONE* **2012**, *7*, e48228. [CrossRef]
21. Nowrouzian, F.L.; Wold, A.E.; Adlerberth, I. *Escherichia coli* strains belonging to phylogenetic group B2 have superior capacity to persist in the intestinal microflora of infants. *J. Infect. Dis.* **2005**, *191*, 1078–1083. [CrossRef] [PubMed]
22. Scheutz, F.; Cheasty, T.; Woodward, D.; Smith, H.R. Designation of O174 and O175 to temporary O groups OX3 and OX7, and six new *E. coli* O groups that include Verocytotoxin-producing *E. coli* (VTEC): O176, O177, O178, O179, O180 and O181. *APMIS* **2004**, *112*, 569–584. [CrossRef] [PubMed]
23. Ballem, A.; Gonçalves, S.; Garcia-Meniño, I.; Flament-Simon, S.C.; Blanco, J.E.; Fernandes, C.; Saavedra, M.J.; Pinto, C.; Oliveira, H.; Blanco, J.; et al. Prevalence and serotypes of Shiga toxin-producing *Escherichia coli* (STEC) in dairy cattle from Northern Portugal. *PLoS ONE* **2020**, *15*, e0244713. [CrossRef] [PubMed]
24. Eklund, M.; Scheutz, F.; Siitonen, A. Clinical isolates of non-O157 Shiga toxin-producing *Escherichia coli*: Serotypes, virulence characteristics, and molecular profiles of strains of the same serotype. *J. Clin. Microbiol.* **2001**, *39*, 2829–2834. [CrossRef]
25. García-Aljaro, C.; Muniesa, M.; Blanco, J.E.; Blanco, M.; Blanco, J.; Jofre, J.; Blanch, A.R. Characterization of Shiga toxin-producing *Escherichia coli* isolated from aquatic environments. *FEMS Microbiol. Lett.* **2005**, *246*, 55–65. [CrossRef]
26. Ori, E.L.; Takagi, E.H.; Andrade, T.S.; Miguel, B.T.; Cergole-Novella, M.C.; Guth, B.; Hernandes, R.T.; Dias, R.; Pinheiro, S.; Camargo, C.H.; et al. Diarrhoeagenic *Escherichia coli* and *Escherichia albertii* in Brazil: Pathotypes and serotypes over a 6-year period of surveillance. *Epidemiol. Infect.* **2018**, *147*, e10. [CrossRef]
27. Wirth, T.; Falush, D.; Lan, R.; Colles, F.; Mensa, P.; Wieler, L.H.; Karch, H.; Reeves, P.R.; Maiden, M.C.; Ochman, H.; et al. Sex and virulence in *Escherichia coli*: An evolutionary perspective. *Mol. Microbiol.* **2006**, *60*, 1136–1151. [CrossRef]
28. Berger, P.; Knödler, M.; Förstner, K.U.; Berger, M.; Bertling, C.; Sharma, C.M.; Vogel, J.; Karch, H.; Dobrindt, U.; Mellmann, A. The primary transcriptome of the Escherichia coli O104:H4 pAA plasmid and novel insights into its virulence gene expression and regulation. *Sci. Rep.* **2016**, *6*, 35307. [CrossRef]
29. Navarro-Garcia, F. *Escherichia coli* O104:H4 pathogenesis: An enteroaggregative *E. coli*/Shiga toxin-Producing *E. coli* explosive cocktail of high virulence. *Microbiol. Spectr.* **2014**, *2*. [CrossRef]
30. Beghain, J.; Bridier-Nahmias, A.; Le Nagard, H.; Denamur, E.; Clermont, O. ClermonTyping: An easy-to-use and accurate in silico method for Escherichia genus strain phylotyping. *Microb Genom.* **2018**, *4*, e000192. [CrossRef]

31. Wilson, K. Preparation of genomic DNA from bacteria. *Curr. Protoc. Mol. Biol.* **2001**, *56*, 2–4. [CrossRef]
32. Oxford Nanopore Technologies. Available online: https://nanoporetech.com/ (accessed on 12 April 2021).
33. Wick, R.R.; Judd, L.M.; Gorrie, C.L.; Holt, K.E. Unicycler: Resolving bacterial genome assemblies from short and long sequencing reads. *PLoS Comput. Biol.* **2017**, *13*, e1005595. [CrossRef]
34. Tatusova, T.; DiCuccio, M.; Badretdin, A.; Chetvernin, V.; Nawrocki, E.P.; Zaslavsky, L.; Lomsadze, A.; Pruitt, K.D.; Borodovsky, M.; Ostell, J. NCBI prokaryotic genome annotation pipeline. *Nucleic. Acids. Res.* **2016**, *44*, 6614–6624. [CrossRef]
35. Joensen, K.G.; Tetzschner, A.M.; Iguchi, A.; Aarestrup, F.M.; Scheutz, F. Rapid and easy in silico serotyping of *Escherichia coli* using whole genome sequencing (WGS) data. *J. Clin. Microbiol.* **2015**, *53*, 2410–2426. [CrossRef]
36. Malberg Tetzschner, A.M.; Johnson, J.R.; Johnston, B.D.; Lund, O.; Scheutz, F. In Silico Genotyping of *Escherichia coli* Isolates for Extraintestinal Virulence Genes by Use of Whole-Genome Sequencing Data. *J. Clin. Micobiol.* **2020**, *58*, e01269-20. [CrossRef]
37. Bortolaia, V.; Kaas, R.S.; Ruppe, E.; Roberts, M.C.; Schwarz, S.; Cattoir, V.; Philippon, A.; Allesoe, R.L.; Rebelo, A.R.; Florensa, A.F.; et al. ResFinder 4.0 for predictions of phenotypes from genotypes. *J. Antimicrob. Chemother.* **2020**, *75*, 3491–3500. [CrossRef]
38. Arndt, D.; Grant, J.R.; Marcu, A.; Sajed, T.; Pon, A.; Liang, Y.; Wishart, D.S. PHASTER: A better, faster version of the PHAST phage search tool. *Nucleic. Acids Res.* **2016**, *44*, W16–W21. [CrossRef]
39. Camacho, C.; Coulouris, G.; Avagyan, V.; Ma, N.; Papadopoulos, J.; Kevin Bealer, K.; Madden, T.L. BLAST+: Architecture and applications. *BMC Bioinform.* **2009**, *10*, 421. [CrossRef]
40. Genomics %G~C Content Calculator—Science Buddies. Available online: https://www.sciencebuddies.org/science-fair-projects/references/genomics-g-c-content-calculator (accessed on 9 November 2011).
41. Darling, A.E.; Mau, B.; Perna, N.T. progressiveMauve: Multiple genome alignment with gene gain, loss and rearrangement. *PLoS ONE* **2010**, *5*, e11147. [CrossRef]
42. Carver, T.J.; Rutherford, K.M.; Berriman, M.; Rajandream, M.A.; Barrell, B.G.; Parkhill, J. ACT: The Artemis Comparison Tool. *Bioinformatics* **2005**, *21*, 3422–3423. [CrossRef]
43. Alikhan, N.F.; Petty, N.K.; Ben Zakour, N.L.; Beatson, S.A. BLAST Ring Image Generator (BRIG): Simple prokaryote genome comparisons. *BMC Genom.* **2011**, *12*, 402. [CrossRef]
44. Wombac. Available online: https://github.com/tseemann/wombac (accessed on 15 November 2021).
45. Huson, D.H.; Bryant, D. Application of Phylogenetic Networks in Evolutionary Studies. *Mol. Biol. Evol.* **2006**, *23*, 254–267. [CrossRef]
46. Molecular Evolution, Phylogenetics and Epidemiology. Available online: http://tree.bio.ed.ac.uk/software/figtree/ (accessed on 15 November 2021).
47. Snippy. Available online: https://github.com/tseemann/snippy (accessed on 15 November 2021).
48. R Core Team. *R: A Language and Environment for Statistical Computing*; R Foundation for Statistical Computing: Vienna, Austria, 2018; Available online: https://www.R-project.org (accessed on 15 February 2022).
49. Wickham, H. *Ggplot2: Elegant Graphics for Data Analysis*; Springer: New York, NY, USA, 2016; Available online: https://ggplot2.tidyverse.org (accessed on 15 February 2022).

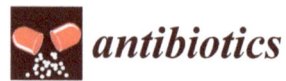 

Article

# First Report of Colistin-Resistant *Escherichia coli* Carrying *mcr-1* IncI2(delta) and IncX4 Plasmids from Camels (*Camelus dromedarius*) in the Gulf Region

Akela Ghazawi [1], Nikolaos Strepis [2], Febin Anes [3], Dana Yaaqeib [1], Amal Ahmed [1], Aysha AlHosani [1], Mirah AlShehhi [1], Ashrat Manzoor [1], Ihab Habib [3], Nisar A. Wani [4], John P. Hays [2] and Mushtaq Khan [1,*]

1. Department of Microbiology and Immunology, College of Medicine and Health Sciences, United Arab Emirates University, Al Ain P.O. Box 15551, United Arab Emirates; akelag@uaeu.ac.ae (A.G.); 201911180@uaeu.ac.ae (D.Y.); 201905030@uaeu.ac.ae (A.A.); 201911679@uaeu.ac.ae (A.A.); 201903821@uaeu.ac.ae (M.A.); 700043295@uaeu.ac.ae (A.M.)
2. Department of Medical Microbiology and Infectious Diseases, Erasmus University Medical Centre (Erasmus MC), P.O. Box 2040 Rotterdam, The Netherlands; n.strepis@erasmusmc.nl (N.S.); j.hays@erasmusmc.nl (J.P.H.)
3. Veterinary Public Health Research Laboratory, Department of Veterinary Medicine, College of Agriculture and Veterinary Medicine, United Arab Emirates University, Al Ain P.O. Box 15551, United Arab Emirates; hfebin@uaeu.ac.ae (F.A.); i.habib@uaeu.ac.ae (I.H.)
4. Reproductive Biotechnology Center, Dubai P.O. Box 299003, United Arab Emirates; nisar.wani@reprobiotech.ae
* Correspondence: mushtaq.khan@uaeu.ac.ae

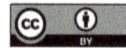

Citation: Ghazawi, A.; Strepis, N.; Anes, F.; Yaaqeib, D.; Ahmed, A.; AlHosani, A.; AlShehhi, M.; Manzoor, A.; Habib, I.; Wani, N.A.; et al. First Report of Colistin-Resistant *Escherichia coli* Carrying *mcr-1* IncI2(delta) and IncX4 Plasmids from Camels (*Camelus dromedarius*) in the Gulf Region. *Antibiotics* **2024**, *13*, 227. https://doi.org/10.3390/antibiotics13030227

Academic Editor: Andrey Shelenkov

Received: 22 January 2024
Revised: 19 February 2024
Accepted: 21 February 2024
Published: 28 February 2024

Copyright: © 2024 by the authors. Licensee MDPI, Basel, Switzerland. This article is an open access article distributed under the terms and conditions of the Creative Commons Attribution (CC BY) license (https://creativecommons.org/licenses/by/4.0/).

**Abstract:** Addressing the emergence of antimicrobial resistance (AMR) poses a significant challenge in veterinary and public health. In this study, we focused on determining the presence, phenotypic background, and genetic epidemiology of plasmid-mediated colistin resistance (*mcr*) in *Escherichia coli* bacteria isolated from camels farmed in the United Arab Emirates (UAE). Fecal samples were collected from 50 camels at a Dubai-based farm in the UAE and colistin-resistant Gram-negative bacilli were isolated using selective culture. Subsequently, a multiplex PCR targeting a range of *mcr*-genes, plasmid profiling, and whole-genome sequencing (WGS) were conducted. Eleven of fifty camel fecal samples (22%) yielded colonies positive for *E. coli* isolates carrying the *mcr-1* gene on mobile genetic elements. No other *mcr*-gene variants and no chromosomally located colistin resistance genes were detected. Following plasmid profiling and WGS, nine *E. coli* isolates from eight camels were selected for in-depth analysis. *E. coli* sequence types (STs) identified included ST7, ST21, ST24, ST399, ST649, ST999, and STdaa2. Seven IncI2(delta) and two IncX4 plasmids were found to be associated with *mcr-1* carriage in these isolates. These findings represent the first identification of *mcr-1*-carrying plasmids associated with camels in the Gulf region. The presence of *mcr-1* in camels from this region was previously unreported and serves as a novel finding in the field of AMR surveillance.

**Keywords:** *mcr-1* gene; plasmids; *Escherichia coli*; camels; United Arab Emirates (UAE)

## 1. Introduction

Antimicrobial resistance (AMR) is a pandemic that is characterized by the continuing global spread of multidrug resistant (MDR) bacteria and accompanying AMR-carrying mobile genetic elements, such as plasmids and transposons. This situation has arisen mainly due to the extensive (inappropriate) overuse of antimicrobials over the last eight decades [1]. The exhaustion of the antibiotic development pipeline, and the resulting shortage of new antibiotics to combat MDR "superbugs" in the foreseeable future, has sparked renewed interest in reviving previously unfavored antibiotics as being potentially effective against MDR pathogens, particularly the previously unfavored polymyxins [1,2].

Colistin is a polymyxin antibiotic whose relatively excessive adverse effects and nephrotoxicity was previously deemed unfavorable for regular parenteral administration. However, the antibiotic has been reintroduced into clinical practice in recent times in order to provide a treatment against globally carbapenem-resistant Enterobacteriaceae, *Pseudomonas*, and *Acinetobacter* infections [3]. However, as the prevalence of these MDR Gram-negative bacteria increased, so did the use of colistin, resulting in the emergence of several novel antimicrobial resistance mechanisms against colistin. Consequently, this antimicrobial has generally lost its efficacy as a last resort for treating infections caused by MDR Gram-negative bacteria worldwide [4]. The already concerning situation has been exacerbated by the identification of mobile colistin resistance genes (*mcr*), predominantly found on plasmids and, in some cases, on bacterial chromosomes [5,6]. In fact, prior to 2016, colistin-resistant bacteria of humans and animals were only attributed to genetic mutations. However, with more extensive colistin use, plasmid-mediated mobile colistin resistance genes have emerged, which have demonstrated rapid dissemination, leading to restrictions in the successful antibiotic therapy of MDR Gram-negative bacterial infections [7,8]. It is now known that multiple variants of the *mcr* gene (*mcr-1* to *mcr-9*) circulate globally in humans, domesticated animals, and livestock, including poultry, pigs, and cows, with the co-occurrence of multiple *mcr* genes within a single colistin-resistant bacterial isolate having been observed [9–11]. In animals and food production, the appearance and evolution of *mcr*-based colistin resistance is intricately linked to the utilization of colistin in the agricultural sector, primarily for promoting animal growth in avian, porcine, and bovine species [12].

With respect to the nations of the Arabian Peninsula, the prevalence of carbapenem-resistant Enterobacterales (CRE) infections has emerged as a significant concern, with reports of CRE colistin resistance rates exceeding 20% [13–16]. However, although the prevalence and diversity of *mcr*-carrying bacterial isolates have previously been documented in camels from Tunisia [17,18], studies have found no presence of *mcr* genes in camels from Kenya (*mcr-1* or *mcr-2*), Nigeria (*mcr-1* to *mcr-8*), or Qatar [19–21]. No reports have yet been made regarding the presence of *mcr* genes in camels from any country in the Gulf region.

Camels play a vital role in arid regions of Asia and Africa, serving as essential livestock resources for milk, meat, and labor, contributing significantly to the agricultural economies of these nations. In many Middle Eastern countries, camel racing is a prestigious and well-organized sport with a multimillion-dollar industry. Additionally, annual camel festivals, featuring beauty contests, offer substantial prizes exceeding USD 22 million. The medicinal value of camel milk has led to the development of advanced camel dairy farms in various countries, meeting the high demand for camel milk and its related products [22]. For these reasons, camels represent an emblem of Emirati heritage occupying a significant position in the country's customs and cultural rituals.

The primary aim of this study was to determine the phenotypic and genetic epidemiology of plasmid-mediated colistin resistance in *E. coli* isolated from camels at a farm in the United Arab Emirates and to compare the genotypic and phenotypic background of these isolates, as well as genotypic aspects of *mcr*-carrying plasmids, with previously published colistin-resistant *E. coli* isolates.

## 2. Results

### 2.1. Detection of mcr Genes, Plasmid Profiling and Antibiotic Susceptibility Profile

Eleven of the fifty camel fecal samples collected (22%) yielded colistin-resistant *E. coli* colonies that were positive for the *mcr-1* gene by PCR. This analysis revealed the exclusive presence of the *mcr-1* gene, with a total of 91 *mcr* gene-positive colonies being identified. After PCR, 14 of the colistin-resistant isolates were subjected to gel electrophoresis and, based on their different plasmid profiles, were subjected to WGS. After quality and contamination checks, a total of nine *E. coli* isolates, derived from eight camels, were available for inclusion, producing sequenced assemblies that matched previously published *E. coli* isolates and plasmids carrying the *mcr-1* gene. Three out of the nine were isolated from "inside" camels, while the remaining six were isolated from "outside" camels. All isolates were resistant to colistin with an MIC of 4 mg/L. Three out of the nine isolates were resistant to more than three classes of antibiotics tested, which is considered multidrug-resistant (Table 1).

Table 1. Antibiotic susceptibility of colistin-resistant, *mcr1*-positive, *E. coli* isolates from camels in the UAE.

| Strains | Camel ID | Colistin MIC (mg/L) | Resistance Detected by Disc Diffusion | |
|---|---|---|---|---|
| | | | Resistant | Intermediate |
| UAE-C1-S1 | 1-inside | 4 | AUG, TET, SXT, AP, DXT | CAZ, CPD, NA |
| UAE-C2-S2 | 2-inside | 4 | NA | CIP, AP |
| UAE-C3-S3 | 3-inside | 4 | - | CIP, NA |
| UAE-C4-S4 | 4-outside | 4 | GM, TET, CIP, SXT, CHL, NA, AP, DXT, TOB | AUG |
| UAE-C5-S5 | 5-outside | 4 | GM, TET, CIP, SXT, CHL, NA, AP, DXT, TOB | AUG |
| UAE-C7-S6 | 7-outside | 4 | NA | CIP, AP |
| UAE-C10-S7 | 10-outside | 4 | - | NA |
| UAE-C10-S8 | 10-outside | 4 | - | NA |
| UAE-C11-S9 | 11-outside | 4 | NA | CIP, AP |

MIC—Minimum Inhibitory Concentration. AUG—Augmentin. AP—Ampicillin. CAZ—Ceftazidime. CHL—Chloramphenicol. CPD—Cefpodoxime. CIP—Ciprofloxacin. DXT—Doxycycline. GM—Gentamicin. NA—Nalidixic acid. SXT—Sulfamethoxazole. TOB—Tobramycin. TET—Tetracycline.

### 2.2. Clonality of the Isolates

Whole-genome sequencing analysis revealed that the nine *E. coli* isolates were assigned to six known sequence types (STs). The most common sequence types (2/9 (22.2%)) among the isolates were ST399, STdaa2, and ST21. These were followed by ST24, ST7, and ST999 as singletons. Core genome multi-locus sequence typing (cgMLST) analysis of the isolates revealed that colistin-resistant *E. coli* isolates UAE-C3-S3/UAE-C10-S8 (STdaa2), UAE-C2-S2/UAE-C7-S6 (ST399), and UAE-C4-S4/UAE-C5-S5 (ST21) possessed identical genotypes. All remaining isolates showed allelic differences in the range of 523–2356 allelic differences (Figure 1). Further phylogenetic analysis based on k-mer analysis of current and publicly available *E. coli* isolates showed that the UAE isolates did not cluster into a single clonal group. Instead, they were associated with several different previously published genotypic clusters of *E. coli* originating from different countries and regions of the world, including clinical, food, and environmental samples (Figure 2).

### 2.3. Antimicrobial Resistance Genes

Detailed examination of the nine *E. coli* isolates listed in Figure 3 showed the presence of the *mcr-1* colistin resistance gene with a 100% identical sequence match between all isolates. Of note, four of these colistin-resistant *E. coli* isolates exhibited an MDR profile, by carrying genes conferring resistance to aminoglycosides, beta-lactams, tetracycline, sulfonamide, and quinolones. Trimethoprim resistance (dfrA5) was detected in a single isolate, while four isolates exclusively possessed the *mcr-1* gene without additional resistance genes. Additionally, a single isolate showed resistance to tetracyclines and quinolones in addition to colistin. The results of in silico AMR gene prediction were consistent with the phenotypic susceptibility results (Table 1).

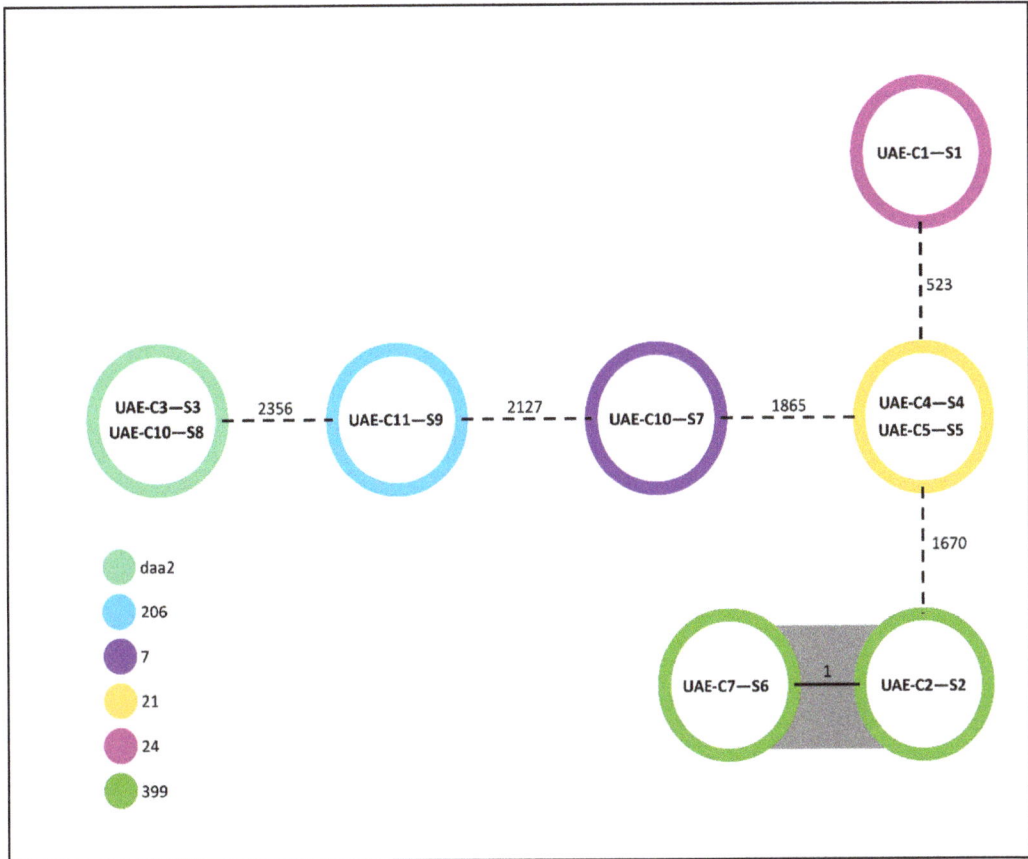

**Figure 1.** Representation of the MLST analysis of the nine *E. coli* genomes with the core genes (cgMLST scheme). The MLST (Pasteur scheme) of the isolates is also indicated. Most of the isolates possessed a high degree of genomic diversity. An exception was the four isolates (two pairs of isolates) that, although deriving from different camels, were observed to have identical genotypes. Nodes represent isolates, numbers indicate allelic differences, and grey clustering indicates identical genotypes. The MLST (Pasteur scheme) is indicated by the colored circles.

### 2.4. Serotype of E. coli Isolates

WGS analysis revealed the presence of four different serotypes among the study isolates (Table 2). Specifically, the serotypes identified were O81 and O49 in conjunction with ST399 and ST21, respectively. It is notable to mention that only two out of nine isolates were of serotype O81. The distribution of phylogroups among the isolates was primarily in phylogroup B1 (five of nine), followed by phylogroup D (two of nine). Regarding the genes responsible for the expression of type 1 fimbriae, an association was observed between the STs and the FimH type.

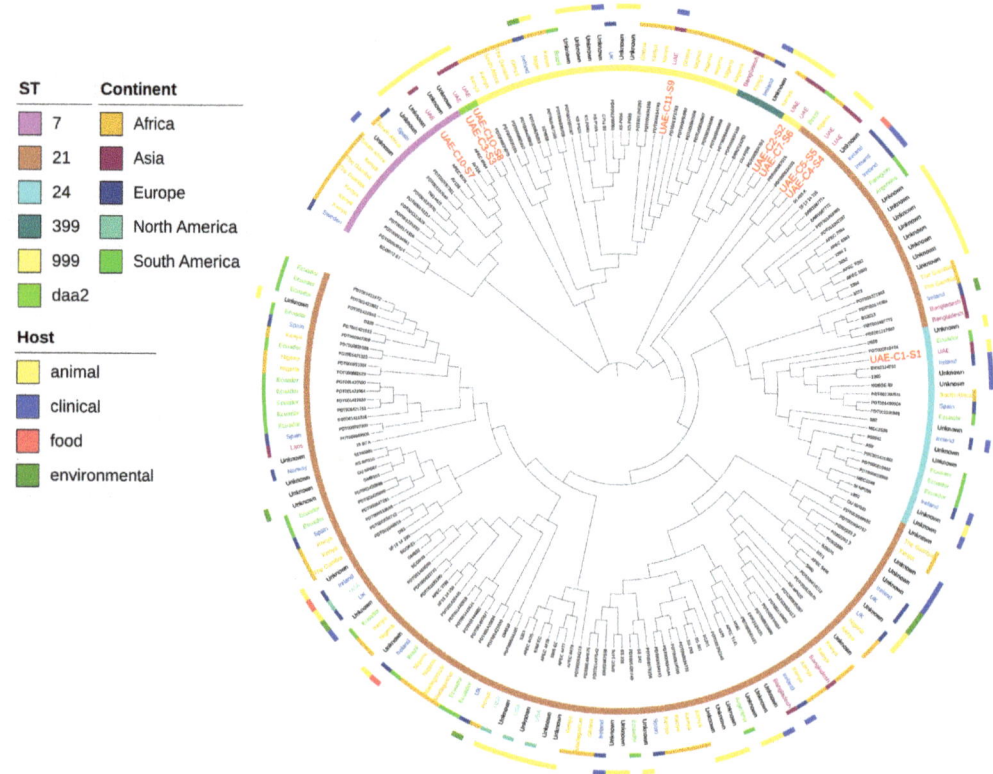

**Figure 2.** Circular visualization of k-mer sequence comparisons (approximately 4.7–5.3 megabases) of the nine colistin-resistant *E. coli* isolates investigated in this study with 184 publicly available *E. coli* genomes. The maximum likelihood tree in the figure describes the SNP differences. From the inner to the outer circle: the inner circle indicates publicly available genomes of *E. coli* with the names from the current UAE study marked in red and larger font size; the second circle indicates sequence type (ST) characterization using an eight-gene comparison scheme; the third circle indicates country of isolation; and the outer circle shows the host from which the *E. coli* was isolated. Gaps in the circles represent *E. coli* genomes with missing country, continent, and/or host metadata.

### 2.5. Virulence Profiles of mcr-1 Producing E. coli Isolates

All genomes were aligned against an *E. coli*-specific virulence gene database and recorded as positive or negative. A total of 44 genes were screened representing different categories (Figure 4). There was a slight difference in the presence of virulence genes based on the ST types. The highest values were recorded in UAE-C1-S1 (ST24), while the lowest were recorded in UAE-C11-S9 (ST 999). The most common genes carried by over 50% of the isolates were genes responsible for long polar fimbriae (*lpfA*), *E. coli* hemolysin (*hlyE*), outer membrane protease (protein protease 7) (*ompT*), tellurium ion resistance protein (*terC*), curlin major subunit (*csgA*), and lipoprotein NlpI precursor (*nlpI*). The aerobactin siderophore genes *iutA* and *iucC* were present only in UAE-C1-S1 (ST24).

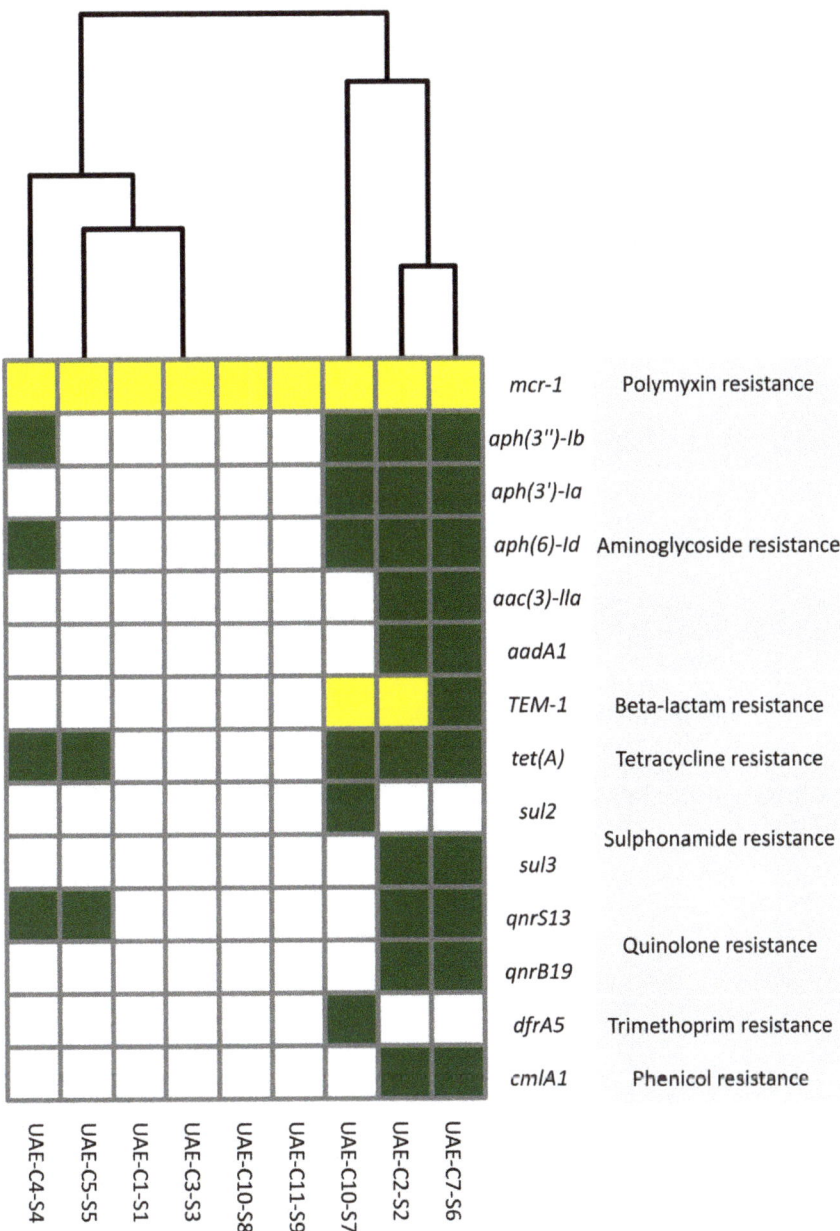

**Figure 3.** Presence of AMR genes as predicted by WGS in *mcr-1*-producing *E. coli* isolates from camels in the UAE. The green squares indicate the presence with >95 and <100 hits with the reference sequence of the CARD database, while the blank squares indicate the absence of the AMR gene. Yellow squares indicate 100% hits with the reference sequence of the CARD database. The clustering of isolates is based on the presence of AMR genes in the respective *E. coli* genomes.

Table 2. WGS serotype and phylogroup prediction of *mcr1* E. coli from the UAE.

| Strains | Sequence Type | Phylogroup | Serotype | FimH Type | CH Type: 4-31 |
|---|---|---|---|---|---|
| UAE-C1-S1 | 24 | B1 | H25, O9 | fimH27 | fumC4-fimH24: 4-27 |
| UAE-C2-S2 | 399 | B1 | H14, O81 | fimH24 | fumC6-fimH24: 6-24 |
| UAE-C3-S3 | daa2 | D | H48, O56 | fimH577 | fumC26-fimH577: 26-577 |
| UAE-C4-S4 | 21 | B1 | H9, O49 | fimH32 | fumC4-fimH32: 4-32 |
| UAE-C5-S5 | 21 | B1 | H9, O49 | fimH32 | fumC4-fimH32: 4-32 |
| UAE-C7-S6 | 399 | B1 | H14, O81 | fimH24 | fumC6-fimH24: 6-24 |
| UAE-C10-S7 | 7 | C | H9, O21 | fimH35 | fumC4-fimH35: 4-35 |
| UAE-C10-S8 | daa2 | D | H48, O56 | fimH577 | fumC26-fimH577: 26-577 |
| UAE-C11-S9 | 999 | A | H5 | fimH41 | fumC7-fimH41: 7-41 |

*2.6. Characterization of mcr-1 Plasmids*

Nine plasmids carrying the *mcr-1* gene were positively detected in fecal samples from eight different camels. Three of these camels were kept in an indoor enclosure while the remaining five were taken outside for various activities. All of the plasmids detected were found to match publicly available plasmid sequences from around the globe. Public plasmids similar to plasmids in this study were hosted in the majority of *E. coli* and *Salmonella* sp. In particular, the *E. coli* isolates UAE-C1-S1, UAE-C2-S2, UAE-C3-S3, UAE-C7-S6, UAE-C10-S7, UAE-C10-S8, and UAE-C11-S9 contain IncI2(delta) plasmids, whereas *E. coli* isolates UAE-C4-S4 and UAE-C5-S5 carried IncX4 plasmids. The IncI2(delta) plasmids had identical genetic backgrounds, with the exception of UAE-C10-S8, which had an additional gene, *repA*. Both IncX4 plasmids had identical genetic backgrounds (Figure 5). When *mcr-1* genome synteny was examined, no integrons were present, although *mcr-1* genome synteny was different between the two different incompatibility types (Inc) (Figure 6).

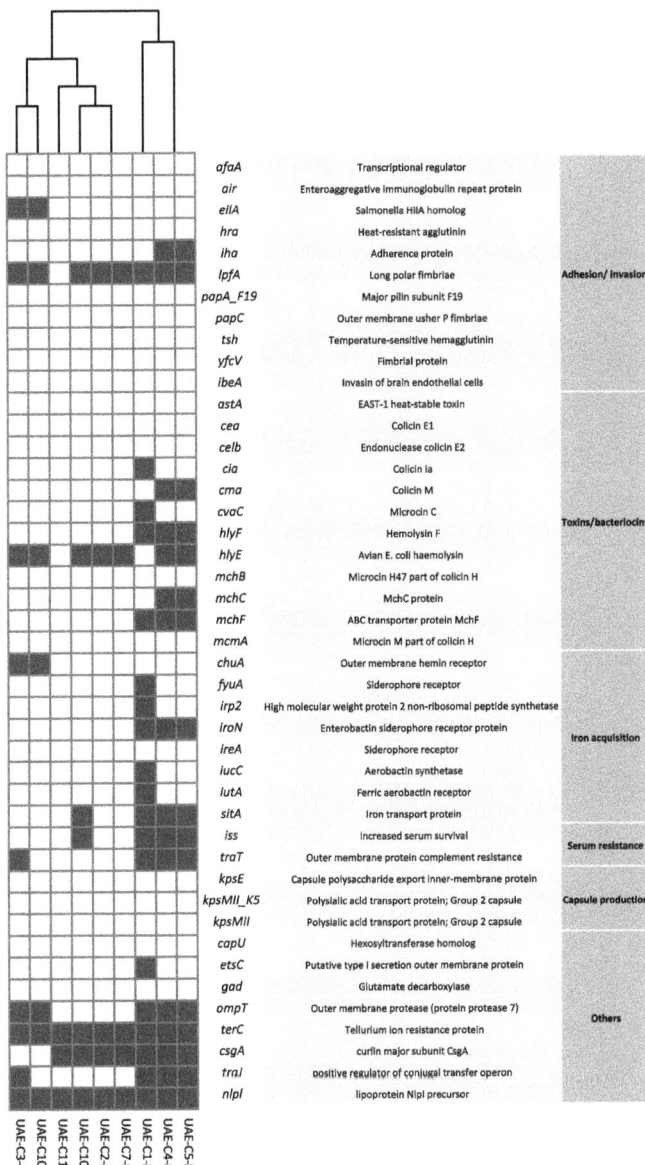

**Figure 4.** Presence of virulence genes predicted by WGS in *mcr-1*-producing *E. coli* isolates from camels in the UAE. The green color indicates the presence while the blank indicates the absence of the gene. The clustering of isolates is based on the presence of virulence genes in their genomes.

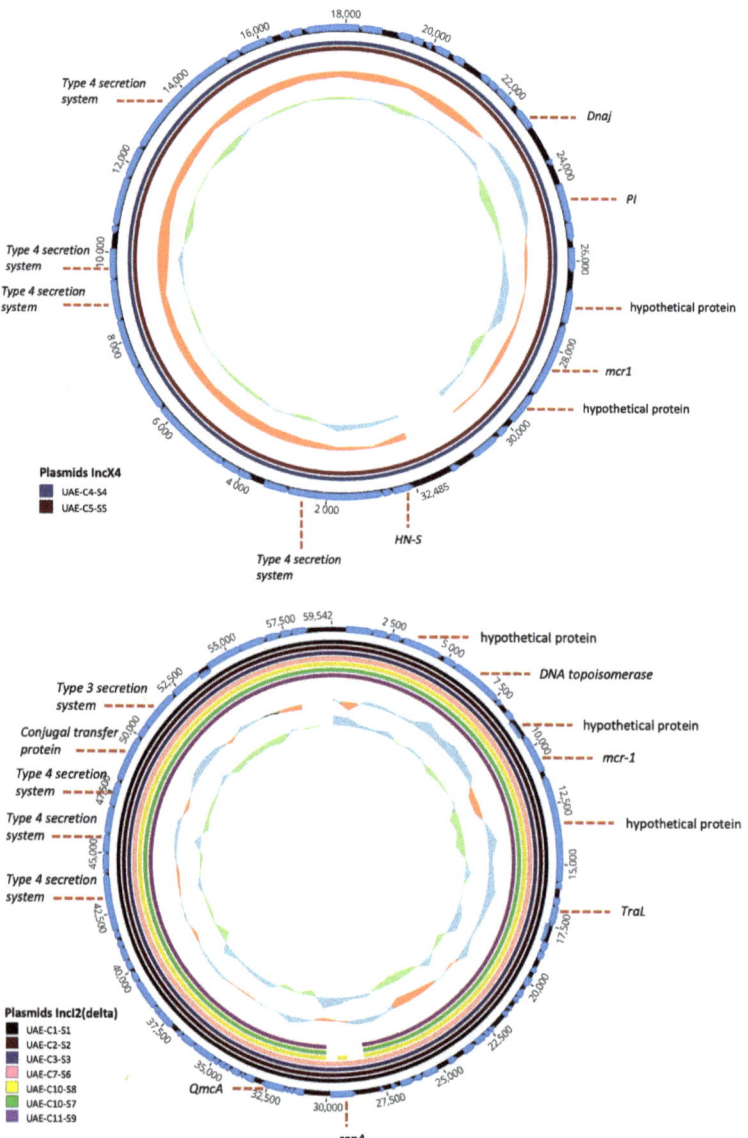

**Figure 5.** Circular representation of *mcr* plasmids based on sequence alignment and gene visualization. Seven IncI2(delta) plasmids with identical genetic backgrounds were identified, except for UAE-C10-S8, which possessed an additional *repA* gene. Additionally, two IncX4 plasmids with identical genetic backgrounds were identified. The inner circle represents the GC skew of the plasmids and the middle circles represent each of the plasmids. The outer circle with the arrows represents nucleotide bases and CDS (genes) of the plasmid that the graph was based upon (for IncI2(delta)—sample UAE-C10-S8 and for IncX4—sample UAE-C4-S4). Annotations of important CDS are included in the Figure.

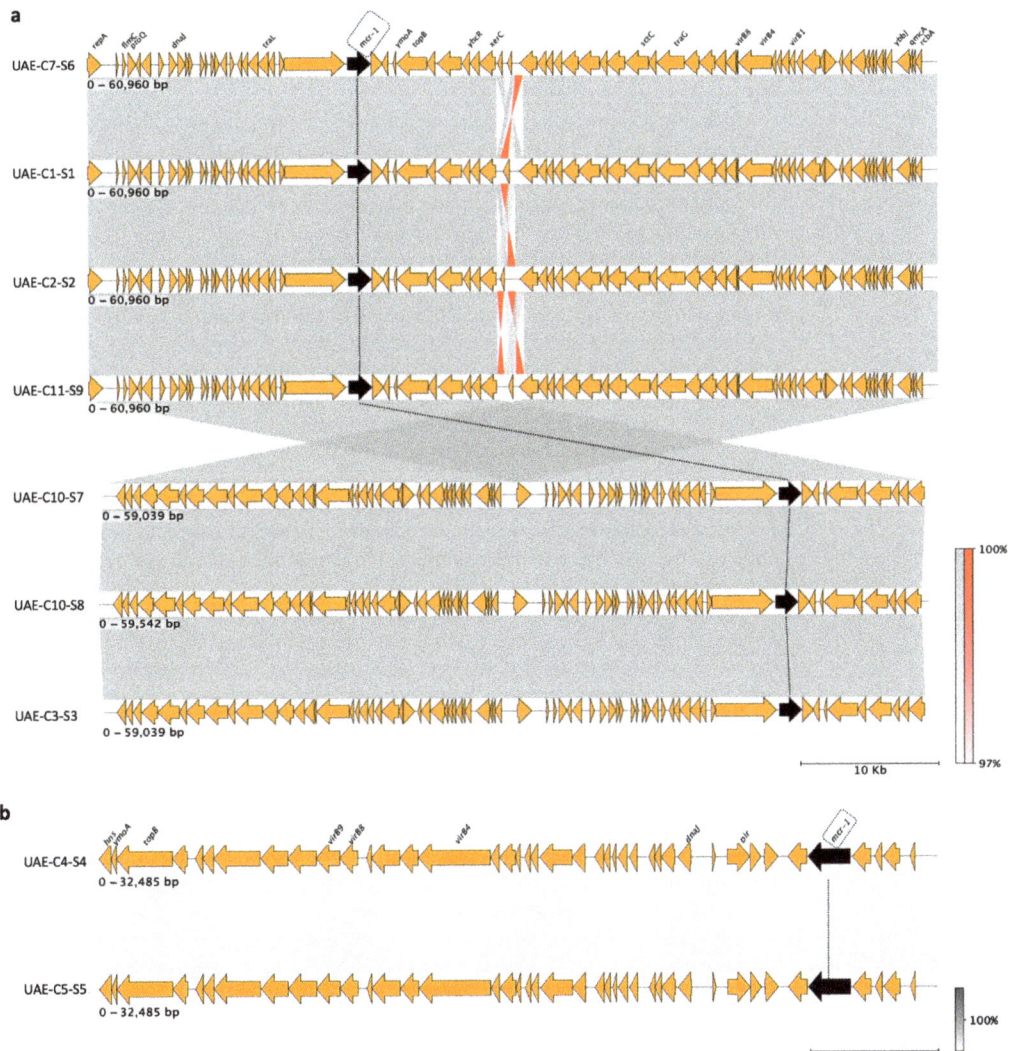

**Figure 6.** Representation of the genomic background of the IncI2(delta) (**a**) and IncX4 (**b**) plasmids carrying the *mcr-1* gene. IncI2(delta) and IncX4 plasmids carrying *mcr-1*, in this study, are observed to have a similar genetic backbone in terms of sequence and gene content. Additionally, the *mcr-1* gene is included in all plasmids in the same region. The *mcr-1* is surrounded by hypothetical proteins and repeat sequences; integron-related genes are absent. Orange arrows indicate genes, the *mcr-1* gene is indicated with a black arrow, and the black dotted line tracks the position among plasmids. The direction of the arrow indicates the direction of the gene. Grey shading among plasmid sequences indicates the sequence identity between them (which was 97–100%). Red shading among them indicates reverse regions in the sequences.

## 3. Discussion

The current publication describes a comprehensive genomic analysis of *mcr-1*-carrying plasmids and their corresponding *E. coli* isolates obtained from camels in the United Arab Emirates (UAE). The study is the first in-depth genomic investigation into colistin resistance and its mechanisms in camels within the UAE and the Gulf region. The results were obtained from a single farm in the UAE using a limited number of samples. Further research is required to determine if more camels in the UAE and Gulf region carry colistin-resistant *mcr* gene-carrying bacteria.

Resistance to polymyxins, including colistin, in Gram-negative enteric bacteria, has historically been rare. The primary mechanism originally involved mutations in bacterial chromosomal genes such as *mgrB*, *phoP/phoQ*, and *pmrA/pmrB*, leading to modifications in bacterial lipopolysaccharides (LPSs) that conferred protection against the polymyxin cationic peptide [23]. This situation has now been complicated by the identification and recognition of the global dissemination of the plasmid-mediated colistin resistance gene *mcr-1* [24]. Additionally, there is a growing appreciation of the problem of polymyxin resistance relating to a "ONE Health" perspective [25]. For example, in veterinary medicine, colistin has been used extensively and in large quantities for decades for the prevention and therapy of infectious diseases in all continents, as well as for growth promotion in some Asian countries, such as China, Japan, India, and Vietnam [26]. The identification of four colistin-resistant *E. coli* isolates with a multidrug-resistant (MDR) profile underscores the complex nature of antimicrobial resistance in this context. The presence of genes conferring resistance to aminoglycosides, beta-lactams, tetracycline, sulfonamide, and quinolones within these isolates highlights the potential for widespread resistance to multiple classes of antibiotics among camel-derived *E. coli* strains. Such MDR phenotypes pose significant challenges for the effective treatment of bacterial infections in both veterinary and public health settings.

It is noteworthy that *mcr-1*-positive Enterobacterales isolates have been previously reported in the UAE; however, these were specifically associated with poultry [27–29], whereas the current study focused on colistin-resistant *E. coli* from camels, indicating a relatively high frequency of *mcr-1*-positive *E. coli* (22%) within a farm camel population in the UAE. In fact, more than seventy-five genotypic sequence types (STs) of *E. coli* have been reported to carry *mcr-1* [25]. Phylogenetic analysis of the nine colistin-resistant *E. coli* isolates investigated in the current study revealed that these nine isolates were not clonally related to each other or to other reported global ST genotypes, with UAE-similar ST genotypes having previously been isolated from several different countries and continents, as well as from animal, clinical, food, and environmental sources (Figure 2). The detection of a higher proportion of *mcr-1*-positive *E. coli* strains from "outside" camels compared to "inside" camels suggests a potential scenario of introduction from external sources. It is conceivable that outside camels, through environmental exposure or contact with other herds, serve as reservoirs or carriers of antibiotic-resistant strains, subsequently introducing them to the farm environment. Furthermore, the identification of resistant strains originating from external sources highlights the importance of stringent biosecurity measures and surveillance protocols to mitigate the risk of introduction and dissemination of antibiotic resistance within animal populations. This collective evidence underscores the need for a ONE Health approach to combatting colistin resistance, specifically in identifying the global dissemination of *E. coli* ST genotypes with the potential to spread *mcr-1*-carrying plasmids across different continents, origins, and environments.

To date, 10 variants of the *mcr* gene have been described in bacteria isolated from human, animal, and environmental sources [30]. These *mcr* genes, particularly *mcr-1*, are carried by various plasmid types in Enterobacterales, including IncI2 (with a size range of 50–250 kb), IncX (30–50 kb), IncHI (75–400 kb), IncY (90–100 kb), IncP (70–275 kb), IncF (45–200 kb), IncN (30–70 kb), and IncQ (8–14 kb) [30]. Over the past decade, IncI2, HI2, and X4 have predominantly served as carriers for *mcr-1* in both human and animal populations, contributing to the escalation of antimicrobial resistance (AMR) in Asia, Europe, and the Middle East. This underscores the significance of the zoonotic transmission of colistin resistance [31].

In the current study, *mcr-1*-positive IncI2 and IncX4 plasmids were isolated. These two plasmid types were closely associated with *mcr-1*-related AMR associated with non-camel livestock in the UAE, as documented in several studies over the past 4 years [27–29]. IncI2 plasmids have been identified in several *mcr-1* cases on various hosts worldwide [32], while the IncX4 plasmid type has been recognized as the primary carrier of the *mcr-1* gene in isolates from healthy individuals in China [33], as well as in Enterobacteriaceae isolates carrying carbapenem and *mcr-1* resistance genes simultaneously from clinical patients in Thailand [34]. Our study identified the presence of *mcr-1* genes on both IncI2 and IncX4 plasmids, which have been recently observed in *E. coli* isolates from food, livestock, and humans across various countries [35,36].

Additionally, IncX4 plasmids are characterized by their genetic stability and their relatively smaller size compared to IncI2 plasmids [37,38]. Further, IncI2 replicon type plasmids are known for their robust competitive and fitness advantage within the host bacterium compared to other plasmid types such as IncHI2 or IncX4 plasmids [32,39]. With respect to the *mcr-1* gene, its presence has been noted to provide fitness advantages to its bacterial host when present on both IncI2 and IncX4 plasmids. This observation suggests that the impact on host strain fitness can vary depending on the combination of host strain and plasmid. This variability could potentially clarify why IncI2 and IncX4 are the predominant carriers of *mcr-1* on a global scale [32]. When compared, the individual *mcr-1*-carrying IncI2(delta) and IncX4 plasmids from this study (Figure 2) were found to have differences in *mcr-1* genome synteny between the two different incompatibility types. However, no integrons were detected, suggesting potential plasmid transmission among the camels themselves, or alternatively, through animal food or exposure to common environments that were shared by the camels on the farm tested.

This study represents the first screening and detailed analysis of *mcr-1*-positive *E. coli* and corresponding plasmids isolated from camels in the United Arab Emirates. Although we were unable to obtain data on antimicrobial use on the farm from which the samples were obtained, this prevalence may indicate the frequent use of colistin and possibly other antimicrobials in the camel industry of this region. The significance of camels in the UAE and the Gulf region is immense, permeating various economic and recreational activities and holding a central place as a cultural heritage. Camels play an indispensable role in daily life, providing essential resources such as meat and milk. Despite this fact (and with the exception of research studying the feces of camel/calves in Tunisia, Kenya, and Nigeria, where colistin-resistant bacteria were found to be devoid of the *mcr* gene), to the best of our knowledge no other studies have reported the existence of bacterial isolates carrying *mcr-1* genes in camels from the Gulf region [17,19,20]. This finding indicates the absence of such research in camels in the Gulf region. This oversight is unfortunate given the critical role camels play in the Gulf region, and highlights the need for more attention and investigation into the antimicrobial resistance patterns associated with these animals.

Based on our findings, further investigations are required to elucidate the precise dynamics behind the dissemination of *mcr-1*-carrying plasmids among international camel populations, including their co-occurrence with, and role in, MDR strains possessing resistance to aminoglycosides, beta-lactams, tetracycline, sulfonamide, and quinolones.

## 4. Materials and Methods

*4.1. Sample Collection*

Samples were collected from a government-owned camel farm located in Dubai, UAE, which could accommodate approximately 300 camels. Camels were divided into two main groups: inside camels—which have resided at the farm for a minimum of five years, and outside camels—which are imported into the farm annually for breeding purposes. These outside camels remained at the farm for the duration of the breeding season or until pregnancy was confirmed, after which time they were returned to their original locations or sent to a larger farm.

During the study period, the farm housed approximately 150 inside camels and 50 outside camels, and to ensure comprehensive representation, we collected 25 fecal samples from each group. Samples were obtained directly from the rectum of each camel using sterile techniques and containers. Collection procedures were performed meticulously to avoid cross-contamination and ensure sample integrity. Given the practical constraints and funding limitations, the sample size was determined to balance feasibility and the need for meaningful insights into the prevalence of the *mcr-1* gene among adult camels at this farm in the UAE. All samples were promptly transported to the microbiology laboratory for processing on the day of collection.

### 4.2. Detection of mcr Genes and Plasmid Profiling

For detection of colistin resistance, one gram of fecal sample was added to 4 mL Tryptic Soy Broth (TSB) containing 1 µg/mL colistin sulphate and 8 µg/mL vancomycin. Following overnight incubation at 37 °C, two McConkey agar plates containing 1µg/mL colistin sulphate were inoculated with 10 µL and 100 µL of the TSB culture and incubated overnight at 37 °C. If there were more than 10 colonies in a sample, then 10 colonies with varying morphologies were chosen for sub-culture [27]. In cases where *mcr*-positive isolates displayed distinctive colony characteristics, one representative of each type was chosen for further investigation for the presence of known mobile colistin resistance determinants using a multiplex PCR targeting *mcr-1, mcr-2, mcr-3, mcr-4, mcr-5* [40], and *mcr-6* to *mcr-9* [41]. To establish the plasmid profiles of the sub-cultured colonies, plasmids were extracted using the alkaline lysis method and plasmids profiled using gel electrophoresis, including reference *E. coli* V517 and *E. coli* 39R861 as plasmid size controls [42]. Plasmid patterns were subsequently compared, and a selection of isolates with different plasmid profiles were used for further analysis.

### 4.3. Antimicrobial Susceptibility Test

The disk diffusion method on Mueller–Hinton agar (Oxoid, Manchester, UK) was employed to perform antimicrobial susceptibility testing (AST) on isolated *E. coli*. The resistant profile of the isolates was assessed against 21 antibiotic discs, including Aztreonam (30 µg), Cefotaxime (30 µg), Amoxicillin-clavulanic acid (30 µg), Ceftazidime (30 µg), Cefpodoxime (10 µg), Trimethoprim-sulfamethoxazole (25 µg), Chloramphenicol (30 µg), Tetracycline (30 µg), Ertapenem (10 µg), Ciprofloxacin (5 µg), Gentamicin (10 µg), Fosfomycin (200 µg), Ampicillin (10 µg), Tobramycin (10 µg), Doxycycline (30 µg), Nalidixic acid (30 µg), Imipenem (10 µg), Meropenem (10 µg), Amikacin (30 µg), and Piperacillin/tazobactam (110 µg). All the antibiotics were purchased from MAST, Liverpool, UK. The zone of inhibition was interpreted based on CLSI guidelines [43]. For colistin, minimum inhibitory concentration (MIC) was determined by broth microdilution (BMD) using Cation-Adjusted Mueller–Hinton Broth (CAMHB) (MAST, Liverpool, UK) and *E. coli* ATCC 25922 as a control strain [43].

### 4.4. Whole-Genome Sequencing

Total DNA extraction was conducted using the Wizard® Genomic DNA Purification Kit (Promega, Madison, WI, USA), in adherence to the manufacturer's instructions. Subsequent sequencing was carried out on the Illumina NovaSeq platform (150 bp paired-end) through a commercial service provided by Novogene (Cambridge, UK). Genome assemblies were generated from the sequencing reads of the isolates using Unicycler v0.48 (https://github.com/rrwick/Unicycler; accessed on 15 November 2023) with default parameters [44]. Quality control of assemblies was assessed based on quast v5.2.0 (https://github.com/ablab/quast; accessed on 20 November 2023) [45]. A contamination check of samples was performed based on Kraken2 (https://github.com/DerrickWood/kraken2; accessed on 20 November 2023) [46]. The identification of antimicrobial resistance (AMR) genes was performed using RGI v6.03 (https://card.mcmaster.ca/analyze/rgi; accessed on 25 November 2023) with default parameters based on the CARD database v3.28 (https://card.mcmaster.ca/analyze/rgi; accessed on 25 November 2023). Plasmid Incompatibility types (Inc types) were identified based on PlasmidFinder v2.10 (https://cge.food.dtu.dk/services/PlasmidFinder/; accessed on 28 November 2023) with an ID threshold of 60%, Enterobacterales database, and default coverage threshold [47]. The virulence genes were detected using VFDB (http://www.mgc.ac.cn/VFs/; accessed on 20 December 2023). The presence of integrons was assessed using IntegronFinder 2.0 (https://github.com/gem-pasteur/Integron_Finder; accessed on 5 December 2023) [48]. Ridom SeqSphere+ v9.00 (https://www.ridom.de/seqsphere/index.shtml; accessed on 28 December 2023) was used for performing cgMLST and MLST typing (scheme Pasteur) for *E. coli* isolates. Public isolates with identical sequence types to those found in this study were obtained from PubMLST [49]. A k-mer analysis was performed for isolates retrieved from PubMLST and this study using kSNP v3.10 [50] with default parameters, and k-mer size of 19 and maximum likelihood tree generation. The generated tree was uploaded to iTOL [51]. Plasmid sequence comparisons and visualizations were performed using Mummer2circos (https://github.com/metagenlab/mummer2circos; accessed on 3 January, 2024) and Geneious (https://www.geneious.com; accessed on 3 January, 2024).

**Author Contributions:** Conceptualization, A.G., J.P.H. and M.K.; Methodology, A.G., N.S., F.A., D.Y., A.A. (Amal Ahmed), A.A. (Aysha AlHosani), M.A. and A.M.; Software, A.G. and N.S.; Formal analysis, A.G., N.S., F.A., D.Y., A.A. (Amal Ahmed), A.A. (Aysha AlHosani), M.A., A.M., I.H. and J.P.H.; Investigation, A.G., I.H., N.A.W. and M.K.; Writing—original draft, A.G., N.S., A.M., I.H., J.P.H. and M.K.; Writing—review and editing, A.G., N.S., A.M., I.H., N.A.W., J.P.H. and M.K.; Project administration, A.G., J.P.H. and M.K.; Funding acquisition, M.K. All authors have read and agreed to the published version of the manuscript.

**Funding:** This research was funded by grants from United Arab Emirates University, UAE (G00003543 and G00004164) awarded to M.K.

**Institutional Review Board Statement:** Not applicable.

**Informed Consent Statement:** Not applicable.

**Data Availability Statement:** The datasets presented in this study can be found in online repositories. The names of the repository/repositories and accession number(s) can be found below: https://www.ebi.ac.uk/ena PRJEB67677 (accessed on 15 November 2023).

**Conflicts of Interest:** The authors declare no conflicts of interest.

# References

1. Lim, L.M.; Ly, N.; Anderson, D.; Yang, J.C.; Macander, L.; Jarkowski, A., III; Forrest, A.; Bulitta, J.B.; Tsuji, B.T. Resurgence of colistin: A review of resistance, toxicity, pharmacodynamics, and dosing. *Pharmacotherapy* **2010**, *30*, 1279–1291. [CrossRef]
2. Bialvaei, A.Z.; Samadi Kafil, H. Colistin, mechanisms and prevalence of resistance. *Curr. Med. Res. Opin.* **2015**, *31*, 707–721. [CrossRef]
3. Dhariwal, A.K.; Tullu, M.S. Colistin: Re-emergence of the 'forgotten' antimicrobial agent. *J. Postgrad. Med.* **2013**, *59*, 208–215. [CrossRef]
4. Capone, A.; Giannella, M.; Fortini, D.; Giordano, A.; Meledandri, M.; Ballardini, M.; Venditti, M.; Bordi, E.; Capozzi, D.; Balice, M.P.; et al. High rate of colistin resistance among patients with carbapenem-resistant Klebsiella pneumoniae infection accounts for an excess of mortality. *Clin. Microbiol. Infect. Off. Publ. Eur. Soc. Clin. Microbiol. Infect. Dis.* **2013**, *19*, E23–E30. [CrossRef]
5. Nang, S.C.; Li, J.; Velkov, T. The rise and spread of *mcr* plasmid-mediated polymyxin resistance. *Crit. Rev. Microbiol.* **2019**, *45*, 131–161. [CrossRef]
6. Caniaux, I.; van Belkum, A.; Zambardi, G.; Poirel, L.; Gros, M.F. MCR: Modern colistin resistance. *Eur. J. Clin. Microbiol. Infect. Dis. Off. Publ. Eur. Soc. Clin. Microbiol.* **2017**, *36*, 415–420. [CrossRef]
7. Sun, J.; Zhang, H.; Liu, Y.H.; Feng, Y. Towards Understanding MCR-like Colistin Resistance. *Trends Microbiol.* **2018**, *26*, 794–808. [CrossRef] [PubMed]
8. Caselli, E.; D'Accolti, M.; Soffritti, I.; Piffanelli, M.; Mazzacane, S. Spread of *mcr*-1-Driven Colistin Resistance on Hospital Surfaces, Italy. *Emerg. Infect. Dis.* **2018**, *24*, 1752–1753. [CrossRef] [PubMed]
9. Sia, C.M.; Greig, D.R.; Day, M.; Hartman, H.; Painset, A.; Doumith, M.; Meunier, D.; Jenkins, C.; Chattaway, M.A.; Hopkins, K.L.; et al. The characterization of mobile colistin resistance (*mcr*) genes among 33000 *Salmonella enterica* genomes from routine public health surveillance in England. *Microb. Genom.* **2020**, *6*, e000331. [CrossRef] [PubMed]
10. García, V.; García-Meniño, I.; Mora, A.; Flament-Simon, S.C.; Díaz-Jiménez, D.; Blanco, J.E.; Alonso, M.P.; Blanco, J. Co-occurrence of *mcr*-1, *mcr*-4 and *mcr*-5 genes in multidrug-resistant ST10 Enterotoxigenic and Shiga toxin-producing Escherichia coli in Spain (2006-2017). *Int. J. Antimicrob. Agents* **2018**, *52*, 104–108. [CrossRef] [PubMed]

11. Hadjadj, L.; Baron, S.A.; Olaitan, A.O.; Morand, S.; Rolain, J.M. Co-occurrence of Variants of *mcr-3* and *mcr-8* Genes in a *Klebsiella pneumoniae* Isolate From Laos. *Front. Microbiol.* **2019**, *10*, 2720. [CrossRef]
12. Callens, B.; Persoons, D.; Maes, D.; Laanen, M.; Postma, M.; Boyen, F.; Haesebrouck, F.; Butaye, P.; Catry, B.; Dewulf, J. Prophylactic and metaphylactic antimicrobial use in Belgian fattening pig herds. *Prev. Vet. Med.* **2012**, *106*, 53–62. [CrossRef]
13. Zowawi, H.M.; Sartor, A.L.; Balkhy, H.H.; Walsh, T.R.; Al Johani, S.M.; AlJindan, R.Y.; Alfaresi, M.; Ibrahim, E.; Al-Jardani, A.; Al-Abri, S.; et al. Molecular characterization of carbapenemase-producing Escherichia coli and Klebsiella pneumoniae in the countries of the Gulf cooperation council: Dominance of OXA-48 and NDM producers. *Antimicrob. Agents Chemother.* **2014**, *58*, 3085–3090. [CrossRef]
14. Sonnevend, Á.; Ghazawi, A.A.; Hashmey, R.; Jamal, W.; Rotimi, V.O.; Shibl, A.M.; Al-Jardani, A.; Al-Abri, S.S.; Tariq, W.U.; Weber, S.; et al. Characterization of Carbapenem-Resistant Enterobacteriaceae with High Rate of Autochthonous Transmission in the Arabian Peninsula. *PLoS ONE* **2015**, *10*, e0131372. [CrossRef]
15. Moubareck, C.A.; Mouftah, S.F.; Pál, T.; Ghazawi, A.; Halat, D.H.; Nabi, A.; AlSharhan, M.A.; AlDeesi, Z.O.; Peters, C.C.; Celiloglu, H.; et al. Clonal emergence of Klebsiella pneumoniae ST14 co-producing OXA-48-type and NDM carbapenemases with high rate of colistin resistance in Dubai, United Arab Emirates. *Int. J. Antimicrob. Agents* **2018**, *52*, 90–95. [CrossRef]
16. Sonnevend, Á.; Ghazawi, A.; Darwish, D.; Barathan, G.; Hashmey, R.; Ashraf, T.; Rizvi, T.A.; Pál, T. In vitro efficacy of ceftazidime-avibactam, aztreonam-avibactam and other rescue antibiotics against carbapenem-resistant Enterobacterales from the Arabian Peninsula. *Int. J. Infect. Dis. IJID Off. Publ. Int. Soc. Infect. Dis.* **2020**, *99*, 253–259. [CrossRef] [PubMed]
17. Rhouma, M.; Bessalah, S.; Salhi, I.; Thériault, W.; Fairbrother, J.M.; Fravalo, P. Screening for fecal presence of colistin-resistant Escherichia coli and *mcr-1* and *mcr-2* genes in camel-calves in southern Tunisia. *Acta Vet. Scand.* **2018**, *60*, 35. [CrossRef] [PubMed]
18. Saidani, M.; Messadi, L.; Mefteh, J.; Chaouechi, A.; Soudani, A.; Selmi, R.; Dâaloul-Jedidi, M.; Ben Chehida, F.; Mamlouk, A.; Jemli, M.H.; et al. Various Inc-type plasmids and lineages of Escherichia coli and Klebsiella pneumoniae spreading bla$_{CTX-M-15}$, bla$_{CTX-M-1}$ and *mcr-1* genes in camels in Tunisia. *J. Glob. Antimicrob. Resist.* **2019**, *19*, 280–283. [CrossRef] [PubMed]
19. Nüesch-Inderbinen, M.; Kindle, P.; Baschera, M.; Liljander, A.; Jores, J.; Corman, V.M.; Stephan, R. Antimicrobial resistant and extended-spectrum ß-lactamase (ESBL) producing *Escherichia coli* isolated from fecal samples of African dromedary camels. *Sci. Afr.* **2020**, *7*, e00274. [CrossRef]
20. Ngbede, E.O.; Poudel, A.; Kalalah, A.; Yang, Y.; Adekanmbi, F.; Adikwu, A.A.; Adamu, A.M.; Mamfe, L.M.; Daniel, S.T.; Useh, N.M.; et al. Identification of mobile colistin resistance genes (*mcr-1.1*, *mcr-5* and *mcr-8.1*) in Enterobacteriaceae and Alcaligenes faecalis of human and animal origin, Nigeria. *Int. J. Antimicrob. Agents* **2020**, *56*, 106108. [CrossRef] [PubMed]
21. Alhababi, D.A.; Eltai, N.O.; Nasrallah, G.K.; Farg, E.A.; Al Thani, A.A.; Yassine, H.M. Antimicrobial Resistance of Commensal *Escherichia coli* Isolated from Food Animals in Qatar. *Microb. Drug Resist.* **2020**, *26*, 420–427. [CrossRef]
22. Wani, N.A. In vitro embryo production (IVEP) in camelids: Present status and future perspectives. *Reprod. Biol.* **2021**, *21*, 100471. [CrossRef]
23. Olaitan, A.O.; Morand, S.; Rolain, J.M. Mechanisms of polymyxin resistance: Acquired and intrinsic resistance in bacteria. *Front. Microbiol.* **2014**, *5*, 643. [CrossRef]
24. Liu, Y.Y.; Wang, Y.; Walsh, T.R.; Yi, L.X.; Zhang, R.; Spencer, J.; Doi, Y.; Tian, G.; Dong, B.; Huang, X.; et al. Emergence of plasmid-mediated colistin resistance mechanism MCR-1 in animals and human beings in China: A microbiological and molecular biological study. *Lancet Infect. Dis.* **2016**, *16*, 161–168. [CrossRef]
25. Biswas, U.; Das, S.; Barik, M.; Mallick, A. Situation Report on *mcr*-Carrying Colistin-Resistant Clones of Enterobacterales: A Global Update Through Human-Animal-Environment Interfaces. *Curr. Microbiol.* **2023**, *81*, 12. [CrossRef]
26. Kempf, I.; Jouy, E.; Chauvin, C. Colistin use and colistin resistance in bacteria from animals. *Int. J. Antimicrob. Agents* **2016**, *48*, 598–606. [CrossRef] [PubMed]
27. Sonnevend, Á.; Alali, W.Q.; Mahmoud, S.A.; Ghazawi, A.; Bharathan, G.; Melegh, S.; Rizvi, T.A.; Pál, T. Molecular Characterization of *MCR-1* Producing *Enterobacterales* Isolated in Poultry Farms in the United Arab Emirates. *Antibiotics* **2022**, *11*, 305. [CrossRef] [PubMed]
28. Habib, I.; Elbediwi, M.; Ghazawi, A.; Mohamed, M.I.; Lakshmi, G.B.; Khan, M. First report from supermarket chicken meat and genomic characterization of colistin resistance mediated by *mcr-1.1* in ESBL-producing, multidrug-resistant Salmonella Minnesota. *Int. J. Food Microbiol.* **2022**, *379*, 109835. [CrossRef] [PubMed]
29. Habib, I.; Elbediwi, M.; Mohamed, M.I.; Ghazawi, A.; Abdalla, A.; Khalifa, H.O.; Khan, M. Enumeration, antimicrobial resistance and genomic characterization of extended-spectrum β-lactamases producing Escherichia coli from supermarket chicken meat in the United Arab Emirates. *Int. J. Food Microbiol.* **2023**, *398*, 110224. [CrossRef] [PubMed]
30. Hussein, N.H.; Al-Kadmy, I.M.S.; Taha, B.M.; Hussein, J.D. Mobilized colistin resistance (*mcr*) genes from 1 to 10: A comprehensive review. *Mol. Biol. Rep.* **2021**, *48*, 2897–2907. [CrossRef]
31. Madec, J.Y.; Haenni, M.; Nordmann, P.; Poirel, L. Extended-spectrum β-lactamase/AmpC- and carbapenemase-producing Enterobacteriaceae in animals: A threat for humans? *Clin. Microbiol. Infect. Off. Publ. Eur. Soc. Clin. Microbiol. Infect. Dis.* **2017**, *23*, 826–833. [CrossRef] [PubMed]
32. Wu, R.; Yi, L.X.; Yu, L.F.; Wang, J.; Liu, Y.; Chen, X.; Lv, L.; Yang, J.; Liu, J.H. Fitness Advantage of *mcr-1*-Bearing IncI2 and IncX4 Plasmids in Vitro. *Front. Microbiol.* **2018**, *9*, 331. [CrossRef]

33. Shen, C.; Zhong, L.L.; Yang, Y.; Doi, Y.; Paterson, D.L.; Stoesser, N.; Ma, F.; El-Sayed Ahmed, M.A.E.; Feng, S.; Huang, S.; et al. Dynamics of *mcr*-1 prevalence and *mcr*-1-positive Escherichia coli after the cessation of colistin use as a feed additive for animals in China: A prospective cross-sectional and whole genome sequencing-based molecular epidemiological study. *Lancet. Microbe* **2020**, *1*, e34–e43. [CrossRef] [PubMed]
34. Paveenkittiporn, W.; Kamjumphol, W.; Ungcharoen, R.; Kerdsin, A. Whole-Genome Sequencing of Clinically Isolated Carbapenem-Resistant Enterobacterales Harboring *mcr* Genes in Thailand, 2016–2019. *Front. Microbiol.* **2021**, *11*, 586368. [CrossRef] [PubMed]
35. Feng, J.; Wu, H.; Zhuang, J.; Luo, J.; Chen, Y.; Wu, Y.; Fei, J.; Shen, Q.; Yuan, Z.; Chen, M. Stability and genetic insights of the co-existence of $bla_{CTX-M-65}$, $bla_{OXA-1}$, and *mcr-1.1* harboring conjugative IncI2 plasmid isolated from a clinical extensively-drug resistant Escherichia coli ST744 in Shanghai. *Front. Public Health* **2023**, *11*, 1216704. [CrossRef] [PubMed]
36. Carhuaricra, D.; Duran Gonzales, C.G.; Rodríguez Cueva, C.L.; Ignacion León, Y.; Silvestre Espejo, T.; Marcelo Monge, G.; Rosadio Alcántara, R.H.; Lincopan, N.; Espinoza, L.L.; Maturrano Hernández, L. Occurrence and Genomic Characterization of *mcr*-1-Harboring Escherichia coli Isolates from Chicken and Pig Farms in Lima, Peru. *Antibiotics* **2022**, *11*, 1781. [CrossRef] [PubMed]
37. Li, R.; Du, P.; Zhang, P.; Li, Y.; Yang, X.; Wang, Z.; Wang, J.; Bai, L. Comprehensive Genomic Investigation of Coevolution of *mcr* genes in Escherichia coli Strains via Nanopore Sequencing. *Glob. Chall.* **2021**, *5*, 2000014. [CrossRef]
38. Rozwandowicz, M.; Brouwer, M.S.M.; Fischer, J.; Wagenaar, J.A.; Gonzalez-Zorn, B.; Guerra, B.; Mevius, D.J.; Hordijk, J. Plasmids carrying antimicrobial resistance genes in Enterobacteriaceae. *J. Antimicrob. Chemother.* **2018**, *73*, 1121–1137. [CrossRef]
39. Li, W.; Liu, Z.; Yin, W.; Yang, L.; Qiao, L.; Song, S.; Ling, Z.; Zheng, R.; Wu, C.; Wang, Y.; et al. MCR Expression Conferring Varied Fitness Costs on Host Bacteria and Affecting Bacteria Virulence. *Antibiotics* **2021**, *10*, 872. [CrossRef]
40. Rebelo, A.R.; Bortolaia, V.; Kjeldgaard, J.S.; Pedersen, S.K.; Leekitcharoenphon, P.; Hansen, I.M.; Guerra, B.; Malorny, B.; Borowiak, M.; Hammerl, J.A.; et al. Multiplex PCR for detection of plasmid-mediated colistin resistance determinants, *mcr*-1, *mcr*-2, *mcr*-3, *mcr*-4 and *mcr*-5 for surveillance purposes. *Euro Surveill. Bull. Eur. Sur Les Mal. Transm.* **2018**, *23*, 17–00672. [CrossRef]
41. Borowiak, M.; Baumann, B.; Fischer, J.; Thomas, K.; Deneke, C.; Hammerl, J.A.; Szabo, I.; Malorny, B. Development of a Novel *mcr*-6 to *mcr*-9 Multiplex PCR and Assessment of *mcr*-1 to *mcr*-9 Occurrence in Colistin-Resistant Salmonella enterica Isolates From Environment, Feed, Animals and Food (2011–2018) in Germany. *Front. Microbiol.* **2020**, *11*, 80. [CrossRef]
42. Kado, C.I.; Liu, S.T. Rapid procedure for detection and isolation of large and small plasmids. *J. Bacteriol.* **1981**, *145*, 1365–1373. [CrossRef]
43. *CLSI Performance Standards for Antimicrobial Susceptibility Testing*, 33rd ed.; CLSI Guideline M100Performance Standards for Antimicrobial Susceptibility Testing; CLSI: Wayne, PA, USA, 2022.
44. Wick, R.R.; Judd, L.M.; Gorrie, C.L.; Holt, K.E. Unicycler: Resolving bacterial genome assemblies from short and long sequencing reads. *PLoS Comput. Biol.* **2017**, *13*, e1005595. [CrossRef]
45. Mikheenko, A.; Prjibelski, A.; Saveliev, V.; Antipov, D.; Gurevich, A. Versatile genome assembly evaluation with QUAST-LG. *Bioinformatics* **2018**, *34*, i142–i150. [CrossRef]
46. Wood, D.E.; Lu, J.; Langmead, B. Improved metagenomic analysis with Kraken 2. *Genome Biol.* **2019**, *20*, 257. [CrossRef]
47. Carattoli, A.; Zankari, E.; García-Fernández, A.; Voldby Larsen, M.; Lund, O.; Villa, L.; Møller Aarestrup, F.; Hasman, H. In silico detection and typing of plasmids using PlasmidFinder and plasmid multilocus sequence typing. *Antimicrob. Agents Chemother.* **2014**, *58*, 3895–3903. [CrossRef] [PubMed]
48. Néron, B.; Littner, E.; Haudiquet, M.; Perrin, A.; Cury, J.; Rocha, E.P.C. IntegronFinder 2.0: Identification and Analysis of Integrons across Bacteria, with a Focus on Antibiotic Resistance in Klebsiella. *Microorganisms* **2022**, *10*, 700. [CrossRef] [PubMed]
49. Jolley, K.A.; Maiden, M.C. BIGSdb: Scalable analysis of bacterial genome variation at the population level. *BMC Bioinform.* **2010**, *11*, 595. [CrossRef]
50. Gardner, S.N.; Slezak, T.; Hall, B.G. kSNP3.0: SNP detection and phylogenetic analysis of genomes without genome alignment or reference genome. *Bioinformatics* **2015**, *31*, 2877–2878. [CrossRef] [PubMed]
51. Letunic, I.; Bork, P. Interactive Tree Of Life (iTOL) v5: An online tool for phylogenetic tree display and annotation. *Nucleic Acids Res.* **2021**, *49*, W293–W296. [CrossRef] [PubMed]

**Disclaimer/Publisher's Note:** The statements, opinions and data contained in all publications are solely those of the individual author(s) and contributor(s) and not of MDPI and/or the editor(s). MDPI and/or the editor(s) disclaim responsibility for any injury to people or property resulting from any ideas, methods, instructions or products referred to in the content.

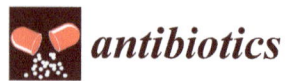 

Article

# Biocide-Resistant *Escherichia coli* ST540 Co-Harboring ESBL, *dfrA14* Confers QnrS-Dependent Plasmid-Mediated Quinolone Resistance

Srinivasan Vijaya Bharathi and Govindan Rajamohan *

Bacterial Signaling and Drug Resistance Laboratory, Council of Scientific and Industrial Research—Institute of Microbial Technology, Sector 39-A, Chandigarh 160036, India
* Correspondence: rmohan@imtech.res.in

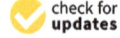

**Citation:** Bharathi, S.V.; Rajamohan, G. Biocide-Resistant *Escherichia coli* ST540 Co-Harboring ESBL, *dfrA14* Confers QnrS-Dependent Plasmid-Mediated Quinolone Resistance. *Antibiotics* **2022**, *11*, 1724. https://doi.org/10.3390/antibiotics11121724

Academic Editor: Andrey Shelenkov

Received: 30 September 2022
Accepted: 29 October 2022
Published: 30 November 2022

**Publisher's Note:** MDPI stays neutral with regard to jurisdictional claims in published maps and institutional affiliations.

**Copyright:** © 2022 by the authors. Licensee MDPI, Basel, Switzerland. This article is an open access article distributed under the terms and conditions of the Creative Commons Attribution (CC BY) license (https://creativecommons.org/licenses/by/4.0/).

**Abstract:** Emerging sequence types of pathogenic bacteria have a dual ability to acquire resistance islands/determinants, and remain renitent towards disinfection practices; therefore, they are considered "critical risk factors" that contribute significantly to the global problem of antimicrobial resistance. Multidrug-resistant *Escherichia coli* was isolated, its genome sequenced, and its susceptibilities characterized, in order to understand the genetic basis of its antimicrobial resistance. The draft genome sequencing of *E. coli* ECU32, was performed with Illumina NextSeq 500, and annotated using a RAST server. The antibiotic resistome, genomic island, insertion sequences, and prophages were analyzed using bioinformatics tools. Subsequently, analyses including antibiotic susceptibility testing, E-test, bacterial growth, survival, and efflux inhibition assays were performed. The draft genome of *E. coli* ECU32 was 4.7 Mb in size, the contigs were 107, and the G+C content was 50.8%. The genome comprised 4658 genes, 4543 CDS, 4384 coding genes, 115 RNA genes, 88 tRNAs, and 3 CRISPR arrays. The resistome characterization of ST540 *E. coli* ECU32 revealed the presence of ESBL, APH(6)-Id, APH(3′)-IIa, *dfrA14*, and QnrS1, with broad-spectrum multidrug and biocide resistance. Comparative genome sequence analysis revealed the presence of transporter and several virulence genes. Efflux activity and growth inhibition assays, which were performed with efflux substrates in the presence of inhibitor PAβN, exhibited significant reduced growth relative to its control. This study discusses the genotypic and phenotypic characterization of the biocide-tolerant multidrug-resistant *E. coli* O9:H30 strain, highlighting the contributory role of *qnrS*-dependent plasmid-mediated quinolone resistance, in addition to innate enzymatic modes of multidrug resistance mechanisms.

**Keywords:** commensal bacteria; reservoirs; drug resistome; active efflux; membrane transporters; outer membrane proteins

## 1. Introduction

Among the different members of genus *Escherichia*, serotypes from bacterial species *E. coli* that belong to *Enterobacteriaceae* are highly pathogenic for humans, birds, and animals. This Gram-negative bacterium is a rod-shaped, facultative anaerobe found in soil, food, environment, and the intestines of animals and humans, with an unmatched capacity to survive in diverse, stressful conditions. *E. coli* produces an arsenal of virulence factors, such as fimbrial adhesins, different iron acquisition systems, heat-labile/stable toxins and hemolysin, capsules, a type III secretion system, and colonization invasion factors. The toxin-producing *E. coli* strains are responsible for causing mild sicknesses, such as diarrhea and vomiting, to severe illnesses such as meningitis, respiratory diseases, pneumonia, and urinary tract infections [1,2]. As per the 2017–2018 GLASS report, *E. coli* was the most frequently reported pathogen with high-level resistance to ciprofloxacin and imipenem. Subsequently, in its 2019–2020 report, focusing on AMR data from 65 different countries, *E. coli* isolates tested from urine samples (from 64% countries) were resistant to ceftriaxone, cefotaxime, ampicillin, and ciprofloxacin, including carbapenems. In 2017, the WHO published its priority list of clinically significant human pathogens, and MDR *E. coli* was classified under the critical threat category, in order to ensure enhanced research activities to control AMR spread, and infection control [3,4].

The major pathotypes of *E. coli* include intestinal (IPEC) and extraintestinal (ExPEC) pathogenic strains. Of the ExPEC *E. coli*, UPEC (uropathogenic *E. coli*) evades the host's innate immunity and colonizes the urinary bladder, kidneys, and is well recognized as a causative agent for urinary tract infections (UTIs), which account for ~80% of urinary infections [5,6].

Recently, India published its first pathogen priority list with a similar frame of objectives, carbapenem and tigecycline resistant *E. coli* topped the critical threat category. According to recent ICMR-AMR data, out of the total 107,387 isolates studied during the year 2019, the relative distribution of *E. coli* remained the highest at 28% ($n$ =30822) in Indian hospitals from different locations. *E. coli* was the most predominant isolate from urine (56%), with strains exhibiting reduced susceptibility to cephalosporins and fluoroquinolones, including imipenem (from 86% in 2016 to 63% in 2019). While ST648, ST2659, and ST540 have been reported to be NDM-5-producing *E. coli* globally, the frequently reported ExPEC sequence types that are linked with UTI cases include ST131, ST73, ST95, and ST69 [7].

Primary susceptibility testing of *E. coli* urinary isolate ECU32 illustrated its antimicrobial resistance behavior, with an innate capability to co-produce multiple resistance determinants. The phylogenetic analysis classified this isolate to the ST540 serotype, one which is usually reported from birds and animals.Therefore, to reach a deeper perspective on its genetic content, genome organization, and phenotypic behaviors, asystematic study was initiated.This study reports the draft genome sequence, analysis, and resistome characterization of ST540 *E. coli* urinary isolate ECU32 from India, co-producing ESBL, APH(6)-Id, APH(3′)-IIa, *dfrA14*, and QnrS1, with broad multidrug and biocide resistance.

## 2. Results and Discussion

### 2.1. Genomic Features and Phylogenetic Analysis of E. coli

The draft genome reads of *E. coli* ECU32 were assembled to a single chromosome of size 4.7 Mb, an N50 spanning 94, 946 bp, L50 being 15, number of contigs being 107, and a G+C content of 50.8% (Assembly: GCA_002872235.1; GenBank: LZGD01000000). Analysis revealed 4658 genes (total), 4543 CDS (total), 4384 coding genes, 115 RNA genes, 8, 3, 2, 5S, 16S, 23S rRNA genes, 88 tRNAs, and 159 pseudogenes (Table 1). Furthermore, PADLOC analysis revealed three CRISPR arrays, including cas_type_I-E array system (Table 2) [8].

Table 1. Genomic features of *E. coli* ECU32.

| Type | Assembly Statistics |
|---|---|
| Genome | *Escherichia coli* ECU32 |
| Size | 4,734,193 |
| GC content | 50.8 |
| Number of coding sequences | 4601 |
| Number of RNAs | 105 |
| Number of subsystems | 595 |
| Contigs generated | 107 |
| Maximum contig length | 239,491 |
| Minimum contig length | 502 |
| Average contig length | 44,244.8 ± 55,998.5 |
| Median contig length | 8912 |
| Total contigs length | 4,734,193 |
| Total number of non-ATGC characters | 663 |

**Table 1.** *Cont.*

| Type | Assembly Statistics |
|---|---|
| Percentage of non-ATGC characters | 0.014 |
| Contigs ≥ 500 bp | 107 |
| Contigs ≥ 1 kbp | 97 |
| Contigs ≥ 10 kbp | 67 |
| Contigs ≥ 1 Mbp | 0 |
| N50 value | 95,844 |
| L50 | 15 |
| Genome coverage | 93.0X |

**Table 2.** Probable CRISPR systems in *E.coli* ECU32 using PADLOC analysis.

| CRISPR System | Protein | Target | Sequence Id | Start | End | Strand |
|---|---|---|---|---|---|---|
| CRISPR_array | CRISPR_array | CRISPR001 | LZGD01000013.1 | 92,385 | 92,901 | - |
| cas_type_I-E | Cas2e | A8A11_20845 | LZGD01000013.1 | 93,006 | 93,291 | - |
| cas_type_I-E | Cas1e | A8A11_20850 | LZGD01000013.1 | 93,292 | 94,210 | - |
| cas_type_I-E | Cas6e | A8A11_20855 | LZGD01000013.1 | 94,225 | 94,825 | - |
| cas_type_I-E | Cas5e | A8A11_20860 | LZGD01000013.1 | 94,811 | 95,486 | - |
| cas_type_I-E | Cas7e | A8A11_20865 | LZGD01000013.1 | 95,488 | 96,580 | - |
| cas_type_I-E | Cas11e | A8A11_20870 | LZGD01000013.1 | 96,592 | 97,075 | - |
| cas_type_I-E | Cas8e | A8A11_20875 | LZGD01000013.1 | 97,067 | 98,576 | - |
| CRISPR_array | CRISPR_array | CRISPR002 | LZGD01000043.1 | 123,708 | 123,910 | - |
| retron_I-C | RT-Toprim_I-C | A8A11_16640 | LZGD01000043.1 | 170,971 | 172,729 | - |
| retron_I-C | msr-msd | NA | LZGD01000043.1 | 172,765 | 172,895 | - |
| RM_type_II | MTase_II | A8A11_21460 | LZGD01000051.1 | 19,587 | 21,006 | + |
| RM_type_II | REase_II | A8A11_21465 | LZGD01000051.1 | 20,986 | 21,457 | + |
| DMS_other | BrxD | A8A11_09690 | LZGD01000074.1 | 2659 | 3976 | + |
| DMS_other | BrxHI | A8A11_09695 | LZGD01000074.1 | 3972 | 6168 | + |
| CRISPR_array | CRISPR_array | CRISPR003 | LZGD01000087.1 | 154,485 | 155,734 | + |

The genomic features of selected ST540 *E. coli* strains were investigated with Indian *E. coli* strains from different available sources in the BacWGSTdb server, while phylogenetic relationshipswere analyzed using the cgMLST approach with the ST540 reference strain. The analysis revealed two major clusters based on the isolation source; the ECU32 strain was found in the second cluster, along with strains predominantly isolated from humans (Figure 1A). Further analysis with only *E. coli* ST540 Indian isolate revealed its clustering with strains of human gut origin (Figure 1B). Overall, the cgMLST analysis revealed that the *E. coli* ECU32 strain was closely related to the human and gut origin multidrug isolates.

Additionally, in the RAST server, functional annotation of the genome revealed the presence of 595 subsystems (39% unassigned). The gene ontology data showed the distribution of genes for different components and functions. The biological processes included genes involved in transcription 5.37%, regulation of transcription 2.62%, transmembrane transport 1.93%, carbohydrate metabolic process 1.77%, cell adhesion 0.85%, cell wall organization 0.83%, and integral component of membrane 20.25%. The cellular components included cytoplasm with 10.22%, and the molecular function included genes with oxidoreductase activity 1.93%, zinc ion binding 2.27%, magnesium ion binding 2.36%, plasma membrane 6.43%, DNA binding 7.99%, ATP binding 8.49%, and transporter activity 2.53% (Figure 1C,D).

The clinical strain belonged to ST540 as the alleles *adk_6*, *fumC_7*, *gyrB_57*, *icd_1*, *mdh_8*, *purA_8*, and *recA_2* exhibited 100% identity to their respective locus, as per MLST typing. Based on Clermon typing, the strain belonged to phylogroup A, a group largely dominated with commensal origins of strains. The *E. coli* ECU32 belongs to serotype H30-H with 100% identity for *fliC* in scaffold8 | size160413, *fimH54* (scaffold11 | size140663), and O9-O antigen (>99% identity to *wzm* and *wzt* in scaffold34 | size42957). These gene clusters were found between *hisI* and *gnd* genes, and belong to group 1 K antigens.

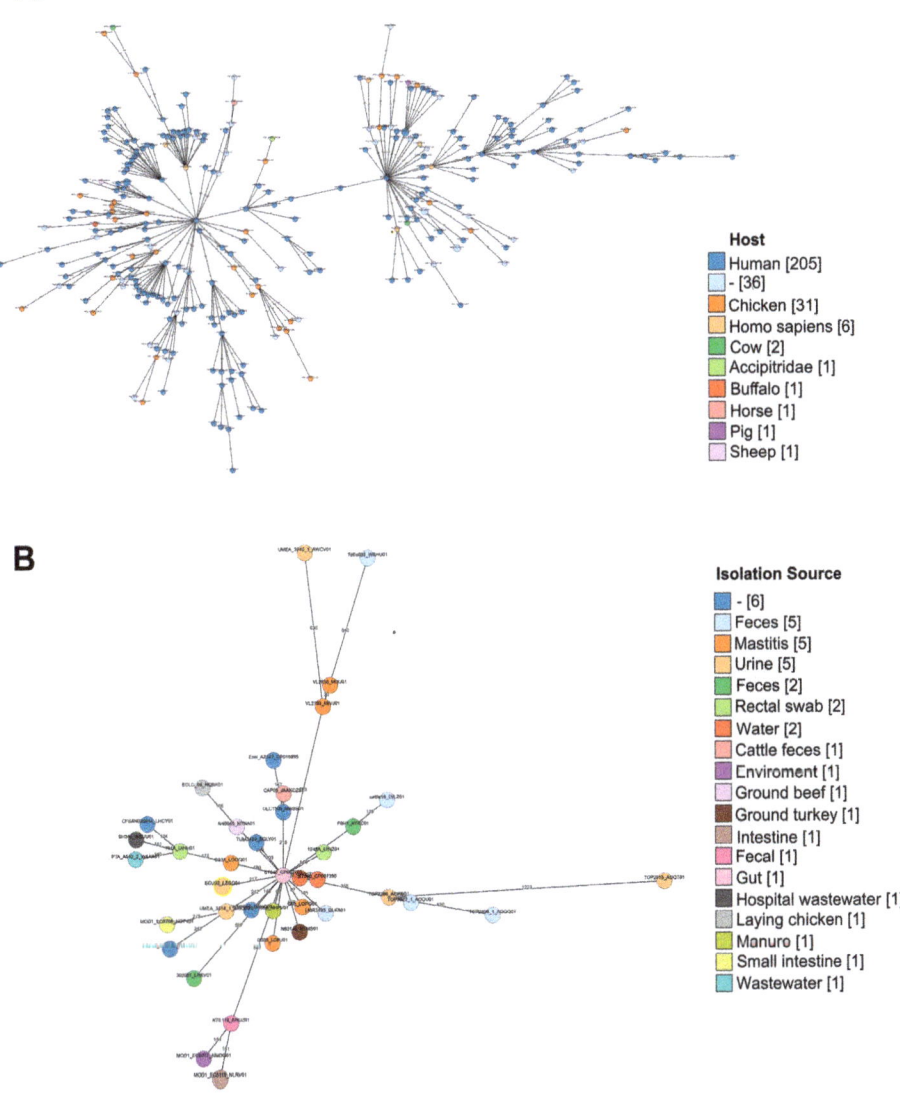

**Figure 1.** *Cont.*

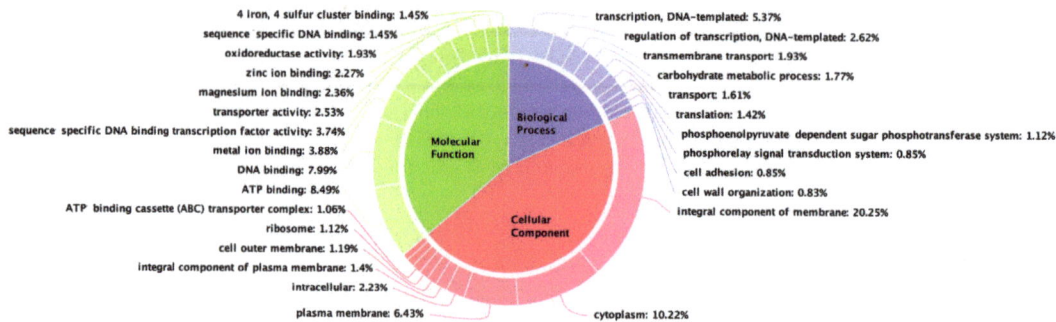

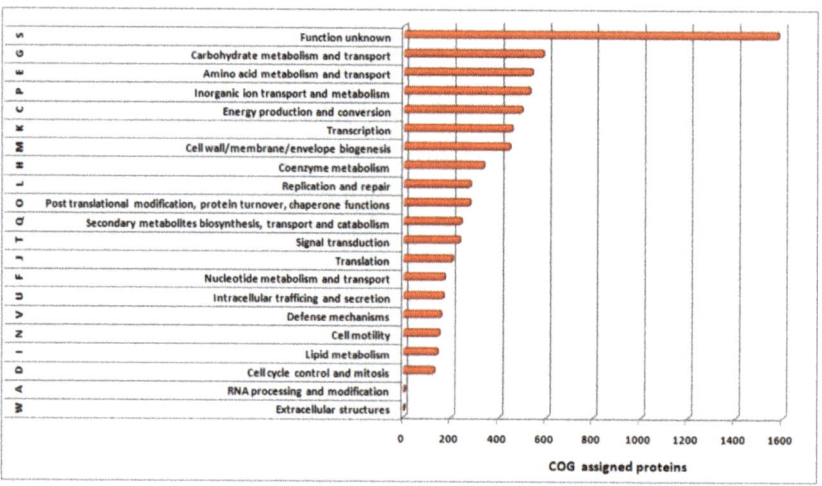

**Figure 1.** (**A**). The core genome multilocus sequence typing-based phylogenetic relationship tree was constructed for all of the available Indian *E. coli* strains in the BacWGSTdb server from different hosts, and ST groups were compared with the reference ST540 *E. coli*_ AZ147 strain. Grape tree displayed the relationship between isolates and comprised two major cluster groups. The *E. coli* ECU32 strain highlighted with a yellow circle with black center was found to be associated with human isolates in the second cluster. The lengths of all branches are scaled logarithmically. The numbers mentioned in square brackets are isolates from a range of hosts. (**B**). Grape tree represents the phylogenetic relationship of available *E. coli* ST540 strains in BacWGSTdb from different isolation sources and countries. The strain name was mentioned along the colored circle, the color indicates the source of isolation, and the isolate counts are mentioned in brackets. The *E. coli* ECU32 strain was highlighted with a yellow circle. The node label represents the allele differences, and the branch lengths are scaled logarithmically. (**C**). Gene ontology annotation of predicted genes was performed using BLAST analysis, and top gene ontologies were classified into cellular components, molecular functions, and biological process. (**D**). Distribution of clusters of orthologous groups (COG) in *E. coli* ECU32. The homologous gene clusters were functionally categorized and classified with COG assignments.

## 2.2. Antimicrobial-Resistant Genes

Upon analyzing the sequence of E. coli strain ECU32 for genetic clusters, a 9852-base-pair genomic island was identified that carried the CRISPR-associated proteins, and the 5540-base-pair genomic island (scaffold94xsize3049) showed the presence of ESBL, the class-A blaTEM beta-lactamase (A8A11_02620).

The 32,081-base-pair genomic island in the strain (scaffold7xsize174057) highlighted the presence of members from the EscJ/YscJ/HrcJ family type III secretion system (from A8A11_10065 to A8A11_10125).

The largest genomic island present in strain ECU32, 131,243bp in size (consisting of scaffold78xsize4056 and scaffold83xsize2691), indicated the presence of aminoglycoside-modifying enzymes APH(3′) (A8A11_04060), APH(6)-Id (A8A11_04065), and class 1 integrase, followed by gene cassette dfrA1 (A8A11_21925). The class-C ampC detected in this study exhibited 97% identity to a homolog found in E. coli O157:H7; 95% to Shigella sonnei; 78% to Enterobacteriaceae bacterium; 73% to Shigella flexneri; 71% to Enterobacter, and 70% to Yersinia ruckeri.

The quinolone resistance gene qnrS1 was found in scaffold57xsize16952 (A8A11_12295) with an adjacent ISKra4-like element (A8A11_12305), while the sulfonamide-resistant dihydropteroate synthase sul2 was found in scaffold78xsize4056 (A8A11_04055). The quinolone resistance determinant exhibited identities to homologs found in Vibrio mytili CAIM 528 (95%); Photobacterium ganghwense strain DSM 22954 (92%); Vibrionales bacterium SWAT-3 (83%); and Photobacterium halotolerans strain MELD1 (66%). The sequence analysis of QnrS1 indicated the conserved pentapeptide sequences, and homology modeling highlighted the differences in loops A and B regions, as shown in Figure S1.

Homologs of well characterized efflux pumps, AcrAB, EmrAB, MdtABC, EmrE, AcrD, and TetA (scaffold82xsize4187; A8A11_05610), were present in the genome; moreover, the marR gene harbored sense mutations at the Y137H and G103S residues. The tetracycline efflux pump exhibited varied identities to homologs found in Aeromonas simiae CIP 107798 (98%), Pseudomonas fluorescens HK44 (97%), E. coli O83:H1 str. NRG 857C (97%), and Clostridium nexile DSM 1787 (78%).

Using the BacWGSTdb server, the resistance genes were assessed amongst ST540 strains from different countries, hosts, and isolation sources, and the ECU32 strain exhibited the presence of diverse resistance genes (Figure 2A).

## 2.3. Virulence and Its Associated Genes

Comparative genome sequence analysis revealed that E. coli strain ECU32, in scaffold21xsize74584, carried ORFs for both the ferric enterobactin ABC transporter system (fepA, fepB, fepC, fepD, fepG, fes), and enterobactin (siderophore) biosynthesis exporter system (entB, entC, entD, entE, entF, entS). Important virulent factors that were identified included the type 1 fimbriae adhesin fimH (scaffold11xsize140663-1, A8A11_14300), hemolysin E hlyE (scaffold22xsize79984, A8A11_04330), invasin of brain endothelial cells, ibeB (scaffold60xsize15487, A8A11_08140), gspC, gspD, gspE, (scaffold35xsize41361), and intimin-like adhesion fdeC (scaffold1xsize239491 with 93% to EC958_0448).

Virulence genes were analyzed and compared with different ST540 strains and pathotypes. The analysis demonstrated the prevalence of virulence genes that are involved in adherence, autotransporter, invasion, non-LEE-encoded TTSS effectors, secretion system, toxin, and others (Figure 2B,C).

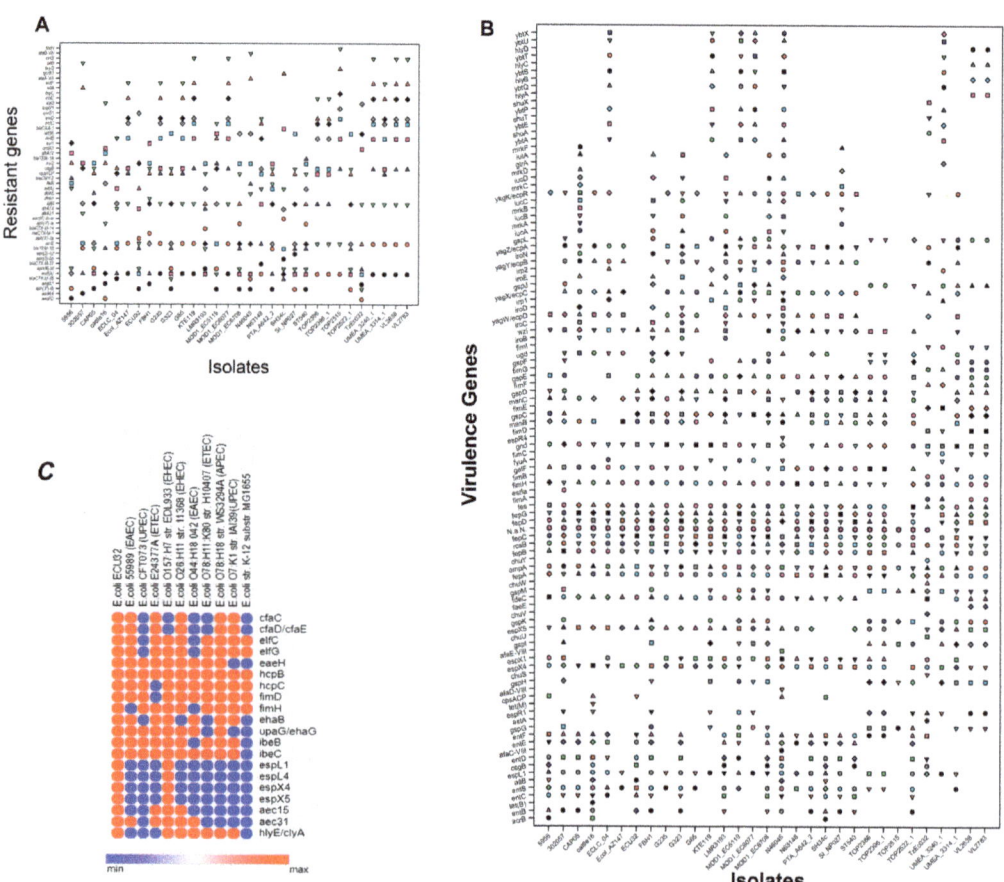

**Figure 2.** (**A**) Prevalence of resistance genes from different Indian *E. coli* ST540 strains, originating from various hosts. The strains used for analysis were strain 5956 (NHPV01, cow); strain 302057 (LRKV01, human); CAP05 (JAAKCZ01, cow); cattle16 (LVLZ01, cow); ECLC_04 (NQBK01, chicken); Ecol_AZ147 (CP018995, human); ECU32 (LZGD01, homo sapiens); FBH1 (AYRC01, human); G235 (LOOQ01, cow); G323 (LOPJ01, cow); G65 (LOPQ01, cow); KTE119 (ANUZ01, human); LMR3193 (QLKA01, human); MOD1_EC5119 (NLRV01, human); MOD1_EC6077 (NMDG01, Serpentes); MOD1_EC6708 (NOTV01, cow); N46045 (NTNA01); N63148 (NTMS01); PTA_A642_2 (WAAK01); SH34c (WSUU01); SI_NP027 (BGHG01, cow); ST540 (CP007265, human); TOP2386(AORB01, human); TOP2396_1 (AOQQ01, human); TOP2515 (AOQT01, human); TOP2522_1(AOQU01, human); TzEc032 (WSHU01, sheep); UMEA_3240_1 (AWCV01, human); UMEA_3314_1 (AWDE01, human); VL2638 (MIXJ01, cow); VL2783 (MIVJ01, cow). The strain accession numbers and hosts are mentioned in parenthesis. (**B**) The diversity of virulence factors are distributed in various Indian ST540 isolates. (**C**) The virulence factors of the ECU32 strain were compared with other *E.coli* pathotypes. The strains were *E. coli* 55989 (enteroaggregative *E. coli*—EAEC) [NC_011748]; *E. coli* CFT073 (uropathogenic *E. coli*—UPEC) [NC_004431]; *E. coli* E24377A (enterotoxigenic *E. coli*—ETEC) [NC_009801]; *E. coli* O157:H7 str. EDL933 (enterohemorrhagic *E. coli*—EHEC) [NC_002655]; *E. coli* O26:H11 str. 11368 (EHEC) [NC_013361]; *E. coli* O44:H18 042 (EAEC) [NC_017626]; *E. coli* O78:H11:K80 str. H10407 (ETEC) [NC_017633]; *E. coli* O78:H18 str. WS3294A (avian pathogenic *E. coli* APEC) [NC_020163]; *E. coli* O7:K1 str. IAI39 (UPEC) [NC_011750]; *E. coli* str. K-12 substr. MG1655 [NC_000913]. Min (blue) and Max (red) indicate absence and presence of virulence genes in a strain, respectively. Accession numbers are listed within the square brackets.

## 2.4. Phenotypic Characterization of Multidrug-Resistant E. coli

The Kirby Bauer assay revealed the *E. coli* strain ECU32 to be multidrug resistant (AMP, AMK, CLI, CST, ERY, KAN, LZD, MET, OXA, PEN, RIF, STR). The minimum inhibitory concentrations of this Indian isolate for different antibiotics, as evaluated by the agar dilution method, were ceftazidime 0.5 µg/mL, ticarcillin >1024 µg/mL, neomycin 4 µg/mL, norfloxacin 16 µg/mL, doxycycline 64 µg/mL, tetracycline 64 µg/mL, nalidixic acid >1024 µg/mL, ampicillin >1024 µg/mL, kanamycin 16 µg/mL, erythromycin >1024 µg/mL, trimethoprim 64 µg/mL, and chloramphenicol 4 µg/mL.

*E. coli*, a common flora in the human gastrointestinal tract, has adaptive survival response strategies under different stress conditions. The growth profile of *E. coli* ECU32 was assessed in the presence of low to high pH concentrations. The strain retained the ability to grow in pH 5.0 to pH 8.0; meanwhile, in pH 10, the strain displayed less (~0.5-fold) growth compared to pH 5.0 (Figure 3A). Concentration-dependent growth of the strain in the presence of the antibiotic norfloxacin was observed. The strain was able to grow in doses upto 64 µg/mL, and exhibited nine-fold lower growth compared to its control (Figure 3B).

However, the *E. coli* ECU32 strain was able to survive in the presence of both oxidative and nitrostative stress-inducing agents, such as hydrogen peroxide, sodium nitroprusside, and sodium nitrite, respectively (Figure 3C–E).

The survival of *E. coli* ECU32 under osmotic stress conditions was determined in the presence of different sodium chloride concentrations. The strain exhibited more than 80% survival upto 0.75 M, and 40% in 1 M of sodium chloride (Figure 3F). Altogether, these observations emphasize the adaptability of *E. coli* under any intracellular stress conditions, and its survival inside the host to cause disease severity.

The *E. coli* ECU32 strain has an ability to cope with different intracellular stress responses. Furthermore, the ability of the strains to survive in the presence of a various range of antimicrobial agents was examined. Analyses revealed a more than 50% survival rate was observed for the strain at 1024 µg/mL for ampicillin, 4 µg/mL for neomycin, and 0.5 µg/mL for tetracycline. Furthermore, the strain was found to have retained the ability to survive in various antimicrobial compounds, such as acriflavine, acridine orange at 256 µg/mL, and saffranine and deoxycholate at 1024 µg/mL (Figure 3G).

In order to detect efflux activity in the *E. coli* strain, MICs for the following efflux-based substrates were initially analyzed: acridine orange 256 µg/mL, acriflavine 64 µg/mL rhodamine >1024 µg/mL, saffranine >1024 µg/mL, deoxycholate >1024 µg/mL, and SDS >1024 µg/mL. Hence, a growth inhibition assay was performed with the *E. coli* strain ECU32, using ampicillin 256 µg/mL, in the presence of known efflux pump inhibitor PAβN, which exhibited an approximatelyfive-fold reduced growth relative to its control. Overall, the assays demonstrated that the strain has the ability to survive under different assails, including antimicrobial compounds. Furthermore, the sequence analysis and phenotypic efflux assays indicated the role of active efflux as the primary mechanism used to confer antimicrobial resistance. In order to substantiate these observations, genomic analysis of the strain further confirmed the presence of well-characterized efflux families, depicting the importance and possible involvement of these pumps in antimicrobial resistance and multiple cellular functions.

The strain was examined for its resistance level towards hospital-based disinfectants, and it exhibited tolerance as follows: benzalkonium chloride 12.8 µg/mL, chlorhexidine <3.2 µg/mL, and triclosan >0.1 µg/mL (Figure 3H(i,ii)), indicating that the urinary strain was broad-spectrum antimicrobial, as well as biocide-resistant. Additionally, the *E. coli* strain ECU32 displayed an ability to form biofilms (ratio 570/600 nm = 0.252), as it harbored genes that are required for adhesion and virulence.

Upon transforming the plasmid preparation from the MDR strain into *E. coli* JM109, transformants were confirmed on ampicillin (>256 µg/mL) and ciprofloxacin (0.5 µg/mL) plates; subsequent PCR detection indicated the presence of quinolone resistance determinant in the transformant, and further sequencing confirmed the role of qnrS-dependent plasmid-mediated resistance in *E. coli* strain ECU32.

It is worthwhile to state here that ST540 has usually been reported in *E. coli* that was isolated from birds and chickens. Identifying the serotype ST540 from a biological sample strictly emphasizes the periodic monitoring of emerging *E. coli* strains at the One-Health Interface. The *E. coli* strains TOP2386 (accession no: AORB01), TOP2396_1 (accession no: AOQQ01), TOP2515 (accession no: AOQT01), TOP2522_1 (accession no: AOQU01), and TUM3433 (accession no: BGLY01), isolated from human samples in USA and Japan, belong to the same ST, as that of *E. coli* strain ECU32. As per the BacWGSTdb server, *E. coli* strain ECU32 (accession no: LZGD01) with ST540 is being reported for the first time in India.

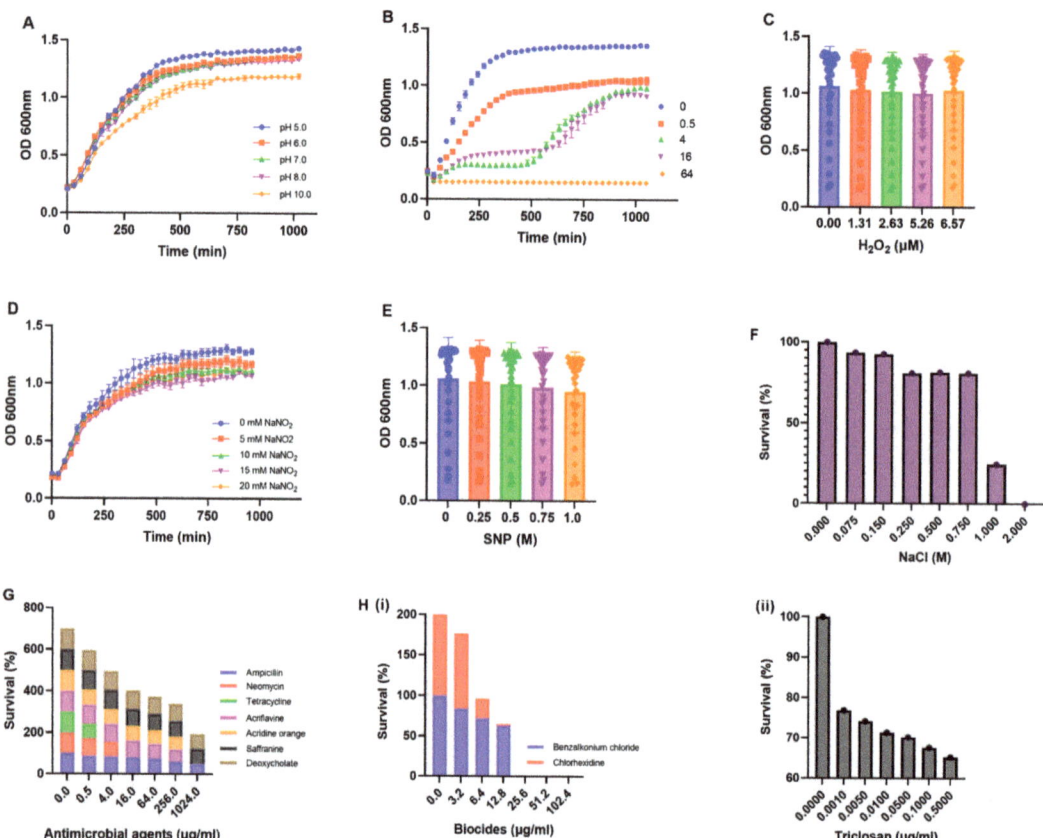

**Figure 3.** Biological characterization of the *E. coli* ECU32 strain. The growth profile of the *E. coli* ECU32 strain was monitored in the presence of different pHs (**A**) and concentrations of norfloxacin (**B**). The growth of the ECU32 strain was monitored in the presence of varied concentrations of oxidative stress-inducing agent—hydrogen peroxide (**C**) and nitrostative stress-inducing agents—sodium nitrite and sodium nitroprusside (**D,E**). The osmotic stress response survival was determined in the presence of sodium chloride concentrations (**F**). The survival ability of the *E. coli* ECU32 strain was determined under different concentrations of antibiotics [ampillicin, neomycin, tetracycline], bile [deoxycholate], structurally unrelated compounds and dyes [acriflavine, acridine orange, saffranine] (**G**), and biocides [benzalkonium chloride, chlorhexidine, and triclosan] (**H(i,ii)**). The mean values of the different independent experiments were used for plotting graphs, using GraphPad Prism.

## 3. Materials and Methods

### 3.1. The Genome Draft Sequence, Annotation and Analysis

The *E. coli* strain, ECU32, selected for this analysis, was obtained in 2013 from a urine sample during our longitudinal study. Draft genome sequencing was carried out with paired-end sequencing technology, Illumina NextSeq 500, and scaffold annotation was performed using a RAST server [9]. Basic local alignment search tool, (BLAST) (GO), was utilized for determining percent identities [10]. The *E. coli* ECU32 genomesequence was compared with available *E. coli* genomes ($n$ =300) that were isolated from India, and core genome multilocus sequence typing (cgMLST) was performed with the selected reference genome (*E. coli_* AZ147 GenBank CP018995 ST540) for phylogenetic analysis. The graph tree and minimum spanning tree were constructed and analyzed, based on cgMLST profiles of Indian *E. coli* isolates. The antibiotic resistome, genomic island, insertion sequences, and prophages were analyzed using bioinformatic tools such as Pathosystems Resource Integration Center tool, Resistance Gene Identifier, Island Viewer 4, Mobile Element Finder, PHAge Search Tool Enhanced Release, and NCBI-BLAST [9–11]. The CRISPR was determined using PADLOC server (https://padloc.otago.ac.nz/ accessed on 26 September 2022). Comprehensive Antibiotic Resistance Database (CARD; https://card.mcmaster.ca/analyze/rgi accessed on 10 May 2021) was used to predict AMR genes and the VR2 profile, in order to identify the associated mobile elements [8,12,13]. Virulence, transposons, and antibiotic resistance genes were determined using the BacWGSTdb server. The distribution of virulence factors in *E. coli* ECU32 with other *E.coli* strains was deciphered using virulence factor database analyzer [14].

### 3.2. Antibiotic Resistance Pattern and Growth Analysis

The antibiotic susceptibility testing, E-test, survival assays, stress response, growth curves, and efflux inhibition assays were performed, as described previously [9,11].

### 3.3. Data Deposition

The *E. coli* ECU32 whole genome sequence was submitted to GenBank NCBI, with accession number LZGD00000000.1.

## 4. Conclusions

Overall, this study highlighted the presence of diverse virulence factors and the antibiotic resistome in ST540 *E. coli* strain ECU32, emphasizing a pressing need to conduct large-scale epidemiological surveillance to monitor the dominant ST/strain that is circulating within the cohort, and also to track the changing patterns in antibiotic susceptibility and resistome amongst swiftly disseminating bacteria such as *E. coli* in India. Emerging STs remain renitent towards hospital sterilization protocols, and havean unprecedented ability to acquire additional resistance determinants; therefore, they are "critical risk factors" that contribute significantly to the global problem of antimicrobial resistance.

**Supplementary Materials:** The following supporting information can be downloaded at: https://www.mdpi.com/article/10.3390/antibiotics11121724/s1, Figure S1: Sequence and homology modelling of QnrS.

**Author Contributions:** S.V.B. and G.R. conceived the idea, designed the strategy, performed the required analysis in this study, and wrote the manuscript. All authors have read and agreed to the published version of the manuscript.

**Funding:** The funding received from ICMR (2020-3673) is highly acknowledged; however, the funders had no role in the study design, data collection, and the analyses; in the decision to publish; or in the preparation of the manuscript.

**Institutional Review Board Statement:** Not applicable.

**Informed Consent Statement:** Not applicable.

**Data Availability Statement:** The genome sequence data have been deposited in NCBI GenBank accession number LZGD01000001 - LZGD01000107.

**Acknowledgments:** All of the authors remain highly grateful to CSIR-IMTECH for excellent support, and the facilities to perform this research. VBS remains grateful to the Department of Science and Technology—SERB (SB/YS/LS-177/2014) and ICMR (2020-3673)—for their excellent grant-in-aid and fellowship.

**Conflicts of Interest:** The authors declare no conflict of interest. The funders had no role in the design of the study; in the collection, analyses, or interpretation of data; in the writing of the manuscript; or in the decision to publish the results.

## References

1. Kaper, J.B.; Nataro, J.P.; Mobley, H.L. Pathogenic *Escherichia coli*. *Nat. Rev. Microbiol.* **2004**, *2*, 123–140. [CrossRef] [PubMed]
2. Nicolas-Chanoine, M.H.; Bertrand, X.; Madec, J.Y. *Escherichia coli* ST131, an intriguing clonal group. *Clin. Microbiol. Rev.* **2014**, *3*, 543–574. [CrossRef] [PubMed]
3. Mendelson, M.; Matsoso, M.P. A global call for action to combat antimicrobial resistance: Can we get it right this time? *S. Afr. Med. J.* **2014**, *7*, 478–479. [CrossRef]
4. World Health Organization. *Prioritization of Pathogens to Guide Discovery, Research and Development of New Antibiotics for Drug-Resistant Bacterial Infections, Including Tuberculosis*; World Health Organization: Geneva, Switzerland, 2017.
5. Denamur, E.; Clermont, O.; Bonacorsi, S.; Gordon, D. The population genetics of pathogenic *Escherichia coli*. *Nat. Rev. Microbiol.* **2021**, *1*, 37–54. [CrossRef] [PubMed]
6. Croxen, M.A.; Law, R.J.; Scholz, R.; Keeney, K.M.; Wlodarska, M.; Finlay, B.B. Recent advances in understanding enteric pathogenic *Escherichia coli*. *Clin. Microbiol. Rev.* **2013**, *4*, 822–880. [CrossRef] [PubMed]
7. Campos, A.C.C.; Andrade, N.L.; Ferdous, M.; Chlebowicz, M.A.; Santos, C.C.; Correal, J.C.D.; Lo Ten Foe, J.R.; Rosa, A.C.P.; Damasco, P.V.; Friedrich, A.W.; et al. Comprehensive Molecular Characterization of *Escherichia coli* Isolates from Urine Samples of Hospitalized Patients in Rio de Janeiro, Brazil. *Front. Microbiol.* **2018**, *9*, 243. [CrossRef] [PubMed]
8. Payne, L.J.; Todeschini, T.C.; Wu, Y.; Perry, B.J.; Ronson, C.W.; Fineran, P.C.; Nobrega, F.L.; Jackson, S.A. Identification and classification of antiviral defence systems in bacteria and archaea with PADLOC reveals new system types. *Nucleic Acids Res.* **2021**, *49*, 10868–10878. [CrossRef] [PubMed]
9. Srinivasan, V.B.; Rajamohan, G. Genome analysis of urease positive *Serratia marcescens*, co-producing SRT-2 and AAC(6′)-Ic with multidrug efflux pumps for antimicrobial resistance. *Genomics* **2019**, *4*, 653–660. [CrossRef]
10. Altschul, S.F.; Gish, W.; Miller, W.; Myers, E.W.; Lipman, D.J. Basic local alignment search tool. *J. Mol. Biol.* **1990**, *215*, 403–410. [CrossRef] [PubMed]
11. Srinivasan, V.B.; Rajamohan, G. Comparative genome analysis and characterization of a MDR *Klebsiella variicola*. *Genomics* **2020**, *5*, 3179–3190. [CrossRef] [PubMed]
12. Alcock, B.P.; Raphenya, A.R.; Lau, T.T.Y.; Tsang, K.K.; Bouchard, M.; Edalatmand, A.; Huynh, W.; Nguyen, A.V.; Cheng, A.A.; Liu, S.; et al. CARD 2020: Antibiotic resistome surveillance with the comprehensive antibiotic resistance database. *Nucleic Acids Res.* **2020**, *48*, D517–D525. [CrossRef] [PubMed]
13. Wang, M.; Goh, Y.X.; Tai, C.; Wang, H.; Deng, Z.; Ou, H.Y. VRprofile2: Detection of antibiotic resistance-associated mobilome in bacterial pathogens. *Nucleic Acids Res.* **2020**, *50*, W768–W773. [CrossRef] [PubMed]
14. Liu, B.; Zheng, D.; Jin, Q.; Chen, L.; Yang, J. VFDB 2019. A comparative pathogenomic platform with an interactive web interface. *Nucleic Acids Res.* **2019**, *47*, D687–D692. [CrossRef] [PubMed]

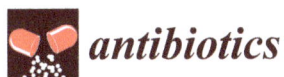 

Article

# Long-Read Whole Genome Sequencing Elucidates the Mechanisms of Amikacin Resistance in Multidrug-Resistant *Klebsiella pneumoniae* Isolates Obtained from COVID-19 Patients

Andrey Shelenkov [1,*], Lyudmila Petrova [2], Anna Mironova [2], Mikhail Zamyatin [2], Vasiliy Akimkin [1] and Yulia Mikhaylova [1]

[1] Central Research Institute of Epidemiology, Novogireevskaya Street 3a, Moscow 111123, Russia
[2] National Medical and Surgical Center Named after N.I. Pirogov, Nizhnyaya Pervomayskaya Street 70, Moscow 105203, Russia
* Correspondence: fallandar@gmail.com

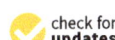

**Citation:** Shelenkov, A.; Petrova, L.; Mironova, A.; Zamyatin, M.; Akimkin, V.; Mikhaylova, Y. Long-Read Whole Genome Sequencing Elucidates the Mechanisms of Amikacin Resistance in Multidrug-Resistant *Klebsiella pneumoniae* Isolates Obtained from COVID-19 Patients. *Antibiotics* **2022**, *11*, 1364. https://doi.org/10.3390/antibiotics11101364

Academic Editor: Maria Lina Mezzatesta

Received: 21 September 2022
Accepted: 4 October 2022
Published: 6 October 2022

**Publisher's Note:** MDPI stays neutral with regard to jurisdictional claims in published maps and institutional affiliations.

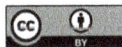

**Copyright:** © 2022 by the authors. Licensee MDPI, Basel, Switzerland. This article is an open access article distributed under the terms and conditions of the Creative Commons Attribution (CC BY) license (https://creativecommons.org/licenses/by/4.0/).

**Abstract:** *Klebsiella pneumoniae* is a Gram-negative, encapsulated, non-motile bacterium, which represents a global challenge to public health as one of the major causes of healthcare-associated infections worldwide. In the recent decade, the World Health Organization (WHO) noticed a critically increasing rate of carbapenem-resistant *K. pneumoniae* occurrence in hospitals. The situation with extended-spectrum beta-lactamase (ESBL) producing bacteria further worsened during the COVID-19 pandemic, due to an increasing number of patients in intensive care units (ICU) and extensive, while often inappropriate, use of antibiotics including carbapenems. In order to elucidate the ways and mechanisms of antibiotic resistance spreading within the *K. pneumoniae* population, whole genome sequencing (WGS) seems to be a promising approach, and long-read sequencing is especially useful for the investigation of mobile genetic elements carrying antibiotic resistance genes, such as plasmids. We have performed short- and long read sequencing of three carbapenem-resistant *K. pneumoniae* isolates obtained from COVID-19 patients in a dedicated ICU of a multipurpose medical center, which belonged to the same clone according to cgMLST analysis, in order to understand the differences in their resistance profiles. We have revealed the presence of a small plasmid carrying *aph(3′)-VIa* gene providing resistance to amikacin in one of these isolates, which corresponded perfectly to its phenotypic resistance profile. We believe that the results obtained will facilitate further elucidating of antibiotic resistance mechanisms for this important pathogen, and highlight the need for continuous genomic epidemiology surveillance of clinical *K. pneumoniae* isolates.

**Keywords:** antimicrobial resistance; *Klebsiella pneumoniae*; COVID-19; plasmids; multidrug resistance; genomic epidemiology; whole genome sequencing

## 1. Introduction

The antimicrobial resistance (AMR) of pathogenic and opportunistic bacteria, especially in clinical settings, has become a major challenge that threatens the success of different protection measures in various medical applications [1]. Currently, drug-resistant infections account for about 700,000 deaths globally, and this number may increase up to several millions in the next decades [2]. According to the pathogens priority list of the World Health Organization (WHO), carbapenem-resistant Enterobacteriaceae were assigned a critical level due to increasing morbidity and mortality caused by them [3]. Within this bacterial family, *Klebsiella pneumoniae* possessing resistance to carbapenems is the most common and dangerous species associated with mortality rates exceeding 30% [4,5]. *K. pneumoniae* is one of the leading causes of healthcare-associated infections worldwide, including sepsis, pulmonary diseases, and urinary tract infections [6].

The global influence of the COVID-19 pandemic on bacterial AMR is yet to be estimated, but some reports have already confirmed the increasing number of infections caused by bacteria producing extended-spectrum beta-lactamases (ESBLs) and carbapenemases [7,8]. The optimal treatment regimen for infections caused by carbapenem-resistant *K. pneumoniae* is yet to be developed [9,10], and the existing options include the administration of colistin, ceftazidime/avibactam, or meropenem/vaborbactam, in high doses [10,11], which are also prone to resistance development and are burdened with substantial toxicity profile [10].

In order to address these challenges appropriately, novel prevention strategies and treatment plans are required, and their development would hardly be possible without the investigation of AMR mechanisms and routes of resistance spreading within the bacterial population. The diffusion of resistance genes is usually attributed to horizontal gene transfer mediated by plasmids, and conjugated plasmids are recognized as important vectors for AMR gene transmission in Gram-negative bacteria [12,13]. In recent years, whole genome sequencing (WGS), especially long-read sequencing, has become a powerful tool for the determination of plasmid structures and AMR gene locations [14–16]. WGS also allows for performing a reliable epidemiological surveillance for outbreak investigations, in which it is vitally important to determine whether particular bacterial isolates belong to an outbreak-causing strain, or not [17].

In this work, we have performed short- and long read sequencing of three carbapenem-resistant *K. pneumoniae* isolates obtained from COVID-19 patients in a dedicated intensive care unit (ICU). Although these isolates constituted the same strain according to cgMLST analysis, their phenotypic AMR profiles were different. Hybrid short- and long-read assembly allowed us to reveal a small plasmid carrying *aph(3′)-VIa* gene providing resistance to amikacin in one of these isolates, which explained the difference in resistance. We believe that the results obtained will contribute to the understanding of antibiotic resistance mechanisms, both in general, and for this important pathogen in particular. Further investigations in this field will ultimately lead to developing better prevention strategies in hospital settings.

## 2. Results

*2.1. Isolate Typing, Resistance Profile, AMR Gene and Plasmid Content Determination*

The typing results revealed the same profile ST395/KL39/O1/O2v1 for all three isolates. cgMLST analysis revealed that the genomic sequences of all isolates were very close (no allele differences between CriePir335 and 336 and six different alleles between either of these isolates and CriePir342). Thus, according to the criterion described previously (less than 18 different cgMLST alleles for *K. pneumoniae* [18]), these isolates were highly likely representing a single strain. Complete cgMLST profiles for the isolates studied are given in Table S1.

All isolates were multidrug-resistant (MDR) and susceptible only to ceftazidime/avibactam and amikacin (except CriePir342). They carried multiple antibiotic resistance determinants, including ESBL-coding genes *blaCTX-M-15*, *blaOXA-48* and *blaTEM-1B* (see Figure 1). The only difference in genomic resistance was revealed for CriePir342, that carried a *aph(3′)-VIa* providing resistance to amikacin [19], which corresponded perfectly with phenotypic data. In general, we have not revealed any discrepancies between phenotypic and genomic resistance profiles. The susceptibility to ceftazidime/avibactam can be attributed to the synergistic effect of this drug.

| Sample id / Antibiotics and resistance genes | Amikacin | Gentamicin | Netilmicin | Cefepime | Ceftazidime | Ceftriaxone | Ertapenem | Imipenem | Meropenem | Amox/Clav | Ampicillin | Cft/Avi | Ciprofloxacin | Levofloxacin | Fosfomycin | Tmp/Smz | Tetracycline | aac(6')-Ib | ant(2'')-Ia | ant(3'')-Ia | aph(3')-VIa | blaCTX-M-15 | blaOXA-1 | blaOXA-48 | blaSHV-182 | blaTEM-1B | catA1 | dfrA1 | oqxA-B | fosA | sul1 | tet(A) |
|---|---|---|---|---|---|---|---|---|---|---|---|---|---|---|---|---|---|---|---|---|---|---|---|---|---|---|---|---|---|---|---|---|
| CriePir335 | S | R | R | R | R | R | R | R | R | R | R | S | R | R | R | R | R | + | + | + | - | + | + | + | + | + | + | + | + | + | + | + |
| CriePir336 | S | R | R | R | R | R | R | R | R | R | R | S | R | R | R | R | R | + | + | + | - | + | + | + | + | + | + | + | + | + | + | + |
| CriePir342 | R | R | R | R | R | R | R | R | R | R | R | S | R | R | R | R | R | + | + | + | + | + | + | + | + | + | + | + | + | + | + | + |

Amox/Clav - amoxicillin/clavulanic acid; Cft/Avi - ceftazidime/avibactam; Tmp/Smz - trimethoprim/sulfamethoxazole;
corresponding classes of antibiotics and resistance genes are filled with the same colors

| Sample id/Plasmids | Col440II | Col(pHAD28) | IncH1b | IncR | IncQ1 |
|---|---|---|---|---|---|
| CriePir335 | + | + | + | + | - |
| CriePir336 | + | + | + | + | - |
| CriePir342 | + | + | + | + | + |

**Figure 1.** Phenotypic and genomic antibiotic resistance profiles of clinical *K. pneumoniae* isolates obtained from COVID-19 patients.

The isolates CriePir335 and CriePir336 possessed the same five plasmids, while CriePir342 included an additional IncQ1 plasmid. This plasmid carried the *aph(3')-VIa* gene mentioned above, which provides resistance to amikacin [19]. Plasmid data are provided in Table 1.

**Table 1.** Plasmid data for the clinical *K. pneumoniae* isolates studied.

| Id | Length | RepliconType | RelaxaseFamily | Plasmid Type |
|---|---|---|---|---|
| 2 | 282,773 | IncH | $MOB_H$, $MPF_T$ | Conjugative |
| 3 | 74,680 | IncR | - | Non-mobilizable |
| 4 | 8351 | IncQ | $MOB_Q$ | Mobilizable |
| 5 | 5010 | ColRNAI | - | Non-mobilizable |
| 6 | 4052 | ColRNAI | $MOB_P$ | Mobilizable |
| 7 | 3511 | ColRNAI | $MOB_P$ | Mobilizable |

We investigated IncQ plasmid more thoroughly to get additional insights into the resistance mechanisms. We revealed a Tn5393 transposon homology, as well as two copies of IS91 insertion sequence, and IS91 family transposase between them, near the *aph(3')-VIa* gene. The plasmid also included the genes encoding replication proteins RepA, RepB and RepC, and mobilization protein genes *mobA* and *mobC*. The plasmid structure is shown in Figure 2.

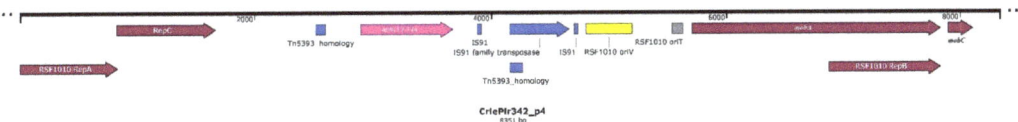

**Figure 2.** The structure of IncQ1 plasmid carrying amikacin resistance gene

### 2.2. Virulence Factors

The three isolates studied included exactly the same set of virulence factors. The list and brief description of important gene clusters are presented in Table 2. The complete list of 87 virulence genes is provided in Table S2. Most genes were located on chromosomes, except for *iucABCD*, *iutA* and *rmpA2*, which were located on IncH1B virulence plasmid.

Table 2. Description of important virulence gene clusters in clinical *K. pneumoniae* isolates studied.

| Gene Cluster | Function | Location |
|---|---|---|
| acrAB | efflux pump genes | Chromosome |
| fimABCDEFGHIK | fimbria production and biofilm formation | Chromosome |
| entABCEF, fepABCDG | enterobactin biosynthesis (siderophore) | Chromosome |
| irp1,2 | iron acquisition system | Chromosome |
| iucABCD, iutA | aerobactin cluster-iron acquisition system | IncH1B plasmid |
| manBC | promoters of capsule synthesis genes | Chromosome |
| mrkABCDFHIJ | fimbria production and biofilm formation | Chromosome |
| rcsAB | exopolysaccharide biosynthesis | Chromosome |
| rmpA2 | regulator of mucoid phenotype | IncH1B plasmid |
| wbbMNO | lipopolysaccharide synthesis | Chromosome |
| ybtAEPQSTU | yersiniabactin cluster-iron acquisition system | Chromosome |

The virulence factor content of CriePir isolates does not allow assigning them to the hypervirulent type since the set of corresponding genes was limited and most heavy metal resistance genes like *pbr* (lead resistance), *pco* (copper), *ter* (tellurite) and *sil* (silver) were missing. However, the isolates deserve additional attention to the presence of mucoid phenotype regulator *rmpA2* and their rapid spread within ICU.

*2.3. Comparison with Reference Isolates of ST395 from Genbank Database*

The isolates obtained were compared to the genomes of ST395 available in Genbank, based on cgMLST. A list of closest matches and their description are provided in Table 3, and the minimum spanning tree for these isolates is shown in Figure 3 All comparisons were made based on genome sequences as the phenotype data were not available.

Table 3. Reference isolates from Genbank, with closest matches to the isolates studied according to cgMLST analysis.

| Genbank Acc. | Number of Allele Differences | Country of Isolation | Isolate Collection Year |
|---|---|---|---|
| GCA_022988285.1 | 8 | Germany | 2016 |
| GCA_022181145.1 | 10 | Finland | 2018 |
| GCA_003401055.1 | 13 | USA | 2013 |
| GCA_013421105.1 | 15 | Russia | 2018 |
| GCA_009661195.1 | 17 | Russia | 2018 |
| GCA_013421315.1 | 18 | Russia | 2018 |
| GCA_017310365.1 | 18 | China | 2015 |

AMR gene content was similar for reference and CriePir isolates, except for *aac(3)-IIa* found in the USA isolate only, *aph(3′)-VIa* revealed in CriePir342 and GCA_013421315 only, and *ant* genes (see Table S3). An important difference was also that GCA_009661195 did not include *blaCTX-M-15* and *blaTEM-1B* beta-lactamase genes, although it possessed IncR plasmid, on which these genes were located in CriePir342.

Virulence factor sets were also quite similar for all isolates, but several noticeable differences were revealed. GCA_003401055 (USA), GCA_009661195 (Russia) and GCA_022988285 (Germany) lack the genes from the *iuc* cluster and *rmpA2*. These genes were located on IncH1B plasmid in CriePir342, and the first two reference isolates did not have this plasmid, while the isolate from Germany did. However, this is not surprising since the plasmid structure has a high degree of plasticity.

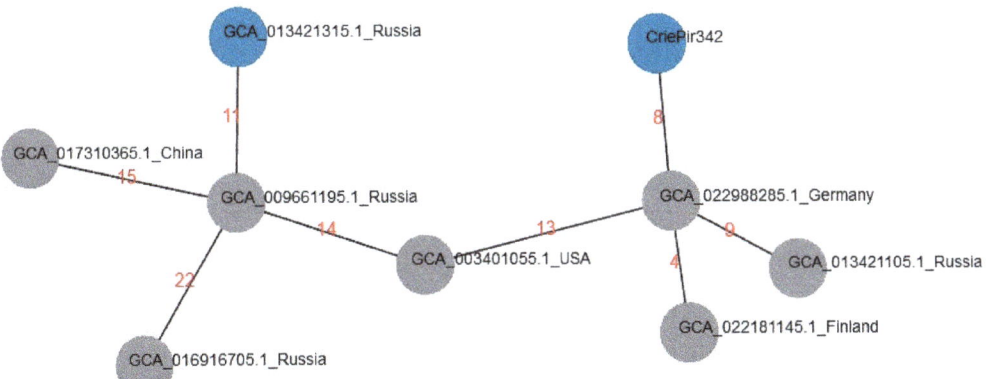

**Figure 3.** Minimum spanning tree based on cgMLST profiles for reference *K. pneumoniae* isolates and CriePir342. Since all our isolates possessed the close profiles, only CriePir342 is indicated. Red numbers show the number of allele differences between the corresponding isolates. The isolates carrying IncQ1 plasmid are colored in blue.

Only the isolate GCA_013421315 included IncQ1 plasmid, which was likely to carry *aph(3′)-VIa*. Unfortunately, the genome record did not contain the plasmid structure, so the direct comparison of plasmid sequences was impossible. However, the contig containing the *aph(3′)-VIa* AMR gene was mapped to the plasmid IncQ1 of CriePir342 with 100% identity (data not shown). At the same time, GCA_013421315 included four additional plasmids in comparison to CriePir342.

The isolates provided in the Table 3 constitute a single strain, or clone, with CriePir342 based on criteria proposed by Schursch et al. [18]. The closest genomic matches to our isolates were revealed in Germany, Finland and the USA. However, the plasmid content of these isolates was different from the one of CriePir342 (see Table S3), namely, the isolates from Finland and Germany did not include IncQ1 plasmid, and the USA isolate possessed two additional plasmids, ColRNAI and IncL.

## 3. Discussion

In this study, a genomic epidemiology investigation of three MDR *K. pneumoniae* isolates from the patients of a dedicated COVID-19 ICU was conducted. Long-read sequencing allowed us to reveal that although these isolates constituted one strain, one of them (CriePir342) had a slightly different resistance profile and possessed additional plasmid encoding *aph(3′)-VIa* providing resistance to amikacin, which corresponded perfectly to its phenotype.

Currently *K. pneumoniae* is the most common cause of nosocomial infections in Russia, accounting for almost 30% of cases in 2020 according to the AMRmap database [20] (https://amrmap.ru/, accessed on 23 August 2022). The isolates studied belonged to the ST395 group, which is known as a high-risk clone with high capacity of drug resistance acquisition [21] and was revealed in different countries, for example, in France [22], Hungary [23] and China [24]. Additionally, ST395/KL39 isolates carrying the *blaOXA-48* gene were recently revealed in Russia, including CriePir234 (GCA_009661195.1) described earlier by us [25], as well as in Finland in the same year, and were also obtained in 2013–2016 in such distant regions of the world as China, Germany and the USA. All these isolates belonged to the same strain as our isolates according to the proposed cgMLST allele difference threshold (≤18, [18]), and contained similar sets of AMR and virulence genes. The AMR determinants included ESBL-encoding genes *blaOXA-48*, *blaCTX-M-15* (except

GCA_009661195.1) and *blaTEM-1B* (except GCA_009661195.1), as well as various other AMR genes sufficient to consider these isolates as multidrug-resistant (MDR). However, only the Russian isolate NNKP343 (GCA_013421315.1) possessed the *aph(3′)-VIa* AMR gene mentioned above.

The virulence gene content was also similar for most isolates, except for the *rmpA2* encoding mucoid phenotype regulator, which was revealed in Russian isolates only, including the CriePir ones. Most virulence genes, except the *iuc* cluster and *rmpA2* mentioned above, were located on the chromosomes, which complies with previous data [25–27]. Another important determinant is a capsule surrounding the surface of *K. pneumoniae*, which serves as a main virulence factor associated with the viscous phenotype [28]. A capsular polysaccharide on the bacterial cell surface plays an important role in the pathogenicity of various bacteria, including *Acinetobacter baumannii* [29] and *K. pneumoniae* [30]. Although the KL39 capsule type is not generally considered as providing hypervirulence characteristics, at least one recent report described the increased virulence for the isolate having this capsule type and O1/O2v1 O-locus, which was found in all the isolates described above [31].

At the same time, the reference isolates exhibited differences in plasmid type and number, both between each other and with our set. For example, all isolates had IncR plasmid encoding, among others, the *blaOXA-1* beta-lactamase gene, but IncF1B was revealed in two Russian isolates only, while large IncHI1B pNDM-MAR-like plasmid carrying both resistance and virulence (*iuc* cluster) traits was revealed in all but two isolates. Last but not the least, IncQ1 plasmid, which carried the amikacin resistance gene in CriePir342, was revealed only in NNKP343 (GCA_013421315.1) reference isolate, thus allowing us to suppose, together with the fact that this isolate exhibited amikacin resistance [32], that this plasmid included *aph(3′)-VIa*. Unfortunately, the exact plasmid structures were not reconstructed in any reference isolates, and thus the direct comparison was not possible. However, additional analysis revealed that the IncQ1 plasmid mentioned above included fragments of the Tn5393 transposon that was known to carry aminoglycoside resistance genes (in our case, aminoglycoside-O-phosphotransferase), and partial sequences of which were more common than the complete transposon in plasmids and genomic islands [33]. We also revealed that this plasmid had a $MOB_Q$ type and was mobilizable, rather than conjugative, which was reported to be a common characteristic of the IncQ1 plasmids [34]. Plasmids of this type are non-self-transmissible, but their host independent replication system allowed them to have a broader host range than any other known replicating components in bacteria [35]. Mobilizable plasmids rely on conjugative plasmids to provide the mating pair formation components, and $MPF_T$ plasmids can serve as helpers in $MOB_Q$ plasmid conjugation [36]. In CriePir342, conjugation could be assisted by large IncH plasmid, but more data are required to prove this hypothesis.

In general, the chromosomal DNA of *K. pneumoniae* carries only inherent resistance genes, and most acquired resistance determinants, including ESBLs, are located on plasmids [6,12,25]. Thus, it is not surprising that differences in plasmid carriage designated the dissimilarities in acquired AMR gene content for CriePir and reference isolates. It should be mentioned that although the reference and our isolates appeared to constitute a single clone, which supposedly spread across the world more than 10 years ago, the acquisition of virulence and AMR determinants through plasmid routes could significantly change the pathogenicity and morbidity of particular isolates. Meanwhile, the plasmid IncQ1 carrying the amikacin resistance gene was revealed in CriePir26 and CriePir28 isolates sequenced by us in 2017 [25]. Although these isolates belonged to a different clone with ST377, the plasmid sequence was completely the same as in CriePir342. Therefore, a continuous genomic epidemiology surveillance of clinical *K. pneumoniae* isolates is required to assess their threat to the patients of particular health care institutions since the determination of a sequence type and clonal lineage appears to be insufficient for this purpose.

The current study is limited to three isolates only since the main goal was to elucidate the difference in the phenotypic resistance profiles for the three *K. pneumoniae* isolates obtained in the same ward during this limited period. This was achieved with the help of third-generation sequencing. During recent years, the increasing use of long-read sequencing greatly facilitated the investigations of outbreaks and exploration of possible resistance transmission routes [37–39], and several bioinformatics protocols were developed for these purposes [15,17,40]. Another possible application of this powerful technology is the investigation of bacterial clone diversity within a particular hospital department or some other healthcare facility [41–43].

At the same time, various factors limit the ability to analyze the putative outbreak genomes in real-time, which, surprisingly, might include not the restrictions imposed by sequencing technologies, but rather data management and bioinformatics, for example, the lack of common outbreak repositories and delays between data collection and computational analysis [44,45]. Thus, creating more sophisticated bioinformatics tools can also advance AMR prevention strategies and the epidemiological surveillance of *K. pneumoniae* and other important pathogens. The development of such tools is one of the future perspectives of our investigations.

## 4. Materials and Methods

*4.1. Sample Collection, Susceptibility Testing, DNA Isolation, and Sequencing*

Three *K. pneumoniae* isolates (named CriePir335 (from urine), CriePir336 (from blood) and CriePir342 (from urine)) were obtained from COVID-19 patients in a dedicated ICU of a multipurpose medical center during the first half of June 2020. The patients were females of 81, 72 and 85 years of age, respectively, with a confirmed diagnosis of COVID-19.

Species identification for the isolates studied was performed using time-of-flight mass spectrometry (MALDI-TOF MS) with the VITEK MS (bioMerieux, Marcy-l'Étoile, France). Antimicrobial susceptibility/resistance was determined by the disc diffusion method using the Mueller-Hinton medium (bioMerieux, Marcy-l'Étoile, France) and disks with antibiotics (BioRad, Marnes-la-Coquette, France), and the minimum inhibitory concentration (MIC) was determined on VITEK 2 Compact 30 analyzer automated system (bioMerieux, Marcy-l'Étoile, France). The antibiotics tested included amikacin, amoxicillin/clavulanic acid, ampicillin, cefepime, ceftazidime, ceftriaxone, ceftazidime/avibactam, ciprofloxacin, ertapenem, fosfomycin, gentamicin, imipenem, levofloxacin, meropenem, netilmicin, tetracycline and trimethoprim/sulfamethoxazole. We used the EUCAST clinical breakpoints, version 11.0 (https://www.eucast.org/clinical_breakpoints/, accessed on 20 December 2020) to interpret the susceptibility/resistance results obtained.

The isolates described above represent a subset of multidrug-resistant (MDR) samples, which were subjected to WGS.

Genomic DNA was isolated using DNeasy Blood and Tissue kit (Qiagen, Hilden, Germany), and Nextera™ DNA Sample Prep Kit (Illumina®, San Diego, CA, USA) was applied for paired-end library preparation and WGS of the isolates on Illumina® Hiseq 2500 platform (Illumina®, San Diego, CA, USA). The same genomic DNA was used to prepare the libraries for the Oxford Nanopore MinION sequencing system (Oxford Nanopore Technologies, Oxford, UK) with the Rapid Barcoding Sequencing kit SQK-RBK004 (Oxford Nanopore Technologies, Oxford, UK). The amount of initial DNA was 400 ng for each sample. The libraries were prepared according to the manufacturer's protocols, and were sequenced on R9 SpotON flow cell with a standard 24 h sequencing protocol using the MinKNOW software (Oxford Nanopore Technologies, Oxford, UK).

*4.2. Data Processing and Genome Assembly*

The base calling of the raw MinION data was performed using the Guppy Basecalling Software version 4.2.2 (Oxford Nanopore Technologies, Oxford, UK), and demultiplexing was performed using the Guppy barcoding software version 4.2.2 (Oxford Nanopore Technologies, Oxford, UK). Hybrid short- and long-read assemblies were obtained using the Unicycler version 0.4.9 (normal mode) [46]. Genome assemblies were submitted to the NCBI Genbank under the project PRJNA839643.

The pipeline described earlier [25] was used for the assembled genome processing and annotation. The Resfinder 4.0 database was used for antimicrobial gene detection (https://cge.cbs.dtu.dk/services/ResFinder/, accessed on 20 August 2022, using default parameters). Virulence factors were revealed by searching in VFDB (http://www.mgc.ac.cn/VFs/main.htm, accessed on 20 August 2022, using default parameters). Plasmids were detected using the PlasmidFinder (https://cge.cbs.dtu.dk/services/PlasmidFinder/, accessed on 20 August 2022, using default parameters).

Isolate typing was performed by MLST using BIGSdb (https://bigsdb.pasteur.fr/klebsiella/, accessed on 25 May 2022). In addition, the types based on capsule synthesis loci (K-loci) and lipooligosaccharide outer core loci (OCL) were also deduced using the Kaptive software v.2.0.3 with default parameters [30].

The detection of cgMLST profiles was performed using the MentaList (https://github.com/WGS-TB/MentaLiST, version 0.2.4, default parameters, accessed on 25 August 2022) [47] using the scheme obtained from cgmlst.org (https://www.cgmlst.org/ncs/schema/schema/2187931/, contained 2,358 loci, last update 25 May 2022). The minimum spanning tree was built using PHYLOViz online (http://online.phyloviz.net, accessed on 20 August 2022).

We used the TnCentral database (https://tncentral.proteininformationresource.org/tn_blast.html, accessed on 20 August 2022) to search for transposon sequences and ISEscan [48] for searching insertion sequences.

## 5. Conclusions

We performed WGS and obtained hybrid short- and long-read assemblies of three MDR ESBL-producing *K. pneumoniae* isolates, representing a single clone, obtained from COVID-19 patients in a dedicated ICU. Bioinformatics analysis allowed us to elucidate the differences in their antibiotic resistance profiles and reveal the possible mechanism of amikacin resistance found in one of the isolates. We believe that our data will facilitate the understanding of transfer mechanisms and developing new strategies for preventing resistance spreading within the clinical *K. pneumoniae* population.

**Supplementary Materials:** The following supporting information can be downloaded at: https://www.mdpi.com/article/10.3390/antibiotics11101364/s1, Table S1: cgMLST profiles for clinical *K. pneumoniae* isolates studied and reference isolates from Genbank.; Table S2: complete list of virulence genes revealed in clinical *K. pneumoniae* isolates studied; Table S3: comparison of antibiotic resistance gene, virulence factor and plasmid content for the reference and CriePir isolates.

**Author Contributions:** Conceptualization, A.S., M.Z. and Y.M.; formal analysis, A.S.; funding acquisition, V.A. investigation, A.S., L.P., A.M. and Y.M.; methodology, A.S., L.P. and Y.M.; project administration, M.Z. and V.A.; resources, L.P., A.M. and Y.M.; software, A.S.; supervision, M.Z. and Y.M.; validation, L.P., A.M. and Y.M.; visualization, A.S.; writing—original draft, A.S.; writing—review and editing, A.S. and Y.M. All authors have read and agreed to the published version of the manuscript.

**Funding:** This research received no external funding.

**Institutional Review Board Statement:** Ethical review and approval were waived for this study since the human samples were routinely collected and patients' data remained anonymous.

**Informed Consent Statement:** Informed consent was obtained from all subjects involved in the study.

**Data Availability Statement:** Genome assemblies were submitted to NCBI Genbank under the project PRJNA839643. Accession numbers are as follows: JAMXKW000000000 (CriePir335), JAMXKV000000000 (CriePir336), JAMXKU000000000 (CriePir342).

**Conflicts of Interest:** The authors declare no conflict of interest.

## References

1. Wang, M.; Earley, M.; Chen, L.; Hanson, B.M.; Yu, Y.; Liu, Z.; Salcedo, S.; Cober, E.; Li, L.; Kanj, S.S.; et al. Clinical outcomes and bacterial characteristics of carbapenem-resistant *Klebsiella pneumoniae* complex among patients from different global regions (CRACKLE-2): A prospective, multicentre, cohort study. *Lancet Infect. Dis.* 2022, *22*, 401–412. [CrossRef]
2. Manesh, A.; Varghese, G.M. Rising antimicrobial resistance: An evolving epidemic in a pandemic. *Lancet Microbe* 2021, *2*, e419–e420. [CrossRef]
3. Tacconelli, E.; Carrara, E.; Savoldi, A.; Harbarth, S.; Mendelson, M.; Monnet, D.L.; Pulcini, C.; Kahlmeter, G.; Kluytmans, J.; Carmeli, Y.; et al. Discovery, research, and development of new antibiotics: The WHO priority list of antibiotic-resistant bacteria and tuberculosis. *Lancet Infect. Dis.* 2018, *18*, 318–327. [CrossRef]
4. Agyeman, A.A.; Bergen, P.J.; Rao, G.G.; Nation, R.L.; Landersdorfer, C.B. A systematic review and meta-analysis of treatment outcomes following antibiotic therapy among patients with carbapenem-resistant *Klebsiella pneumoniae* infections. *Int. J. Antimicrob. Agents* 2020, *55*, 105833. [CrossRef]
5. Li, Y.; Li, J.; Hu, T.; Hu, J.; Song, N.; Zhang, Y.; Chen, Y. Five-year change of prevalence and risk factors for infection and mortality of carbapenem-resistant *Klebsiella pneumoniae* bloodstream infection in a tertiary hospital in North China. *Antimicrob. Resist. Infect. Control* 2020, *9*, 79. [CrossRef]
6. Gorrie, C.L.; Mirceta, M.; Wick, R.R.; Judd, L.M.; Lam, M.M.C.; Gomi, R.; Abbott, I.J.; Thomson, N.R.; Strugnell, R.A.; Pratt, N.F.; et al. Genomic dissection of *Klebsiella pneumoniae* infections in hospital patients reveals insights into an opportunistic pathogen. *Nat. Commun.* 2022, *13*, 3017. [CrossRef]
7. Saini, V.; Jain, C.; Singh, N.P.; Alsulimani, A.; Gupta, C.; Dar, S.A.; Haque, S.; Das, S. Paradigm Shift in Antimicrobial Resistance Pattern of Bacterial Isolates during the COVID-19 Pandemic. *Antibiotics* 2021, *10*, 954. [CrossRef]
8. Lai, C.C.; Chen, S.Y.; Ko, W.C.; Hsueh, P.R. Increased antimicrobial resistance during the COVID-19 pandemic. *Int. J. Antimicrob. Agents* 2021, *57*, 106324. [CrossRef]
9. Pitout, J.D.; Nordmann, P.; Poirel, L. Carbapenemase-Producing *Klebsiella pneumoniae*, a Key Pathogen Set for Global Nosocomial Dominance. *Antimicrob. Agents Chemother.* 2015, *59*, 5873–5884. [CrossRef]
10. Spaziante, M.; Oliva, A.; Ceccarelli, G.; Venditti, M. What are the treatment options for resistant *Klebsiella pneumoniae* carbapenemase (KPC)-producing bacteria? *Expert Opin. Pharmacother.* 2020, *21*, 1781–1787. [CrossRef]
11. Tsuji, B.T.; Pogue, J.M.; Zavascki, A.P.; Paul, M.; Daikos, G.L.; Forrest, A.; Giacobbe, D.R.; Viscoli, C.; Giamarellou, H.; Karaiskos, I.; et al. International Consensus Guidelines for the Optimal Use of the Polymyxins: Endorsed by the American College of Clinical Pharmacy (ACCP), European Society of Clinical Microbiology and Infectious Diseases (ESCMID), Infectious Diseases Society of America (IDSA), International Society for Anti-infective Pharmacology (ISAP), Society of Critical Care Medicine (SCCM), and Society of Infectious Diseases Pharmacists (SIDP). *Pharmacotherapy* 2019, *39*, 10–39. [CrossRef] [PubMed]
12. Wang, X.; Zhao, J.; Ji, F.; Chang, H.; Qin, J.; Zhang, C.; Hu, G.; Zhu, J.; Yang, J.; Jia, Z.; et al. Multiple-Replicon Resistance Plasmids of Klebsiella Mediate Extensive Dissemination of Antimicrobial Genes. *Front. Microbiol.* 2021, *12*, 754931. [CrossRef]
13. Meng, M.; Li, Y.; Yao, H. Plasmid-Mediated Transfer of Antibiotic Resistance Genes in Soil. *Antibiotics* 2022, *11*, 525. [CrossRef] [PubMed]
14. Shaidullina, E.; Shelenkov, A.; Yanushevich, Y.; Mikhaylova, Y.; Shagin, D.; Alexandrova, I.; Ershova, O.; Akimkin, V.; Kozlov, R.; Edelstein, M. Antimicrobial Resistance and Genomic Characterization of OXA-48- and CTX-M-15-Co-Producing Hypervirulent *Klebsiella pneumoniae* ST23 Recovered from Nosocomial Outbreak. *Antibiotics* 2020, *9*, 862. [CrossRef]
15. Peter, S.; Bosio, M.; Gross, C.; Bezdan, D.; Gutierrez, J.; Oberhettinger, P.; Liese, J.; Vogel, W.; Dorfel, D.; Berger, L.; et al. Tracking of Antibiotic Resistance Transfer and Rapid Plasmid Evolution in a Hospital Setting by Nanopore Sequencing. *mSphere* 2020, *5*, 4. [CrossRef] [PubMed]
16. Bird, M.T.; Greig, D.R.; Nair, S.; Jenkins, C.; Godbole, G.; Gharbia, S.E. Use of Nanopore Sequencing to Characterise the Genomic Architecture of Mobile Genetic Elements Encoding blaCTX-M-15 in Escherichia coli Causing Travellers' Diarrhoea. *Front. Microbiol.* 2022, *13*, 862234. [CrossRef]
17. Ferreira, F.A.; Helmersen, K.; Visnovska, T.; Jorgensen, S.B.; Aamot, H.V. Rapid nanopore-based DNA sequencing protocol of antibiotic-resistant bacteria for use in surveillance and outbreak investigation. *Microb. Genom.* 2021, *7*, 000557. [CrossRef] [PubMed]
18. Schurch, A.C.; Arredondo-Alonso, S.; Willems, R.J.L.; Goering, R.V. Whole genome sequencing options for bacterial strain typing and epidemiologic analysis based on single nucleotide polymorphism versus gene-by-gene-based approaches. *Clin. Microbiol. Infect.* 2018, *24*, 350–354. [CrossRef]
19. Lambert, T.; Gerbaud, G.; Courvalin, P. Characterization of transposon Tn1528, which confers amikacin resistance by synthesis of aminoglycoside 3′-O-phosphotransferase type VI. *Antimicrob. Agents Chemother.* 1994, *38*, 702–706. [CrossRef] [PubMed]
20. Kuzmenkov, A.Y.; Trushin, I.V.; Vinogradova, A.G.; Avramenko, A.A.; Sukhorukova, M.V.; Malhotra-Kumar, S.; Dekhnich, A.V.; Edelstein, M.V.; Kozlov, R.S. AMRmap: An Interactive Web Platform for Analysis of Antimicrobial Resistance Surveillance Data in Russia. *Front. Microbiol.* 2021, *12*, 620002. [CrossRef]
21. Dogan, O.; Vatansever, C.; Atac, N.; Albayrak, O.; Karahuseyinoglu, S.; Sahin, O.E.; Kilicoglu, B.K.; Demiray, A.; Ergonul, O.; Gonen, M.; et al. Virulence Determinants of Colistin-Resistant *K. pneumoniae* High-Risk Clones. *Biology* 2021, *10*, 436. [CrossRef]

22. Muggeo, A.; Guillard, T.; Klein, F.; Reffuveille, F.; Francois, C.; Babosan, A.; Bajolet, O.; Bertrand, X.; de Champs, C.; CarbaFrEst, G. Spread of *Klebsiella pneumoniae* ST395 non-susceptible to carbapenems and resistant to fluoroquinolones in North-Eastern France. *J. Glob. Antimicrob. Resist.* **2018**, *13*, 98–103. [CrossRef]
23. Kovacs, K.; Nyul, A.; Mestyan, G.; Melegh, S.; Fenyvesi, H.; Jakab, G.; Szabo, H.; Janvari, L.; Damjanova, I.; Toth, A. Emergence and interhospital spread of OXA-48-producing *Klebsiella pneumoniae* ST395 clone in Western Hungary. *Infect. Dis.* **2017**, *49*, 231–233. [CrossRef]
24. Cienfuegos-Gallet, A.V.; Zhou, Y.; Ai, W.; Kreiswirth, B.N.; Yu, F.; Chen, L. Multicenter Genomic Analysis of Carbapenem-Resistant *Klebsiella pneumoniae* from Bacteremia in China. *Microbiol. Spectr.* **2022**, *10*, e0229021. [CrossRef] [PubMed]
25. Shelenkov, A.; Mikhaylova, Y.; Yanushevich, Y.; Samoilov, A.; Petrova, L.; Fomina, V.; Gusarov, V.; Zamyatin, M.; Shagin, D.; Akimkin, V. Molecular Typing, Characterization of Antimicrobial Resistance, Virulence Profiling and Analysis of Whole-Genome Sequence of Clinical *Klebsiella pneumoniae* Isolates. *Antibiotics* **2020**, *9*, 261. [CrossRef] [PubMed]
26. Muraya, A.; Kyany'a, C.; Kiyaga, S.; Smith, H.J.; Kibet, C.; Martin, M.J.; Kimani, J.; Musila, L. Antimicrobial Resistance and Virulence Characteristics of *Klebsiella pneumoniae* Isolates in Kenya by Whole-Genome Sequencing. *Pathogens* **2022**, *11*, 545. [CrossRef] [PubMed]
27. Lery, L.M.; Frangeul, L.; Tomas, A.; Passet, V.; Almeida, A.S.; Bialek-Davenet, S.; Barbe, V.; Bengoechea, J.A.; Sansonetti, P.; Brisse, S.; et al. Comparative analysis of *Klebsiella pneumoniae* genomes identifies a phospholipase D family protein as a novel virulence factor. *BMC Biol.* **2014**, *12*, 41. [CrossRef] [PubMed]
28. Zhu, J.; Wang, T.; Chen, L.; Du, H. Virulence Factors in Hypervirulent *Klebsiella pneumoniae*. *Front. Microbiol.* **2021**, *12*, 642484. [CrossRef] [PubMed]
29. Arbatsky, N.P.; Shneider, M.M.; Dmitrenok, A.S.; Popova, A.V.; Shagin, D.A.; Shelenkov, A.A.; Mikhailova, Y.V.; Edelstein, M.V.; Knirel, Y.A. Structure and gene cluster of the K125 capsular polysaccharide from *Acinetobacter baumannii* MAR13-1452. *Int. J. Biol. Macromol.* **2018**, *117*, 1195–1199. [CrossRef] [PubMed]
30. Wick, R.R.; Heinz, E.; Holt, K.E.; Wyres, K.L. Kaptive Web: User-Friendly Capsule and Lipopolysaccharide Serotype Prediction for Klebsiella Genomes. *J. Clin. Microbiol.* **2018**, *56*, e00197-18. [CrossRef]
31. Arena, F.; Menchinelli, G.; Di Pilato, V.; Torelli, R.; Antonelli, A.; Henrici De Angelis, L.; Coppi, M.; Sanguinetti, M.; Rossolini, G.M. Resistance and virulence features of hypermucoviscous *Klebsiella pneumoniae* from bloodstream infections: Results of a nationwide Italian surveillance study. *Front. Microbiol.* **2022**, *13*, 983294. [CrossRef]
32. Alekseeva, A.E.; Brusnigina, N.F.; Gordinskaya, N.A.; Makhova, M.A.; Kolesnikova, E.A. Molecular genetic characteristics of resistome and virulome of carbapenem-resistant *Klebsiella pneumoniae* clinical strains. *Klin. Lab. Diagn.* **2022**, *67*, 186–192. [CrossRef] [PubMed]
33. Partridge, S.R.; Kwong, S.M.; Firth, N.; Jensen, S.O. Mobile Genetic Elements Associated with Antimicrobial Resistance. *Clin. Microbiol. Rev.* **2018**, *31*, e00088-17. [CrossRef]
34. Orlek, A.; Phan, H.; Sheppard, A.E.; Doumith, M.; Ellington, M.; Peto, T.; Crook, D.; Walker, A.S.; Woodford, N.; Anjum, M.F.; et al. Ordering the mob: Insights into replicon and MOB typing schemes from analysis of a curated dataset of publicly available plasmids. *Plasmid* **2017**, *91*, 42–52. [CrossRef]
35. Meyer, R. Replication and conjugative mobilization of broad host-range IncQ plasmids. *Plasmid* **2009**, *62*, 57–70. [CrossRef] [PubMed]
36. Loftie-Eaton, W.; Rawlings, D.E. Diversity, biology and evolution of IncQ-family plasmids. *Plasmid* **2012**, *67*, 15–34. [CrossRef]
37. Prussing, C.; Snavely, E.A.; Singh, N.; Lapierre, P.; Lasek-Nesselquist, E.; Mitchell, K.; Haas, W.; Owsiak, R.; Nazarian, E.; Musser, K.A. Nanopore MinION Sequencing Reveals Possible Transfer of bla KPC-2 Plasmid Across Bacterial Species in Two Healthcare Facilities. *Front. Microbiol.* **2020**, *11*, 2007. [CrossRef] [PubMed]
38. Greig, D.R.; Jenkins, C.; Gharbia, S.E.; Dallman, T.J. Analysis of a small outbreak of Shiga toxin-producing Escherichia coli O157:H7 using long-read sequencing. *Microb. Genom.* **2021**, *7*, 000545. [CrossRef]
39. Roberts, L.W.; Harris, P.N.A.; Forde, B.M.; Ben Zakour, N.L.; Catchpoole, E.; Stanton-Cook, M.; Phan, M.D.; Sidjabat, H.E.; Bergh, H.; Heney, C.; et al. Integrating multiple genomic technologies to investigate an outbreak of carbapenemase-producing Enterobacter hormaechei. *Nat. Commun.* **2020**, *11*, 466. [CrossRef]
40. Steinig, E.; Duchene, S.; Aglua, I.; Greenhill, A.; Ford, R.; Yoannes, M.; Jaworski, J.; Drekore, J.; Urakoko, B.; Poka, H.; et al. Phylodynamic Inference of Bacterial Outbreak Parameters Using Nanopore Sequencing. *Mol. Biol. Evol.* **2022**, *39*, 3. [CrossRef]
41. de Siqueira, G.M.V.; Pereira-Dos-Santos, F.M.; Silva-Rocha, R.; Guazzaroni, M.E. Nanopore Sequencing Provides Rapid and Reliable Insight Into Microbial Profiles of Intensive Care Units. *Front. Public Health* **2021**, *9*, 710985. [CrossRef]
42. Shelenkov, A.; Petrova, L.; Zamyatin, M.; Mikhaylova, Y.; Akimkin, V. Diversity of International High-Risk Clones of *Acinetobacter baumannii* Revealed in a Russian Multidisciplinary Medical Center during 2017–2019. *Antibiotics* **2021**, *10*, 1009. [CrossRef] [PubMed]
43. Mustapha, M.M.; Srinivasa, V.R.; Griffith, M.P.; Cho, S.T.; Evans, D.R.; Waggle, K.; Ezeonwuka, C.; Snyder, D.J.; Marsh, J.W.; Harrison, L.H.; et al. Genomic Diversity of Hospital-Acquired Infections Revealed through Prospective Whole-Genome Sequencing-Based Surveillance. *mSystems* **2022**, *7*, e0138521. [CrossRef] [PubMed]
44. Hodcroft, E.B.; De Maio, N.; Lanfear, R.; MacCannell, D.R.; Minh, B.Q.; Schmidt, H.A.; Stamatakis, A.; Goldman, N.; Dessimoz, C. Want to track pandemic variants faster? Fix the bioinformatics bottleneck. *Nature* **2021**, *591*, 30–33. [CrossRef]

45. Viehweger, A.; Blumenscheit, C.; Lippmann, N.; Wyres, K.L.; Brandt, C.; Hans, J.B.; Holzer, M.; Irber, L.; Gatermann, S.; Lubbert, C.; et al. Context-aware genomic surveillance reveals hidden transmission of a carbapenemase-producing *Klebsiella pneumoniae*. *Microb. Genom.* **2021**, *7*, 000741. [CrossRef] [PubMed]
46. Wick, R.R.; Judd, L.M.; Gorrie, C.L.; Holt, K.E. Unicycler: Resolving bacterial genome assemblies from short and long sequencing reads. *PLoS Comput. Biol.* **2017**, *13*, e1005595. [CrossRef] [PubMed]
47. Feijao, P.; Yao, H.T.; Fornika, D.; Gardy, J.; Hsiao, W.; Chauve, C.; Chindelevitch, L. MentaLiST-A fast MLST caller for large MLST schemes. *Microb. Genom.* **2018**, *4*, 2. [CrossRef] [PubMed]
48. Xie, Z.; Tang, H. ISEScan: Automated identification of insertion sequence elements in prokaryotic genomes. *Bioinformatics* **2017**, *33*, 3340–3347. [CrossRef]

MDPI AG
Grosspeteranlage 5
4052 Basel
Switzerland
Tel.: +41 61 683 77 34

*Antibiotics* Editorial Office
E-mail: antibiotics@mdpi.com
www.mdpi.com/journal/antibiotics

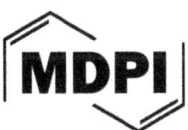

Disclaimer/Publisher's Note: The title and front matter of this reprint are at the discretion of the . The publisher is not responsible for their content or any associated concerns. The statements, opinions and data contained in all individual articles are solely those of the individual Editor and contributors and not of MDPI. MDPI disclaims responsibility for any injury to people or property resulting from any ideas, methods, instructions or products referred to in the content.

www.ingramcontent.com/pod-product-compliance
Lightning Source LLC
LaVergne TN
LVHW070613100526
838202LV00012B/634